Periodontal and Gingival Health and Diseases

I dedicate this book to my wife Galia, and my children Lilach, Ravit, and Dicla, in whom I contemplate my future.

Enrique Bimstein

To the memory of my beloved wife, Harriet L. Needleman, for her unyielding love and support.

Howard L. Needleman

Dedicated to the children this book will help, to my wife Hema, and to my children Naavin and Tarin.

Nadeem Karimbux

To my wife Barbara and my sons Charles and William, thank you for your continuous love and support.

Thomas E. Van Dyke

Periodontal and Gingival Health and Diseases

Children, Adolescents, and Young Adults

Edited by

Enrique Bimstein CD
Professor in Pediatric Dentistry,
Hebrew University–Hadassah School of Dental Medicine
founded by the Alpha Omega Fraternity,
Jerusalem, Israel

Howard L. Needleman DMD
Clinical Professor in Growth and Development (Pediatric Dentistry),
Harvard School of Dental Medicine,
Associate Dentist-in-Chief, Children's Hospital,
Boston, Massachusetts, USA

Nadeem Karimbux DMD, MMSc
Assistant Professor in Periodontology,
Harvard School of Dental Medicine, Boston,
Massachusetts, USA

Thomas E. Van Dyke DDS, PhD
Professor in Periodontology and Oral Biology;
Director, Graduate Periodontology;
Director, Clinical Research Center,
Boston University School of Dental Medicine,
Boston, Massachusetts, USA

MARTIN ■ DUNITZ

© 2001 Martin Dunitz Ltd, a member of the Taylor & Francis group

First published in the United Kingdom in 2001 by
Martin Dunitz Ltd
The Livery House
7–9 Pratt Street
London NW1 0AE

Tel: +44 (0)20 7482 2202
Fax: +44 (0)20 7267 0159
E-mail: info.dunitz@tandf.co.uk
Website: http://www.dunitz.co.uk

Reprinted 2002

A CIP catalogue record for this book is available from the British Library

ISBN 1–85317–781–4

Distributed in the United States by:
Thieme Medical Publishers Inc
333 Seventh Avenue
New York, NY 10001
USA
Tel: 1 212 760 0888

Distributed in the rest of the world by:
Thomson Publishing Services
Cheriton House
North Way
Andover, Hampshire SP10 5BE, UK
Tel: +44 (0)1264 332424
E-mail: salesorder.tandf@thomsonpublishingservices.co.uk

Composition by Scribe Design, Gillingham, Kent, UK
Printed and bound in Singapore by Kyodo Pte Ltd

CONTENTS

CONTRIBUTORS

Rina Adut DMD, MPH
Department of Community Dentistry, Hebrew
University–Hadassah School of Dental Medicine
founded by the Alpha Omega Fraternity,
Jerusalem, Israel

Gary C. Armitage DDS, MS
Professor and Chairman, Division of
Periodontology, University of California San
Francisco, School of Dentistry, San Francisco,
California, USA

Adrian Becker BDS, LDS, DDO
Clinical Associate Professor in Orthodontics,
Department of Orthodontics, Hebrew
University–Hadassah School of Dental Medicine
founded by the Alpha Omega Fraternity,
Jerusalem, Israel

Enrique Bimstein CD
Professor in Pediatric Dentistry, Hebrew
University–Hadassah School of Dental Medicine
founded by the Alpha Omega Fraternity,
Jerusalem, Israel

Andrew J. Delima DMD, DSc
Department of Periodontology and Oral
Biology, School of Dental Medicine, Boston
University, USA

Thomas C. Hart DDS, PhD
Associate Professor, Department of Oral
Medicine, University of Pittsburgh School of
Dental Medicine, University of Pittsburgh,
Pittsburgh, USA

Nadeem Karimbux DMD, MMSc
Assistant Professor in Periodontology,
Harvard School of Dental Medicine, Boston,
Massachusetts, USA

David Kohavi DMD
Associate Professor. Director of the Oral Implant
Center, Department of Prosthodontics, Hebrew
University–Hadassah School of Dental Medicine
founded by the Alpha Omega Fraternity,
Jerusalem, Israel

Angelo J. Mariotti BS, DDS, PhD
Associate Professor of Periodontology, Department
of Periodontology, College of Dentistry, Ohio State
University, Columbus, Ohio, USA

Howard L. Needleman DMD
Clinical Professor in Growth and Development
(Pediatric Dentistry), Harvard School of Dental
Medicine, Associate Dentist-in-Chief, Children's
Hospital, Boston, Massachusetts, USA

Hubert N. Newman BDentSc, MDS, FRCPath,
CBiol, FIBiol, MA, PhD, ScD
President (1999–2001), International Academy of
Periodontology; President-Elect (2000–2001),
British Society of Periodontology; Emeritus
Professor of Periodontology and Preventive
Dentistry at Eastman Dental Institute; Honorary
Professor, University College, London, UK

Roy C. Page DDS, PhD
Professor of Periodontics, Director of the
Regional Clinical Dental Research Center,
Associate Dean, School of Dentistry; Professor
of Pathology, School of Medicine, University of
Washington, Seattle, Washington, USA

Harvey A. Schenkein DDS, PhD
Paul Tucker Goad Professor, Clinical Research
Center for Periodontal Disease, Virginia,
Commonwealth University School of Dentistry,
Richmond, Virginia, USA

Harold D. Sgan-Cohen DMD MPH
Senior Lecturer, Department of Community
Dentistry, Hebrew University–Hadassah School
of Dental Medicine founded by the Alpha
Omega Fraternity, Jerusalem, Israel

Stephen Shusterman BA, DMD
Dentist-in-Chief, Children's Hospital, Boston,
Massachusetts, USA; Associate Clinical Professor
of Growth and Development (Pediatric
Dentistry), Harvard School of Dental Medicine,
Boston, Massachusetts, USA

Thomas J. Sims PhD
Immunology Research Scientist, School of
Dentistry, University of Washington, Seattle,
Washington, USA

Bengt E. Sjödin DDS, Odont Dr
Associate Professor Periodontics, Comprehensive
Dental Clinic, Institute of Odontology, Karolinska
Institute, Stockholm, Sweden

Jørgen Slots DDS, DMD, PhD, MS, MBA
Professor and Chairperson of the Department
of Periodontology, Associate Dean for
Research, University of Southern California
School of Dentistry, Los Angeles, California,
USA

Miriam Ting BDS, MS
Clinical Assistant Professor in Periodontology,
Department of Periodontology, University of
Southern California School of Dentistry, Los
Angeles, California, USA

Maurizio S. Tonetti DMD, PhD, MMSc
Professor and Head of Periodontology, Eastman
Dental Institute and Hospital, University
College, London, UK

Thomas E. Van Dyke DDS, PhD
Professor in Periodontology and Oral Biology;
Director, Graduate Periodontology; Director,
Clinical Research Center, Boston University
School of Dental Medicine, Boston,
Massachusetts, USA

Narawat Wara-aswapati DDS, DMSc
Instructor in Periodontology, Department of
Periodontology, Harvard School of Dental
Medicine; Department of Periodontology,
Faculty of Dentistry, Khon Kaen University,
Khon Kaen, Thailand

PREFACE

As we enter the first century of the third millennium, we cannot but admire the overwhelming influence of silicon chip technology on almost every aspect of our life. The practice of medicine and dentistry, and medical and dental research, are today characterized by efficient and sophisticated diagnostic, therapeutic, and research tools, causing unbounded admiration in those of us who were born and raised in a computerless society.

Despite the power of these advances, health-care providers should be astute enough not to become a mere extension of sophisticated appliances. Excellence in medical or dental practice and research is not based on silicon chips, but on human kindness, awareness, and understanding. Attesting to this fact is the vast repository of manuscripts that were published years ago, when clinicians' and researchers' word-processing devices were pencils, pens, scissors, transparent sticky tape, and, in some cases, a typewriter.

The current obsession with years, centuries, and millennia may lead us to ask which perspective of time should influence the reasoning of health-care providers, particularly those who treat children and adolescents. Clinicians treat today a disease that was initiated yesterday, and do their best to solve the present problem. At the same time, they must seize the opportunity to enable children and adolescents to grow in health and enjoy freedom from disease. We must always remember that all patients, but especially children and adolescents, have a future and not only a past and present. Too often we are terrorized by warnings of hazards to our health; instead, we should take a positive attitude towards maintaining health. In dentistry, simple awareness about oral hygiene will lead most children and adolescents to conserve the treasure of oral health.

Gingival and periodontal diseases in childhood and adolescence are rarely sensational, yet they may be the beginning of deterioration. Prevention, early diagnosis, and treatment of disease are always important, and particularly so in patients who are prone to diseases, or who unfortunately have systemic conditions that reduce their natural defenses. The fact that gingival and periodontal disease may influence systemic health—and not only the reverse—is being widely recognized. Moreover, the clinician must not miss the real possibility of diagnosing a gingival or periodontal problem that unveils a concealed systemic disease.

While it is intriguing to contemplate where technological development will lead the future of dental practice and research, we should not forget that there is still much basic information to clarify, to learn, and to teach about gingival and periodontal health and diseases in children and adolescents. It is our responsibility to ensure the future health of our young patients.

Enrique Bimstein
Jerusalem, Israel

PART I

Introduction

1
Introduction

Howard L. Needleman, Hubert N. Newman, and Enrique Bimstein

It has been over a quarter of a century since the state of knowledge concerning the classification, etiology, diagnosis, and treatment of gingival and periodontal diseases in children and adolescents has been compiled into a single work. In 1974, Drs. Paul Baer and Sheldon Benjamin co-authored, along with contributors, an original and landmark textbook entitled *Periodontal Disease in Children and Adolescents* (Baer and Benjamin, 1974). In their introduction they stated that the book had been written to fill a void. They astutely pointed out that while textbooks on periodontology were generally in agreement that the onset of periodontal disease frequently occurred during childhood or adolescence, minimal attention was given to the specific periodontal problems associated with this critical period of life. Their book firmly established the relevance and significance of periodontal diseases in children and adolescents.

Gingival and periodontal diseases comprise the most widespread infections of humankind and many of these first manifest themselves in childhood. As early as 1938, MacCall stated that there was a lack of appreciation of the fact that the foundation of virtually all periodontal disease is laid in childhood, citing Wordsworth: "The child is the father of the man" (MacCall, 1938). In 1975, Greene stated that because periodontal diseases in their destructive stages peak in middle age, we are inclined to think that they are adult diseases (Greene, 1975). However, periodontal diseases may have their inception during childhood and reach destructive stages while those affected are still in their teens.

As we enter the twenty-first century of the Common Era, an update of the Baer and Benjamin work is long overdue. Tremendous strides have been made in such fields as molecular biology, genetics, immunology, and microbiology, which have influenced our understanding of all aspects of periodontology and have also emphasized the relevance of gingival and periodontal diseases in children and adolescents. These advances are documented in an ever-expanding range of research articles and review manuscripts, from which it is difficult to assimilate all of the relevant information. As a result, practitioners may be unaware of the current state of knowledge of gingival and periodontal diseases as they relate to children, adolescents, and young adults. Using outdated information or knowledge based on adult gingival and periodontal diseases in managing children can result in inappropriate diagnosis and treatment with unfortunate long-term consequences.

This increase in information on the nature of gingival and periodontal diseases in children, adolescents, and young adults, in conjunction with the renewed field of evidence-based medicine and dentistry, has led to a shift in emphasis from mechanical treatment to a pharmacological, regenerative approach (Barnett, 1997). While periodontal surgery is likely to remain an extremely important part of treatment, we have now reached the age of periodontal medicine (Newman, 1994).

The purpose of this book is to establish the importance of periodontal diseases in young patients. In addition, it is intended to enhance cooperation between dentists and to encourage the early detection, diagnosis, and treatment of periodontal diseases in children, adolescents, and young adults.

Epidemiological data indicate that gingival and periodontal diseases in this age group are more prevalent and severe than previously believed, especially in susceptible individuals, families, and certain ethnic groups (Armitage, 1986; Stamm, 1986; Aass et al., 1988; Bimstein et al., 1988a, 1989, 1994; Löe and Brown, 1991;

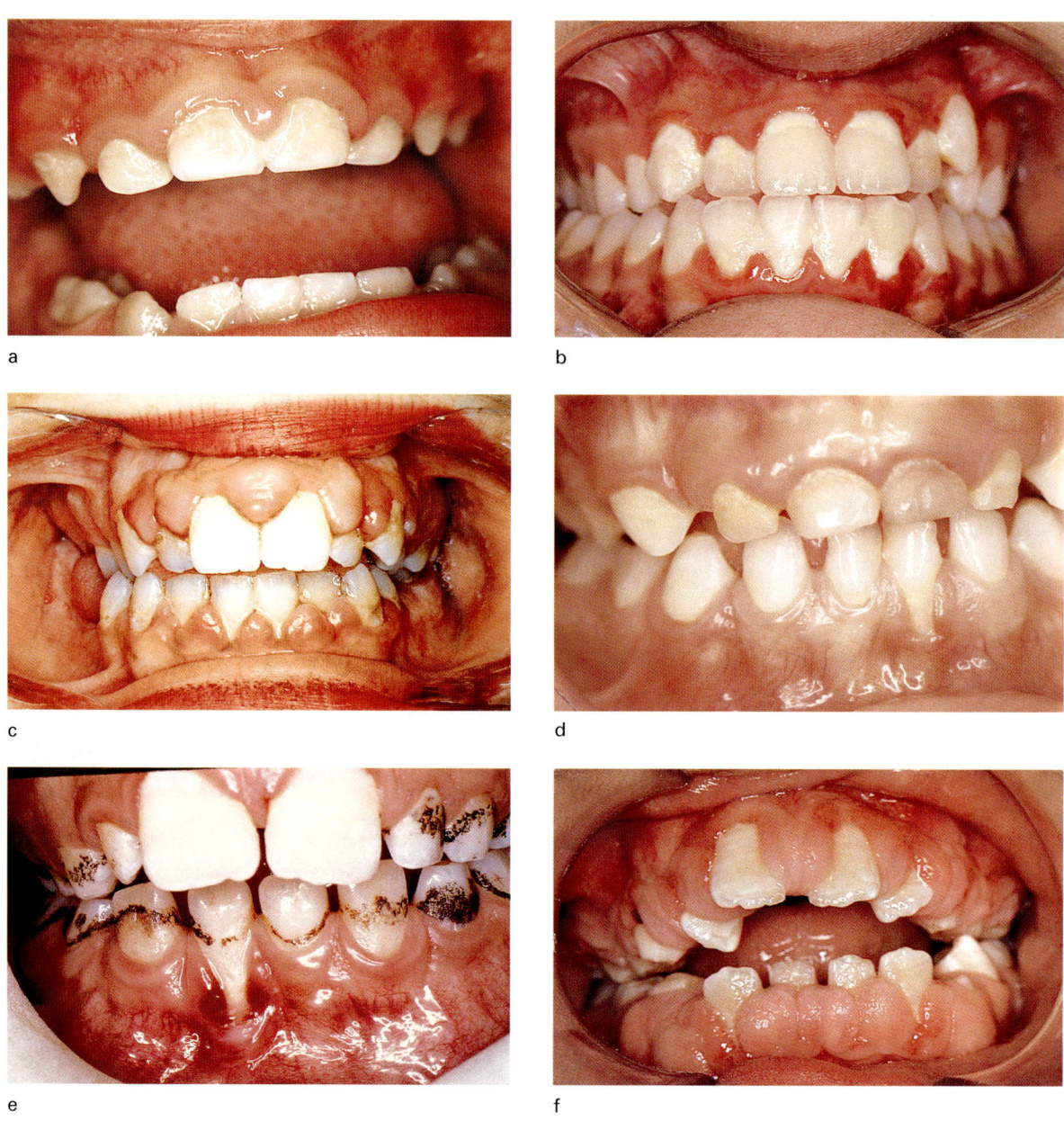

Figure 1.1

Gingivitis and mucogingival defects. (a) Gingivitis in the deciduous dentition. (b) Gingivitis in the permanent dentition of an adolescent. (c) Puberty gingivitis. (d) Mucogingival defect in a mandibular central deciduous incisor. (e) Mucogingival defect in a permanent mandibular incisor of a child (with permission of *ASDC J Dent Child*, from Bimstein et al., 1988b). (f) Gingival enlargement as a side-effect of immunosuppresive therapy.

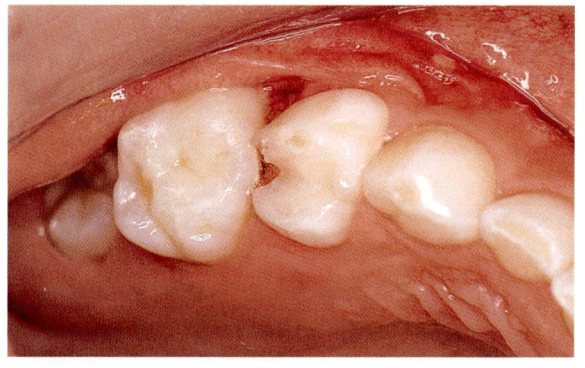

a

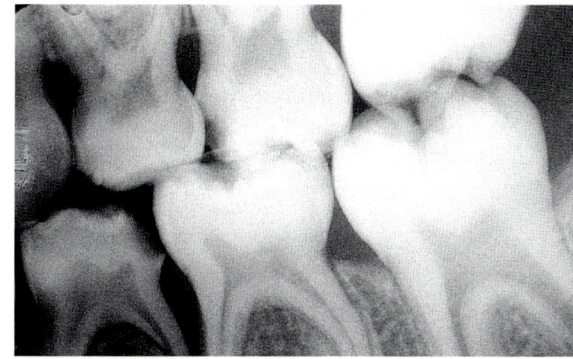

b

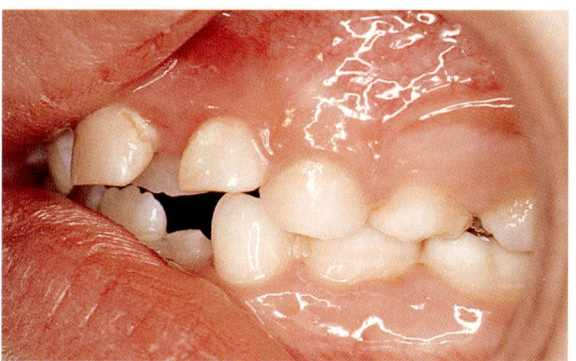

c

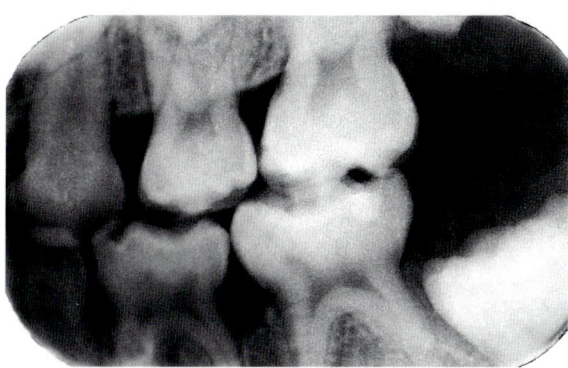

d

Figure 1.2

Childhood periodontitis (a) An inflamed interdental papilla between the maxillary deciduous molars, adjacent to carious proximal contact loss, may indicate the presence of periodontitis. (b) Bite-wing radiograph in which periodontitis, attributable to food impaction, is evident between the first and second deciduous molars. (c) Healthy-appearing oral structures of a 9-year-old patient with localized periodontitis in the deciduous dentition. (d) Bite-wing radiograph of the area in (c). Periodontitis is evident at the distal root of the mandibular first deciduous molar. (e) Localized periodontitis in the deciduous dentition of an 8-year-old patient with slight gingival inflammation on the buccal surface of the mandibular first deciduous molar. The interdental papilla between the maxillary deciduous molars does not completely fill the interdental space as would be normal.

continued overleaf

Schenkein et al., 1993; Matsson et al., 1995, 1997; Brown et al., 1996). Reported prevalence values of gingival and periodontal diseases in children and adolescents vary extensively, depending on definitional criteria and method of examination. Nevertheless, epidemiological data indicate that gingivitis of varying severity is a universal finding in children and adolescents (Figure 1.1a–c), and in certain age groups and populations affects almost every child (Armitage, 1986; Stamm, 1986; Bimstein et al., 1989). It should be emphasized that mucogingival problems (Figure 1.1d, e), attachment loss and periodontitis (Figure 1.2a–i), and periodontal abscesses (Figure 1.3a–e)

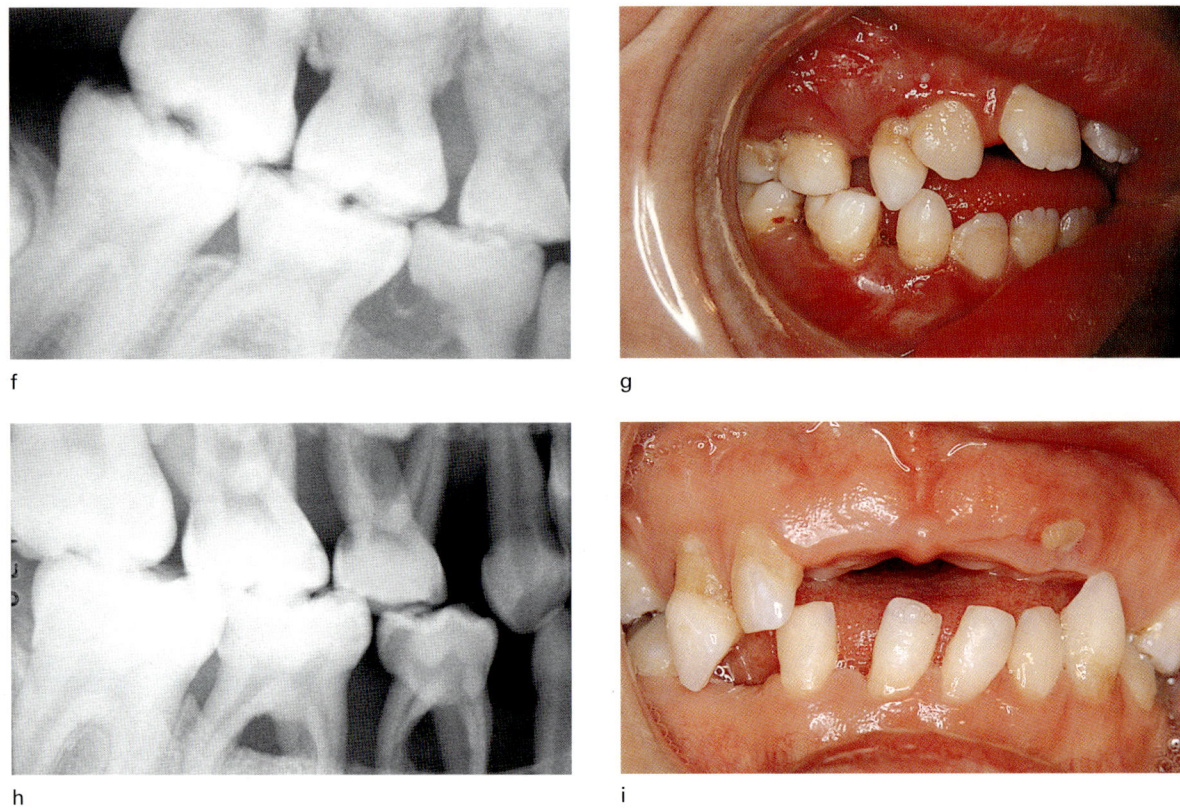

f

g

h

i

Figure 1.2 *continued*

(f) Bite-wing radiograph of the area in (e). Periodontitis is evident at the distal roots of the mandibular and maxillary first deciduous molars. The distal root of the first mandibular deciduous molar has been abnormally resorbed (with permission of *Pediatric Dentistry*, from Bimstein et al., 1977). (g) Generalized periodontitis affecting the deciduous teeth of the mixed dentition of a 9-year-old child with extensive attachment loss. (h) Radiograph of the area in (g). Generalized periodontitis is evident on all the deciduous teeth (with permission of *Pediatric Dentistry*, from Bimstein et al., 1997). (i) Early exfoliation of the anterior deciduous teeth and extensive alveolar bone support as a result of generalized periodontitis in a child with history of extreme malnutrition and vitamin D deficiency rickets. Further periodontal destruction was subsequently prevented by an adequate diet, treatment and oral hygiene.

are not problems confined uniquely to adolescents or adults; they may begin in childhood and show a high prevalence in certain populations (Watanabe, 1990; Van der Velden, 1991). Basic research and epidemiological data have also elucidated numerous risk factors (ethnicity, systemic host factors, microbial composition of the dental plaque, and heredity) that are potential markers to identify individuals, families, or populations at special risk of periodontal diseases (Aass et al., 1994; Watson et al., 1994;

Asikainen et al., 1996; Ellwood et al., 1997; Shapira et al., 1997; Tinoco et al., 1998).

Preventive periodontics

The key to preventive periodontics in relation to common gingival and periodontal diseases is in the maintenance of high individual standards of oral hygiene. This should be reinforced by

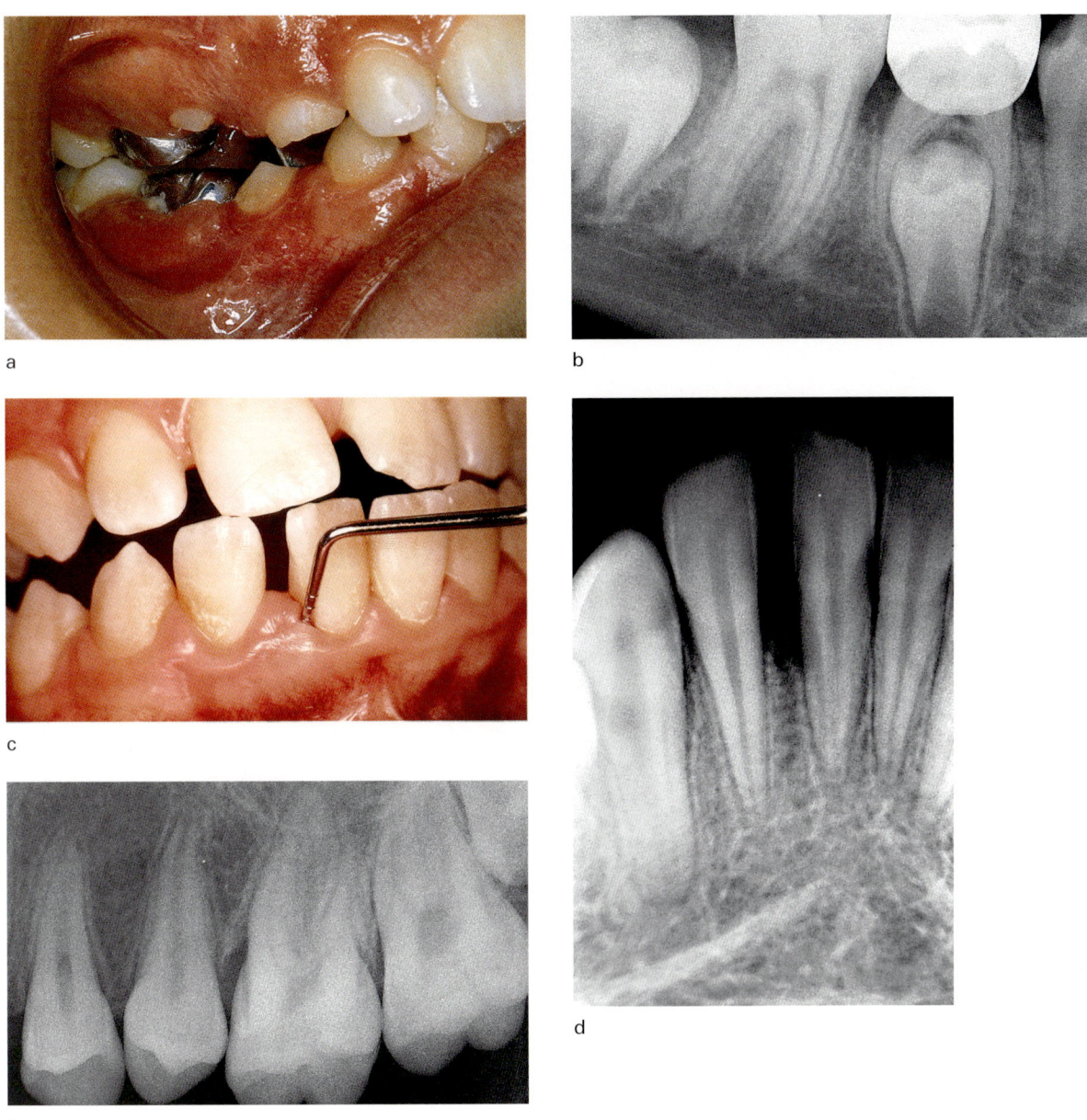

Figure 1.3

Periodontal abscesses. (a) Periodontal abscess around a stainless steel preformed crown on the second mandibular deciduous molar of a 9-year-old child. (a) Periapical radiograph of the area in (a). (c) Periodontal abscess in the mandibular incisor area of a 13-year-old adolescent (courtesy of Professor Eliezer Eidelman). (d) Periapical radiograph of the area in (c) (courtesy of Professor Eliezer Eidelman). (e) Periapical radiograph of the same adolescent shown in (c–d). Periodontitis developed a few years later on the mesial surface of a maxillary permanent molar (courtesy of Professor Eliezer Eidelman).

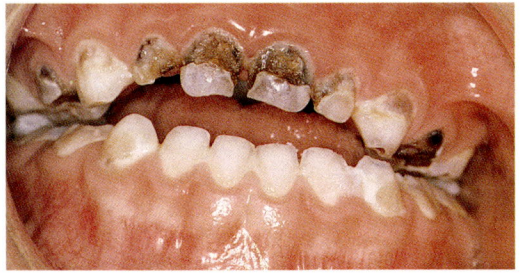

a

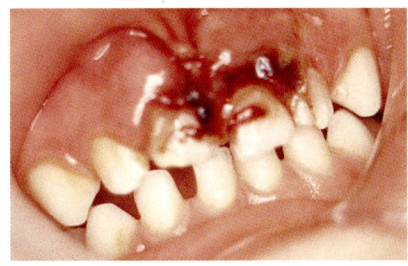

b

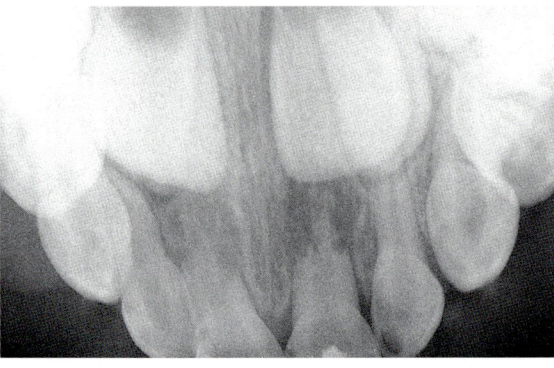

c

Figure 1.4

(a) Early childhood caries (courtesy of Professor Benny Peretz). (b) Trauma to the deciduous dentition. (c) External root resorption and periodontal destruction in a maxillary deciduous incisor due to a traumatic injury (courtesy of Dr Gideon Holan). (d) External root resorption and periodontal destruction in a maxillary permanent incisor due to a traumatic injury (courtesy of Dr Gideon Holan).

d

periodic professional services, with special emphasis on prophylaxis. It seems strange, perhaps ironic, that such a complicated and destructive disease can be significantly influenced by one of the oldest and simplest dental regimens. It also appears that diet has a significant effect on the periodontium. Indeed, one of the fundamental reasons why gingival and periodontal diseases are so widespread is attributable to the softer texture of the diet in modern civilized societies; this results in an accumulation of plaque and a stagnant and increasingly anaerobic bacterial population

(Newman, 1974, 1990). Experimentally, diets rich in sugar lead to increased development of gingivitis, despite similar levels of plaque initially (Egelberg, 1965). It is also well known that many types of malnutrition have an impact on periodontal health (Figure 1.2i) (Ferguson and Wall, 1995).

Awareness and diagnosis

Identification of individuals at high risk should improve the efficiency of efforts to prevent or

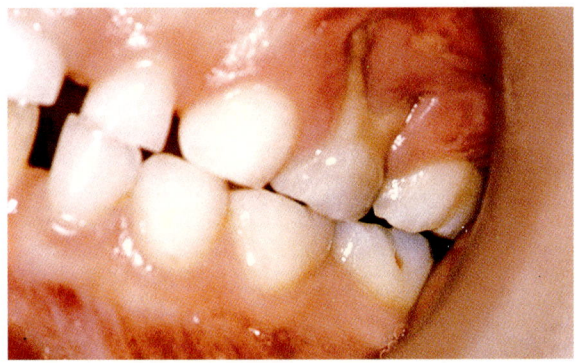

a

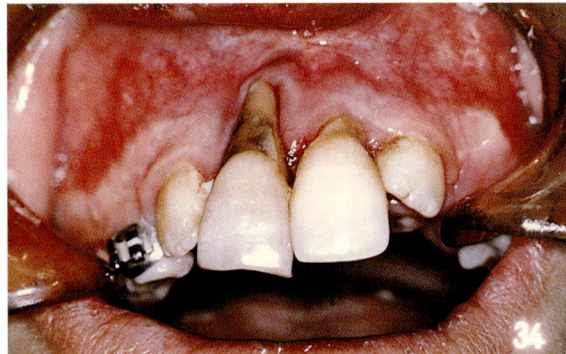

b

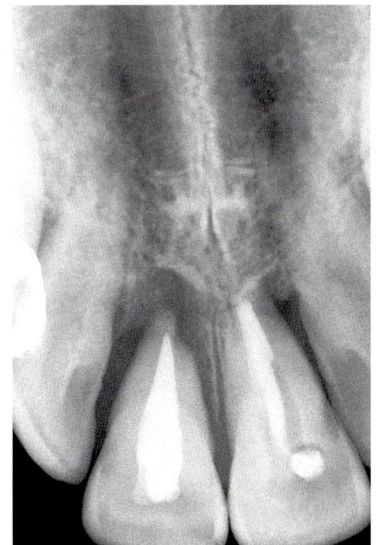

c

Figure 1.5

(a) A fingernail picking habit resulted in periodontal destruction on the first decid-uous molar (with permission of *Acta Odontol Pediatr*, from Bimstein, 1987). (b) Periodontal destruction of the alveolar bone surrounding the maxillary permanent central incisors due to apical migration of an unmonitored orthodontic elastic used to close the diastema. (c) Periapical radiograph of the area shown in (b).

control the disease. Risk factors are particularly relevant to (a) clinicians who seek early detection and appropriate management, (b) scientists researching the etiology and pathogenesis of the disease, (c) public health policy-makers who can help develop rational and effective preventive and treatment strategies and reduce risk factors, and (d) industries which can develop and market reliable diagnostic, preventive and therapeutic products, especially for high-risk populations.

Without an ingrained suspicion of gingival and periodontal diseases and their manifestations in children, clinicians may not detect the early stages of these diseases until they present in a more fulminant form, missing the opportunity for early intervention and prevention of

advanced disease. The control and prevention of these entities in childhood or adolescence would have major implications for oral health through-out life. Most cases of gingival and periodontal disease in children do not have an obvious or pathognomonic clinical appearance because of their slow rate of progression within the life span of the primary and mixed dentitions (Van der Velden, 1991).

The clinician's attention is usually drawn to more dramatic and obvious clinical entities such as dental caries (Figure 1.4a), trauma (Figure 1.4b) and periodontal destruction due to trauma (Figure 1.4c, d), overzealous tooth brushing, habits such as nail picking (Figure 1.5a), or inappropriate dental treatments (Zilberman et al.,

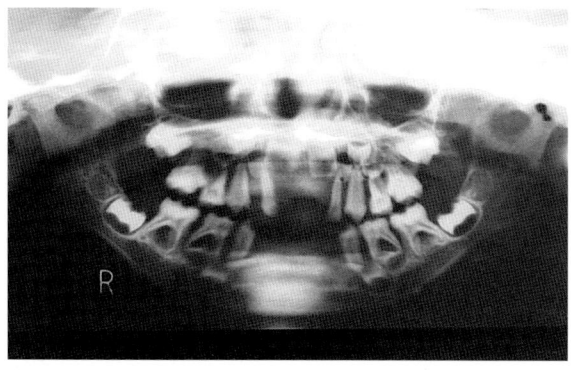

a

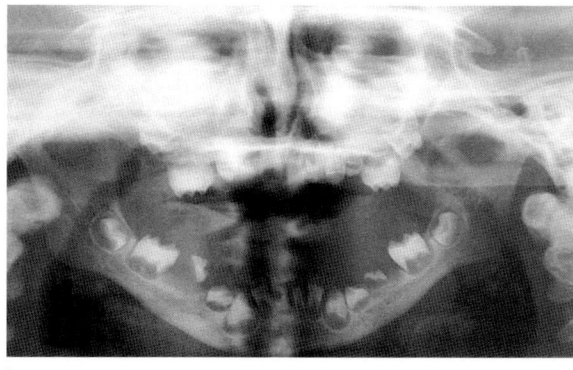

b

Figure 1.6

(a) Panoramic radiograph of a child with periodontitis affecting numerous deciduous teeth. Extraction of the afffected teeth was recommended. (b) Panoramic radiograph of the same child as in (a). Since the extractions were not performed, the alveolar bone resorption continued and damaged the developing permanent teeth.

1976) (Figures 1.5b, c). Moreover, gingival and periodontal diseases in young individuals tend to be localized rather than generalized, often without marked gingival change, making them more difficult to identify (Figures 1.1a–b, 1.2a–f, 1.3c). Failure to diagnose these diseases and to control plaque and host factors responsible for gingival and periodontal disease in childhood can lead to severe adverse effects on speech, comfort, eating, oral, and systemic health (Figures 1.6a, b). Conversely, correct diagnosis and early intervention may obviate the need for extraction and complex periodontal or prosthodontic therapies. For all of these reasons, children and adolescents must routinely receive a thorough periodontal examination and preventive care, as recommended by the American Academy of Periodontology (1996).

Treatment outcomes

To optimize treatment outcomes, it is best to diagnose gingival and periodontal diseases as near to their inception as possible, usually during childhood. Clinicians must take into consideration such factors as the biological changes that take place during childhood and adolescence, i.e., the structural and functional changes in the periodontium during the eruption and exfoliation of teeth; the establishment and maturation of the oral microflora; and the gradual development of the immune defense system (Bimstein and Matsson, 1999). Treatment now goes beyond home maintenance and surgery, and includes such elements as new antimicrobial regimens, guided tissue regeneration, new drug delivery systems, and modification of host factors. General dentists, periodontists, pediatric dentists, oral pathologists, orthodontists, and oral and maxillofacial surgeons must all be familiar with these advances to optimize the treatment of young patients with incipient or obvious periodontal problems.

Periodontal–systemic relationships

The relationships between gingival, periodontal, and systemic diseases are increasingly recognized as relevant to the overall health of all age groups (Newman, 1994, 1996). The fact that gingival and periodontal diseases are widespread often obscures the fact that systemic diseases can manifest in the periodontium. It requires a trained eye to recognize these problems and thus the responsibility for detecting systemic disease through gingival and periodontal manifestations

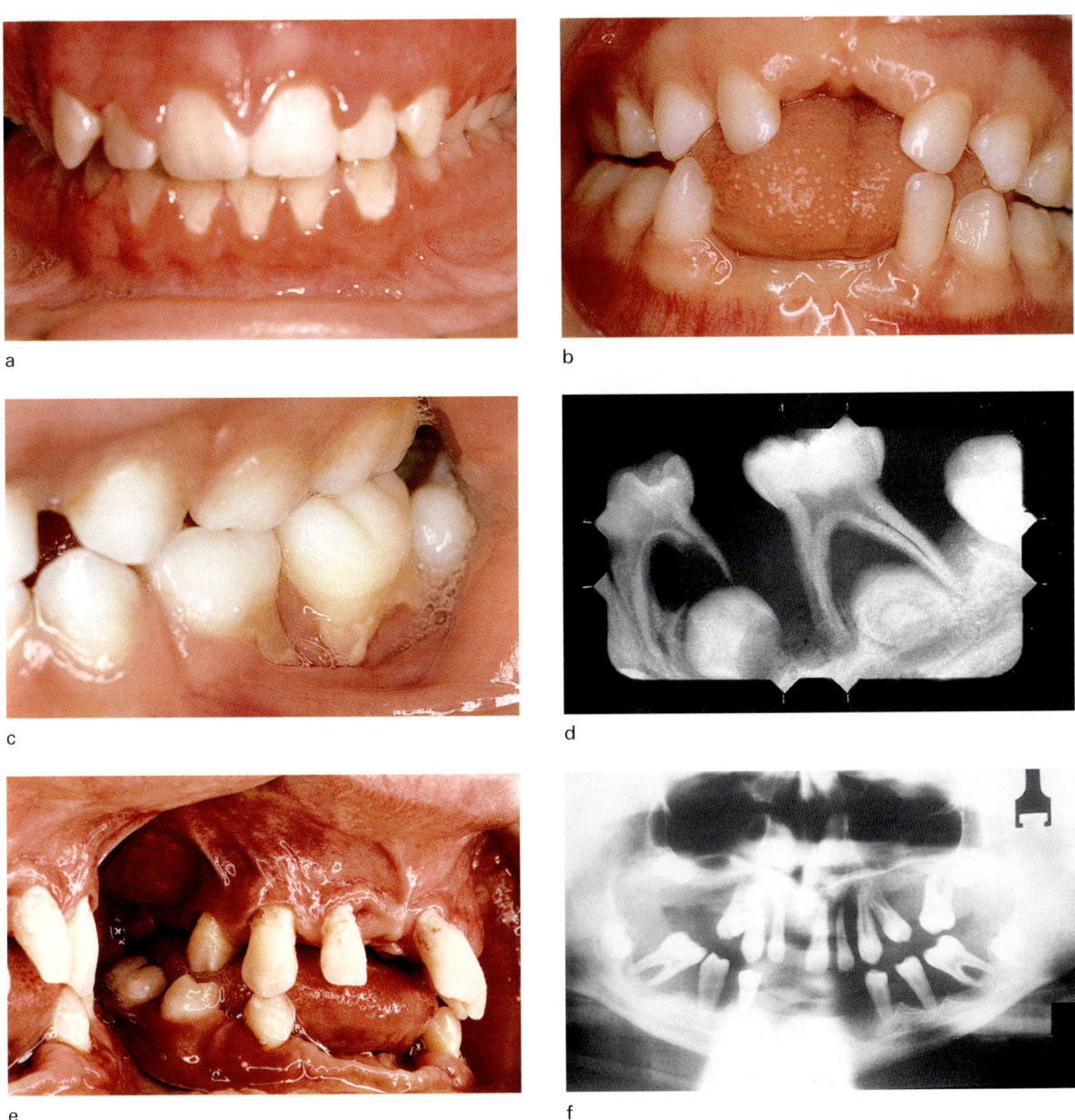

Figure 1.7

(a) Extensive gingival hypertrophy and erythema due to leukemic infiltrate in an 11-year-old girl with acute myelogenous leukemia. (b) Early shedding of the deciduous anterior incisors of a 4-year-old girl who was diagnosed to have hypophosphatasia after the early shedding of these teeth. (c) Gingival and alveolar bone destruction around the primary molars of a 7-year-old child with histiocytosis. (d) Periapical radiograph of a 4-year-old child with histiocytosis in which extensive alveolar bone loss is evident. The deciduous mandibular molars appear to "float" in the radiolucent area (courtesy of Dr Evelyn Mamber). (e) A 14-year-old girl with Papillon–Lefèvre syndrome. Extensive attachment and alveolar bone loss and early loss of permanent teeth are evident (with permission of the *Journal of Periodontology*, from Bimstein et al., 1990). (f) Panoramic radiograph of the child in (e) demonstrating extensive alveolar bone loss around all teeth (with permission of the *Journal of Periodontology*, from Bimstein et al., 1990).

rests with the dental profession. An important example is childhood malignancy such as acute myelogenous leukemia. Although relatively rare, acute myelogenous leukemia often affects the periodontium and gingival abnormalities may constitute the earliest discernible manifestation of the disease (Felix and Lukens, 1986; Lee, 1986) (Figure 1.7a). Other examples include host response deficiencies including leukocyte adhesion deficiency, hypophosphatasia (Figure 1.7b), histiocytosis (Figures 1.7c, d), diabetes, and genetic syndromes such as Papillon–Lefèvre syndrome (Figures 1.7e, f) (Bruckner et al., 1962; Izumi et al., 1989; Bimstein et al., 1990; Modeer et al., 1990; Stabholz et al., 1991; Meyle, 1994; Plagman et al., 1994; Waltrop et al., 1995; Santos et al., 1996; Biasi et al., 1999). Rare as they may be individually, collectively these disease entities are numerous enough to emphasize the need to pay greater attention to periodontal abnormalities in children and adolescents.

Systemic conditions may also affect the presentation and severity of existing periodontal disease. This is demonstrated by the relationship between gingival and periodontal diseases and normal hormonal changes which are common during puberty (Figure 1.1c) (Sutcliffe, 1972; Delaney et al., 1986; Mombelli et al., 1989, 1995). In general, with similar amounts of plaque, older children tend to have more pronounced gingival inflammation (Matsson, 1978, 1993; Matsson and Goldberg, 1985; Bimstein and Ebersole, 1989). Based on the amount of plaque and the age of the child, the clinician should be able to diagnose disproportionate gingival responses to a given level of dental plaque accumulation. More dramatically, the immunosuppression of patients who have undergone successful organ transplantation often results in significant periodontal problems (Ross et al., 1989; Allman et al., 1994; da Fonseca, 1998) (Figure 1.1f). With the ever-increasing success of transplantation, this is becoming a common clinical problem in both hospital and private practice.

Periodontal disease or manipulation of the periodontium can directly affect the systemic status of an individual. The subject of focal infection is currently receiving renewed interest at an international level. Researchers are investigating many serious systemic disorders that are thought to have an infective origin in dental plaque (Shurin et al., 1979; Crossner et al., 1990;

Newman, 1996; Beck and Offenbacher, 1998; Beck et al., 1998, 1999; Offenbacher et al., 1998a, b). To emphasize the importance of this for our young patients, one has only to consider the possible sequel of bacterial endocarditis in children with congenital or rheumatic heart disease.

Classification

The classification of gingival and periodontal diseases has changed frequently as our understanding of gingival and periodontal disease processes has increased. This has often led to the use of non-standardized, conflicting, or inaccurate classification systems, which in turn have led to incorrect diagnostic criteria, resulting in inaccurately high prevalence values (Bimstein and Matsson, 1999). It is hoped the classification system used in this book will be accepted internationally since it is based on the findings of recent clinical and cellular/molecular biological research and the relationships between systemic, gingival, and periodontal conditions. In addition, this classification system is consistent with recommendations of the World Workshop on the Classification of Periodontal Diseases (2000). It simplifies the nomenclature and takes into consideration the clinical expression and basic etiology of periodontal diseases in children, adolescents, and young adults.

Gingival disease is separated in this book from periodontal disease to help distinguish those entities that are generally solely confined to the supporting soft tissues. Periodontal disease is divided into two broad categories: those that are associated with systemic disease and those that are not. Entities not associated with systemic disease in children, adolescents, and young adults are further subdivided into acute periodontal abscesses, periodontitis, aggressive periodontitis, and necrotizing periodontitis.

Organizational policies and dental providers

General dentists, pediatric dentists and pediatricians have an important role to play in the early diagnosis and treatment of oral diseases (including gingival and periodontal diseases), extending the longevity of the permanent dentition and improving the quality of life of our patients. The American Academy of Periodontology (1996) and the American Academy of Pediatric Dentistry (1999b, c) have published guidelines entitled *Periodontal Diseases of Children and Adolescents* and *Guidelines for Periodontal Therapy*. These policy statements clearly indicate the recognition of this issue and a desire to make their combined memberships aware of the need for gingival and periodontal evaluations in childhood and adolescence. Furthermore, according to the American Dental Association Commission on Dental Accreditation (1985) curriculum guidelines for predoctoral pediatric dentistry, all US graduating dentists must be trained to identify normal and abnormal soft tissues and supporting structures in the child and adolescent, and to describe applicable therapeutic intervention, including surgery, for gingival and periodontal problems. The American Dental Association Commission on Dental Accreditation (1999) accreditation standards for advanced specialty education programs in pediatric dentistry require all pediatric dentists completing their advanced training to have the "ability to diagnose the various periodontal diseases of childhood and adolescence, and to treat and/or refer cases of periodontal diseases to the appropriate specialist."

Pediatric dentistry is an age-defined specialty which "provides both primary and comprehensive preventive and therapeutic oral health care for infants and children through adolescence, including those with special care needs" (American Academy of Pediatric Dentistry, 1999a). Therefore, pediatric dentistry is not limited to a technique or to a type of orofacial disease. This necessitates that pediatric dentists be expert in all aspects of oral health and disease in this population and be able to make appropriate referrals. The training, and thus the clinical practice of pediatric dentistry, has traditionally focused on the management of childhood behavior, caries, developing malocclusion, and traumatic incidents. Incipient gingival and periodontal disease are not easy to detect; all too often only the most flagrant and clinically obvious entities are readily diagnosed. Depending on both the complexities of the

diagnosis and the necessary therapy, it may be appropriate for the pediatric dentist to refer the patient to the periodontist. Because it is often difficult to decide when to refer children to a specialist, one of the goals of this book is to help pediatric dentists become better equipped to diagnose and treat periodontal diseases in children and adolescents, as well as to make appropriate referrals.

Periodontists, while they may be expected to have expertise in the full range of gingival and periodontal diseases and treatments, typically have little experience with young patients during training, and may feel uncomfortable when confronted with behavioral management issues and clinical entities not often encountered in training or practice. This book will help the periodontist become more confident in recognizing, diagnosing and treating periodontal disease in children and adolescents.

Another objective of this book is the fostering of cooperation and interaction between all dentists, especially between the pediatric dentist and the periodontist. This includes evaluation, diagnosis, and treatment of gingival and periodontal diseases in these groups. While it is clear that both professionals should be able to identify gingival and periodontal problems in children and adolescents, the decision as to who should perform the treatment depends on each professional's level of training (predoctoral, postdoctoral, and/or continuing education), interest and experience in managing a particular gingival or periodontal disease entity or procedural technique, and behavior management skills. In some cases it may be necessary for the pediatric dentist and the periodontist to work as a team to ensure that the child receives optimal dental care.

The purpose of this book is not only to bridge the gaps between pediatric dentists and periodontists, but between general dentists and all dental specialists. Since most children are treated by generalists and not by pediatric dentists or periodontists, the generalist is in an ideal position to detect and either manage or appropriately refer the child patient with gingival and periodontal problems. The orthodontist frequently encounters gingival and periodontal problems which develop during treatment, or needs the periodontist's help in orthodontic treatment of such problems as severe gingivitis, mucogingival defects, or impacted permanent teeth. Oral pathologists and oral and maxillofacial surgeons are often confronted with specific oral mucosal, gingival, or alveolar features and/or systemic problems in the child and adolescent which may be associated with periodontal problems. This book is also directed at these specialists since gingival and periodontal diseases are not a major focus during their training.

References

Aass AM, Albandar J, Aasenden R et al (1988) Variation in prevalence of radiographic alveolar bone loss in subgroups of 14-year-old schoolchildren in Oslo. *J Clin Periodontol* **15**: 130–3.

Aass AM, Rossow I, Preus HR, Gjermo P (1994) Incidence of early periodontitis in a group of young individuals during 8 years: associations with selected potential predictors. *J Periodontol* **65**: 814–19.

Allman SD, McWhorter AG, Seale S (1994) Evaluation of cyclosporin-induced gingival overgrowth in the pediatric transplant patient. *Pediatr Dent* **16**: 36–40.

American Academy of Pediatric Dentistry (1999a) Definition of Pedaitric Dentistry. *Pediatr Dent* (special issue: Reference Manual), **21**: 4.

American Academy of Pediatric Dentistry (1999b) Guidelines for periodontal therapy. *Pediatr Dent* (special issue: Reference Manual), **21**: 57–9.

American Academy of Pediatric Dentistry (1999c) Periodontal disease of children and adolescents. *Pediatr Dent* (special issue: Reference Manual), **21**: 81–5.

American Academy of Periodontology, Committee on Research Science and Therapy (1996) Periodontal diseases in children and adolescents. *J Periodontol* **67**: 57–62.

American Dental Association Commission on Dental Accreditation (1985) Curriculum guidelines for pre-doctoral pediatric dentistry. *J Dent Educ* **49**: 607–10.

American Dental Association Commission on Dental Accreditation (1999) *Accreditation Standards for Advanced Specialty Education Programs*, pp. 17, 19. Chicago: American Dental Association.

Armitage GC (1986) Periodontal diseases of children and adolescents. *Cal Dent Assoc J* **14**: 57–61.

Asikainen S, Chen C, Slots J (1996) Likelihood of transmitting *Actinobacillus actinomycetemcomitans* and *Porphyromonas gingivalis* in families with periodontitis. *Oral Microbiol Immunol* **11**: 387–94.

Baer PN, Benjamin SD (1974) *Periodontal Disease in Children and Adolescents*. Philadelphia: JB Lippincott.

Barnett ML (1997) Molecular approaches to oral therapeutics: dentistry in the next millenium? *J Dent Res* **76**: 1236–8.

Beck JD, Offenbacher S (1998) Oral health and systemic disease: periodontitis and cardiovascular disease. *J Dent Educ* **62**: 859–70.

Beck JD, Offenbacher S, Wijlliams R, et al (1998) Periodontitis: a risk factor for coronary heart disease? *Ann Periodontol* **3**: 127–41.

Beck JD, Pankow J, Tyroler HA, Offenbacher S (1999) Dental infections and atherosclerosis. *Am Heart J* **138**: 528–33.

Biasi D, Bambara LM, Carletto A et al. (1999) Neutrophil migration, oxidative metabolism and adhesion in early onset periodontitis. *J Clin Periodontol* **26**: 563–8.

Bimstein, E (1987) Periodontal considerations in the child dental patient. *Acta Odontol Pediatr* **8**: 13–19.

Bimstein E, Ebersole J (1989) The age-dependent reaction of the periodontal tissues to dental plaque. *ASDC J Dent Child* **56**: 358–62.

Bimstein E, Matsson L (1999) Growth and development considerations in the diagnosis of gingivitis and periodontitis in children. *Pediatr Dent* **21**: 186–91.

Bimstein E, Sela MN, Shapira L (1997) Clinical and microbial considerations for the treatment of an extended kindred with seven cases of prepubertal periodontitis: a two year follow up. *Pediatr Dent* **19**: 396–403.

Bimstein E, Delaney JE, Sweeney EA (1988a) Radiographic assessment of the alveolar bone height in children and adolescents. *Pediatr Dent* **10**: 199–204.

Bimstein E, Machtei E, Becker A (1988b) The attached gingiva in children: diagnostic, developmental and orthodontic considerations for its treatment. *ASDC J Dent Child* **55**: 351–6.

Bimstein E, Shanzer Y, Sgan Cohen H (1989) Prevalence and severity of gingivitis in children aged 13–14 years in Jerusalem. *Commun Dent Oral Epidemiol* **17**: 331–2.

Bimstein E, Lustman J, Sela MN, et al (1990) Periodontitis associated with Papillon Lefèvre Syndrome. *J Periodontol* **61**: 373–7.

Bimstein E, Tressure ET, Williams SM, Dever JG (1994) Alveolar bone loss in 5-year-old New-Zealand children: its prevalence and relationship to caries prevalence, socio-economic status and ethnic origin. *J Clin Periodontol* **21**: 447–50.

Brown LJ, Brunelle JA, Kingman A (1996) Periodontal status in the United States, 1988–1991: prevalence, extent, and demographic variation. *J Dent Res* **75**: 672–83.

Bruckner RJ, Rickles NH, Porter DR (1962) Hypophosphatasia with premature shedding of teeth and aplasia of cementum. *Oral Surg Oral Med Oral Path* **15**: 1351–69.

Crossner CG, Carlsson J, Sjödin B et al. (1990) Periodontitis in the primary dentition associated with *Actinobacillus actinomycetemcomitans* infection and leukocyte dysfunction. *J Clin Periodontol* **17**: 264–7.

da Fonseca MA (1998) Pediatric bone marrow transplantation: oral complications and recommendations for care. *Pediatr Dent* **20**: 386–94.

Delaney J, Ratzan SK, Kornman KS (1986) Subgingival microbiota associated with puberty: studies of pre-, circum-, and postpubertal human females. *Pediatr Dent* **8**: 268–75.

Egelberg J (1965) Local effect of diet on plaque formation and development of gingivitis in dogs. I. Effect of hard and soft diets. *Odont Rev* **16**: 31–61.

Ellwood R, Worthington HV, Cullinan MP et al. (1997) Prevalence of suspected periodontal pathogens identified using ELISA in adolescents of different ethnic origins. *J Clin Periodontol* **24**: 141–5.

Ferguson MM, Wall JG (1995) The effects of hormones and nutritional factors on the periodontal ligament. In: Berkowitz BKB, Moxham BJ, Newman HN (eds.) *The Periodontal Ligament in Health and Disease.* London: Mosby-Wolfe, pp. 417–32.

Felix DE, Lukens J (1986) Oral symptoms as a chief sign of acute monoblastic leukemia: report of case. *J Am Dent Assoc* **13**: 899–902.

Greene JC (1975) The case for preventive periodontics. *ASDC J Dent Child* **42**: 24–7.

Izumi Y, Sugiyama S, Shinozuka O et al. (1989) Defective neutrophil chemotaxis in Down's syndrome patients and its relationship to periodontal destruction. *J Periodontol* **60**: 238–42.

Lee SB (1986) Periodontal manifestations of leukemia. *J Indiana Dent Assoc* **65**: 23–4.

Löe H, Brown LJ (1991) Early onset periodontitis in the United States of America. *J Periodontol* **62**: 608–16.

MacCall JO (1938) Gingival and periodontal disease in children. *J Periodontol* **9**: 7–15.

Matsson L (1978) Development of gingivitis in preschool children and young adults. A comparative experimental study. *J Clin Periodontol* **5**: 24–34.

Matsson L (1993) Factors influencing the susceptibility to gingivitis during childhood—a review. *Int J Paed Dent* **3**: 119–27.

Matsson L, Goldberg P (1985) Gingival inflammatory reaction in children at different ages. *J Clin Periodontol* **12**: 98–103.

Matsson L, Hjersing K, Sjödin B (1995) Periodontal conditions in Vietnamese immigrant children in Sweden. *Swed Dent J* **19**: 73–81.

Matsson L, Sjödin B, Blomquist HK (1997) Periodontal health in adopted children of Asian origin living in Sweden. *Swed Dent J* **21**: 177–84.

Meyle J (1994) Leukocyte adhesion deficiency and prepubertal periodontitis. *Periodontol 2000* **6**: 26–36.

Modeer T, Barr M, Dahllof G (1990) Periodontal disease in children with Down's syndrome. *Scand J Dent Res* **98**: 228–34.

Mombelli A, Gusterbi FA, van Oosten MAC, Lang NP (1989) Gingival health and gingivitis development during puberty. A 4-year longitudinal study. *J Clin Periodontol* **16**: 451–6.

Mombelli A, Rutar A, Lang NP (1995) Correlation of the periodontal status 6 years after puberty with clinical and microbiological conditions during puberty. *J Clin Periodontol* **22**: 300–5.

Newman (1974) Diet, attrition, plaque and dental disease. *Br Dent J* **136**: 491–7.

Newman HB (1990) Plaque and chronic inflammatory periodontal disease—a question of ecology. *J Clin Periodontol* **17**: 533–41.

Newman HN (1994) Periodontal Medizine. *Parodontologiel* **1**: 61–4.

Newman HN (1996) Focal infection. *J Dent Res* **75**: 1912–19.

Offenbacher S, Beck JD, Lieff S, Slade G (1998a) Role of periodontitis in systemic health: spontaneous preterm birth. *J Dent Educ* **62**: 852–8.

Offenbacher S, Jared HL, O'Reilly PG et al. (1998b) Potential pathogenic mechanisms of periodontitis associated pregnancy complications. *Ann Periodontol* **3**: 233–50.

Plagman HC, Kocher T, Kuhrau N, Caliebe A (1994) Periodontal manifestation of hypophosphatasia. A family case report. *J Clin Periodontol* **21**: 710–16.

Ross PJ, Nazif MM, Zullo T et al (1989) Effects of Cyclosporin A on gingival status following liver transplantation. *ASDC J Dent Child* **56**: 56–9.

Santos R, Shanfeld J, Casamassimo P (1996) Serum antibody response to *Actinobacillus actinomycetemcomitans* in Down's syndrome. *Spec Care Dent* **16**: 680–3.

Schenkein HA, Burmesteir JA, Koertge TE et al. (1993) The influence of race and gender on periodontal microflora. *J Periodontol* **64**: 292–6.

Shapira L, Schlesinger M, Bimstein E (1997) Possible autosomal-dominant inheritance of prepubertal periodontitis in an extended kindred. *J Clin Periodontol* **24**: 388–93.

Shurin SB, Socransky SS, Sweeney E, Stossel TP (1979) A neutrophil disorder induced by capnocytophaga, a dental micro-organism. *New Engl J Dent* **301**: 849–54.

Stamm JW (1986) Epidemiology of gingivitis. *J Clin Periodontol* **13**: 360–6.

Stabholz A, Mann J, Sela M et al. (1991) Caries experience, periodontal treatment needs, salivary pH, and *Streptococcus mutans* counts in preadolescent Down syndrome population. *Spec Care Dent* **11**: 203–8.

Sutcliffe PA (1972) Longitudinal study of gingivitis and puberty. *J Periodont Res* **7**: 52–8.

Tinoco EM, Sivakumar M, Preus HR (1998) The distribution and transmission of *Actinobacillus actinomycetemcomitans* in families with localized juvenile periodontitis. *J Clin Periodontol* **25**: 99–105.

Van der Velden U (1991) The onset age of periodontal destruction. *J Clin Periodontol* **18**: 380–3.

Waltrop TC, Hallmon WW, Mealey BL (1995) Observations of root surfaces from patients with early-onset periodontitis and leukocyte adhesion deficiency. *J Clin Periodontol* **22**: 168–78.

Watanabe K (1990) Prepubertal periodontitis: a review of diagnostic criteria, pathogenesis, and differential diagnosis. *J Periodont Res* **25**: 31–48.

Watson MR, Bretz WA, Loesche WJ (1994) Presence of *Treponema denticola* and *Porphyromonas gingivalis* in children correlated with periodontal disease of their parents. *J Dent Res* **70**: 1636–40.

World Workshop on the Classification of Periodontal Diseases (2000) *Periodontol 2000.* (in press)

Zilberman Y, Shteyer A, Azaz B (1976) Iatrogenic exfoliation of teeth by the incorrect use of orthodontic elastic bands. *J Am Dent Assoc* **93**: 89–93.

2
The normal gingiva and periodontium

Enrique Bimstein

The components of the gingival and periodontal structures are the same in childhood, adolescence, and adulthood. However, the clinical and radiographic images of the gingiva and periodontium of children and adolescents differ from those seen in adults, owing to the significant changes that take place during growth and development. The clinician should be able to differentiate these normal images from disease, in order to prevent erroneous diagnosis, unnecessary therapeutic procedures, or exaggerated disease prevalence values. Moreover, when treatment is considered, the inherent healing capability and potential benefit from the growth and developmental changes in children and adolescents should be taken into account (Bimstein and Matsson, 1999).

Baer and Benjamin (1974), in their book *Periodontal Disease in Children and Adolescents*, wrote that, "The periodontium during childhood and puberty is in constant state of change owing to the exfoliation and eruption of teeth. This makes a general description of the normal periodontium difficult because it varies with the age of the patient." They quote Zappler (1948), who described "the gingiva in children as more reddish, lacking stippling, flabbier, rounded and rolled and with a greater sulcular depth; the cementum as being thinner, less dense and with a tendency to hyperplasia; the periodontal membrane as wider, with less dense fiber bundles, and with greater blood supply; the alveolar bone with a thinner lamina dura, fewer trabeculae, larger marrow spaces, decreased degree of calcification and greater blood and lymph supply." Unfortunately, since that time few studies have investigated the normal characteristics of the periodontium in children, adolescents, and young adults. Consequently, these classic studies have been repeatedly quoted in the dental literature during the intervening years.

Comprehensive descriptions of the histological development and the general morphology of the periodontium have been published elsewhere (Grant et al., 1979; Bernick and Grant, 1982; Lindhe and Karring, 1997). This chapter concentrates on growth and development changes that are relevant to the diagnosis and treatment of gingival and periodontal diseases in children and adolescents.

Tooth formation, eruption, and shedding

After the tooth enamel is fully formed, the basal lamina of the ameloblasts and the cells of the outer enamel epithelium create the reduced enamel epithelium. As the erupting tooth approaches the oral epithelium, the cells of the outer layer of the reduced enamel epithelium and of the basal layer of the oral epithelium show increased mitotic activity. When the tooth enters the oral cavity the reduced enamel epithelium and the oral epithelium fuse, and as eruption progresses, all the former enamel epithelium is gradually replaced by junctional epithelium (Lindhe and Karring, 1997).

The free gingival margin in the recently erupted tooth is often rounded in such a way that a very small invagination or sulcus is formed (Figure 2.1). When a periodontal probe is inserted into this invagination towards the cementoenamel junction (CEJ), the gingival tissue is separated from the tooth and a "gingival pocket" or "gingival crevice" is artificially opened (Lindhe and Karring, 1997). In newly erupted teeth this crevice is several millimeters

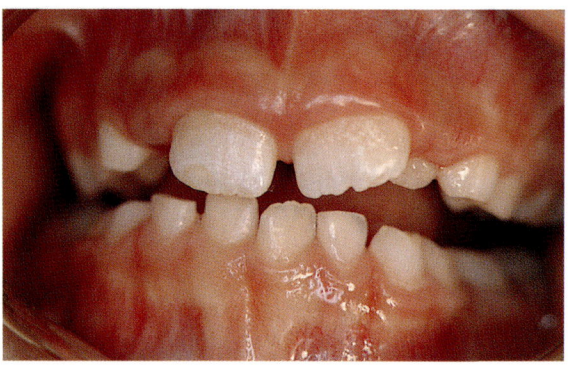

Figure 2.1

Newly erupted anterior permanent teeth with rounded marginal gingiva and shallow gingival sulci. A normal diastema is present between the maxillary central incisors with a saddle-shaped interdental papilla. Minimal to no attached gingiva is evident in the erupting teeth. Stippling is evident.

deep, and this depth will gradually decrease during the eruption process. The crevice depth of a newly erupted permanent tooth is significantly larger than that of its deciduous predecessor which is usually 1–2 mm just before its shedding. (Rosenblum, 1966; Kleiner and Garcia-Godoy, 1982; Bimstein and Eidelman, 1983, 1988; Tenenbaum and Tenenbaum, 1986; Peretz et al., 1996). The clinical significance of this difference is described later.

In the radicular area during the tooth bud formation, the collagen fibers produced by the fibroblasts in the loose connective tissue of the tooth bud are, during the process of their maturation, embedded into the newly formed cementum, immediately apical to the CEJ (Lindhe and Karring, 1997). Therefore, the "normal" position of the attachment apparatus has the apical end of the junctional epithelium at the CEJ and the most coronal periodontal ligament fibers located immediately apical to it (Figures 2.2a, b).

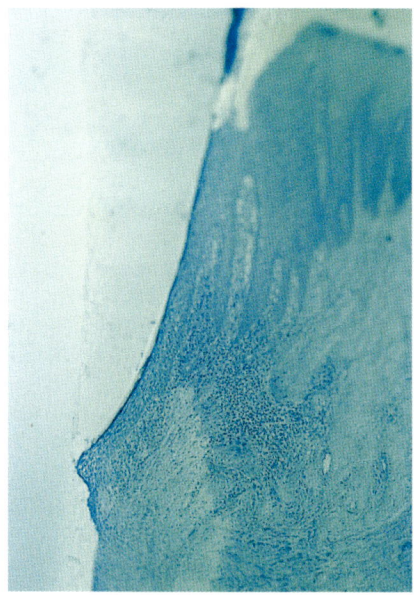

a

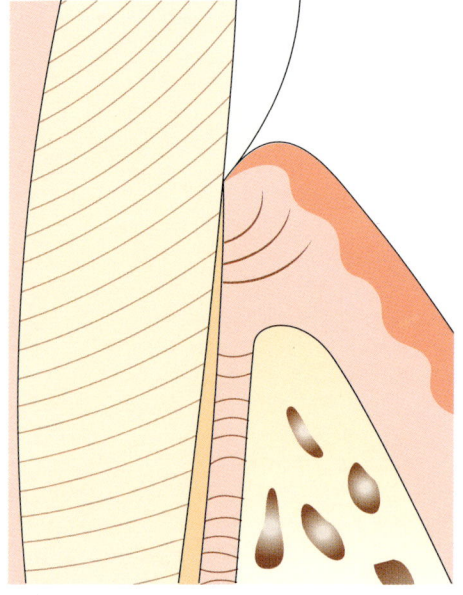

b

Figure 2.2

Human deciduous tooth with the apical end of the junctional epithelium normally located at the cementoenamel junction. (a) Histological section (with permission of *J Clin Periodontal*, Bimstein et al., 1988). (b) Diagrammatic presentation.

Apical migration of the junctional epithelium

There is clear evidence—clinical (Jamison, 1963), in vitro (Keszthelyi and Szabo, 1987), and histological (Bimstein et al., 1985, 1988, 1994a)—that apical migration of the epithelial attachment is not a rare phenomenon in the human deciduous teeth. While some authors have related this migration solely to periodontal disease, others have also linked it to physiologic processes. Jamison (1963) found clinical evidence of attachment loss in the deciduous dentition of 25.2% of 159 children, and concluded that they had "destructive periodontal disease". However, in the same article, he points out that he used this term to describe the condition in which the bottom of the gingival sulcus is located apical to the CEJ, a situation that may be a physiologic phenomenon preceding the exfoliation of the primary teeth.

Keszthelyi and Szabo (1987) measured the distance from the CEJ to the most coronal attachment fibers on extracted, stained human primary teeth. They reported such a distance to be present in two-thirds of the tooth surfaces (mean 0.26 ± 0.32 mm), and concluded that periodontitis in the primary dentition is not a rare phenomenon. Histological findings, however, indicate that changes in the junctional epithelium of human deciduous teeth are not always related to disease; they may be related to at least two additional parameters:

- Normal shedding: Bernick et al. (1951) indicated that apical migration of the epithelial attachment aids in the eventual shedding of the deciduous teeth. Soskolne and Bimstein (1977) found that the junctional epithelium migrates under the resorbing surface as it reaches the junctional epithelium (Figure 2.3).
- Continuous eruption: apical migration is characterized by elongation of the junctional epithelium, with no change in the histologic sulcus depth; it has no significant correlation with the adjacent tissue inflammation (Bimstein et al., 1985, 1988, 1994a) (Figure 2.4a, b). Therefore, it has been proposed that apical migration in the deciduous teeth may be related to continuous eruption of the tooth, as described for the permanent dentition

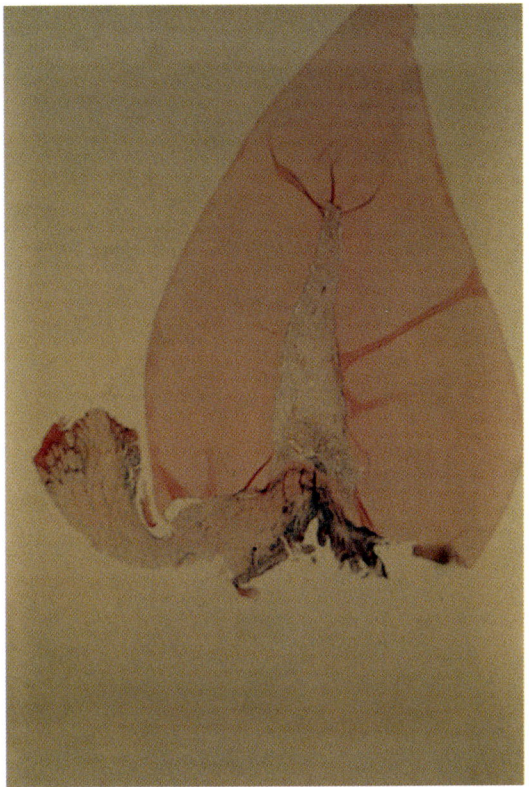

Figure 2.3

Histologic section of a deciduous human tooth with its junctional epithelium migrating under the resorbing surface (with permission of *Archives of Oral Biology*, Soskolne and Bimstein, 1977).

(Gargiulo et al., 1961; Newman and Levers, 1979; Levers and Darling, 1983). It is noteworthy that the values for the extent of the migration in a histologic study by Bimstein et al. (1988)—mean 0.28 ± 0.06 mm, affecting 53% of the teeth—were found to be similar to those reported by Keszthelyi and Szabo (1987) in their study in vitro.

Apical migration of the junctional epithelium in the primary dentition should therefore be considered a biologic feature that is related to a combination of factors. It is inadequate to attribute it solely to physiologic processes or periodontal disease.

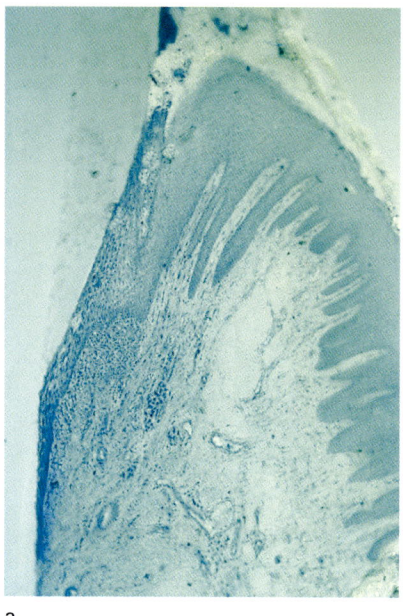

a

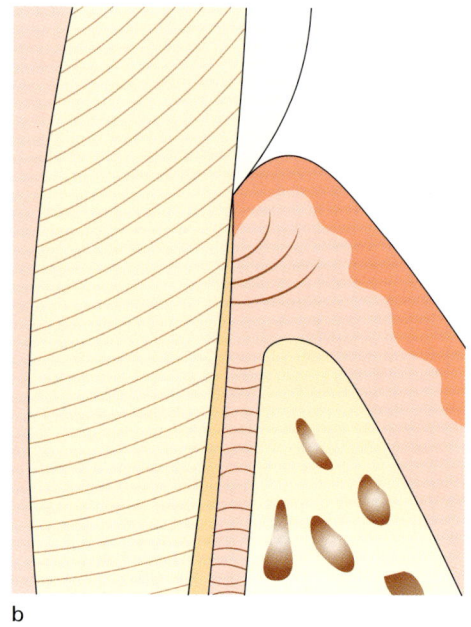

b

Figure 2.4

Human deciduous tooth in which apical migration of the junctional epithelium, apical to the cementoenamel junction, is evident. (a) Histologic section. (b) Diagrammatic presentation.

Gingival characteristics

The normal gingiva, composed of the free or marginal gingiva and the attached gingiva, is bounded by the mucogingival junction and by the gingival margin (Figure 2.5). It is important to be aware that these tissues have an age-dependent reactivity to plaque: for similar amounts of plaque accumulation, the degree of severity of gingivitis increases from early childhood, through childhood, adolescence, and adulthood (Matsson, 1978, 1993; Matsson and Goldberg, 1985; Bimstein and Matsson, 1999). With experience, the clinician must learn to recognize the degree of gingivitis appropriate to a given age and amount of dental plaque (Figure 2.6). Unexpectedly severe gingival inflammation indicates the presence of local or systemic factors that exacerbate the gingival response to dental plaque.

Gingival color

The normal gingival color in children has been described as either pink (Parfitt, 1973; Baer and Benjamin, 1974) or red (Magnusson et al., 1981). This inconsistency has been attributed to a normal change in gingival color with age. The color of the gingiva varies normally according to the degree of vascularity, epithelial keratinization, pigmentation, and thickness of the epithelium. With age, the amount of blood vessels decreases relative to the amount of connective tissue and the gingiva changes from red to pink (Grant et al., 1979; Lindhe and Karring, 1989). However, factors such as individual patient characteristics and the examiner's subjectivity significantly complicate the evaluation of the normal gingival color. Moreover, physiologic pigmentation of the gingiva (Figure 2.7) may vary according to ethnic group (Grant et al., 1979; Bimstein, 1987; Lindhe and Karring, 1997).

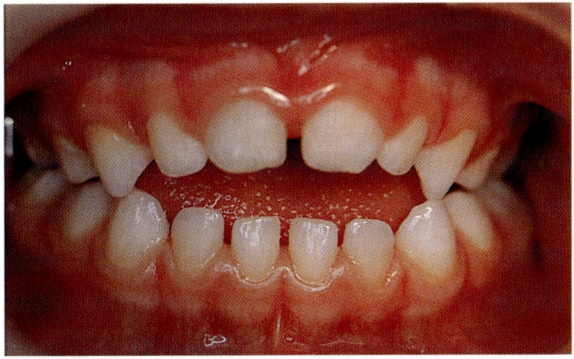

a

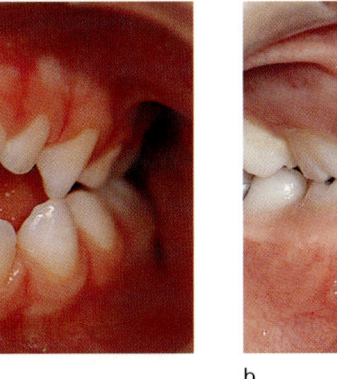

b

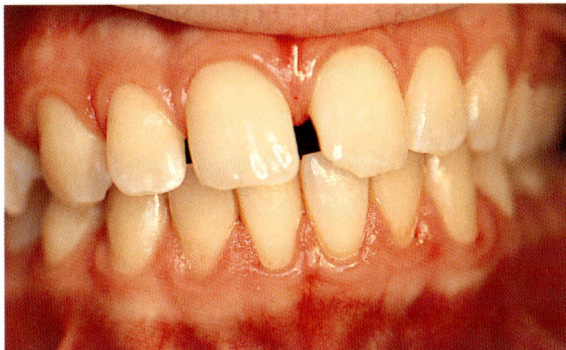

c

Figure 2.5

(a) A deciduous dentition demonstrating a wide band of attached gingiva bounded by a rounded marginal gingiva and the mucogingival junction. The interdental papillae have a saddle shape in areas with no proximal contacts and completely fill the interdental spaces in sites with proximal contact. (b) A mixed dentition demonstrating a minimal to non-existent band of the attached gingiva in areas of newly erupted anterior mandibular permanent teeth. The attached gingiva is significantly wider in the adjacent deciduous teeth. The interdental papillae completely fill the interdental spaces in sites with proximal contact. (c) The permanent dentition of an adolescent demonstrating a significantly wider band of attached gingiva adjacent to the anterior mandibular permanent teeth than that seen in (b). The interdental papilla at the diastema between the maxillary central permanent incisors has a saddle shape. In other sites with proximal contact, the papilla completely fills the interdental space.

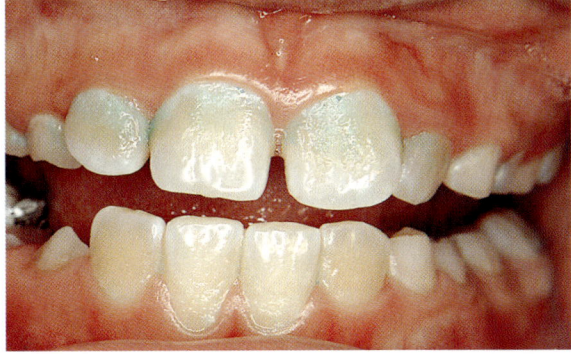

Figure 2.6

A mixed dentition exhibiting green staining of the dental plaque due to a long period of absence of adequate oral hygiene; however, gingival inflammation is minimal. The interdental papillae completely fill the interdental spaces in sites with proximal contacts. Stippling is evident.

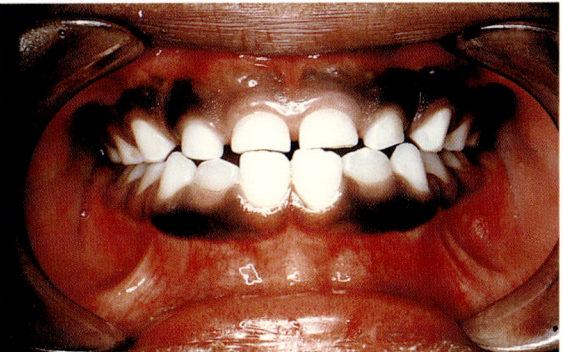

Figure 2.7

Physiologic pigmentation concomitant to dark skin. The interdental papillae have a saddle shape in sites with no proximal contacts, and completely fill the interdental spaces in sites with proximal contact in the deciduous dentition. Stippling is evident.

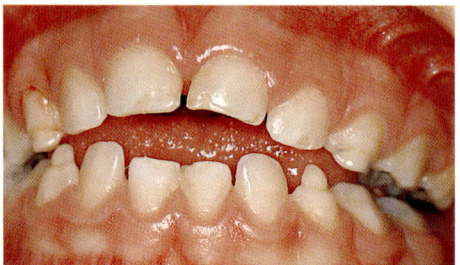

Figure 2.8

A deciduous dentition demonstrating rounded marginal gingiva, wide bands of attached gingiva and stippling. The interdental papillae completely fill the interdental spaces in sites with proximal contacts.

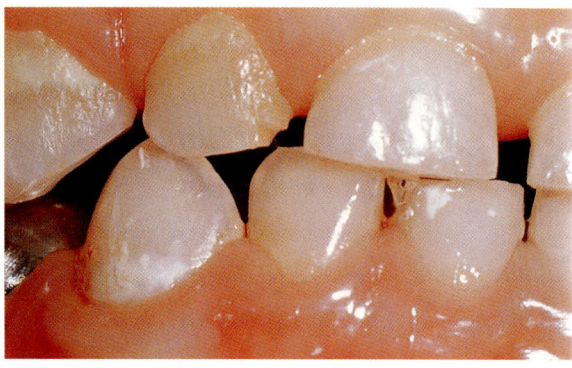

Figure 2.9

Rounded marginal gingiva of deciduous teeth.

Stippling

The surface of the gingiva is characterized by an "orange peel" appearance known as stippling (Figures 2.1, 2.5c, 2.6, 2.7), which reflects the contour of the epithelial connective tissue boundary in health (Grant et al., 1979). Stippling has been described as "fine" or "coarse", as variable between individuals and ages, and as being finer in females than in males (Wentz et al., 1952; Rosenberg and Massler, 1967). As part of the early signs of inflammation stippling is obliterated (Grant et al., 1979); however, the clinician must take into consideration that stippling starts to be evident at age 2–3 years, and that its absence has been described as normal also at older ages (Magnusson et al., 1981; Lindhe and Karring, 1989).

The free or marginal gingiva

The free gingiva has a dull surface and firm consistency. It comprises the gingival tissue at the vestibular and lingual/palatal aspects of the teeth, and the interdental gingiva or interdental papillae. On the vestibular and lingual side, the free gingiva extends from the gingival margin in an apical direction to the free gingival groove which is located at a level corresponding to the CEJ. Variations in gingival contour, thickness, and height are dependent on the presence of diastema, degree of eruption, and missing teeth (Grant et al., 1979). In adults, the gingiva tends to slope coronally to a round or a thin edge; in the primary dentition, owing to the normal cervical crown constriction, the marginal gingiva tends to be rounded (Grant et al., 1979; Magnusson et al., 1981; MacDonald et al., 1994; Figures 2.5a, 2.7–2.10). In addition, it has been reported that during the period of eruption of the permanent teeth the gingiva is thicker and has rounded margins (MacDonald et al., 1994) (see Figure 2.1).

The shape of the interdental gingiva (interdental papilla) is determined by the contact relationship between the teeth, the width of the proximal tooth surfaces, and the course of the CEJ, and should normally fill the interproximal spaces (Figures 2.5b, c, 2.6–2.8, 2.10). However, when normal spaces are evident between teeth, the papilla has a "saddle" shape and remains healthy because of increased keratinization (Figures 2.5a, c, 2.7, 2.9). This feature may appear both in adults and children, but it is more characteristic in children, both in the primary dentition in which primate spaces are common, and during the eruption of permanent teeth (Figure 2.1). In both cases when the spaces close

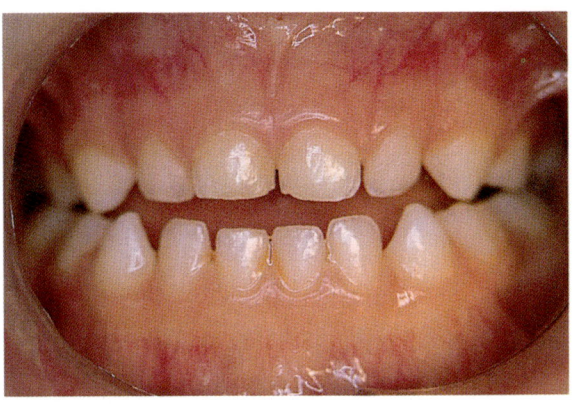

a

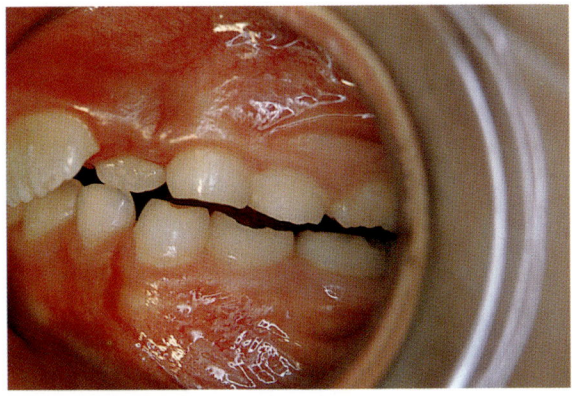

b

Figure 2.10

(a) Deciduous anterior teeth with no interdental spaces. The interdental papillae completely fill the interdental spaces. The marginal gingiva has a rounded appearance. (b) Deciduous molars with no interdental spaces. The interdental papillae completely fill the interdental spaces. The marginal gingiva has a rounded appearance.

during normal development, the interdental papilla will completely occupy the interdental space (Baer and Benjamin, 1974; Grant et al., 1979; Magnusson et al., 1981; Bimstein, 1987).

Attached gingiva

The coronal demarcation of the attached gingiva is the free gingival groove or (when the groove is absent) a horizontal plane at the level of the CEJ. The apical demarcation of the attached gingiva is the mucogingival junction where it becomes continuous with the alveolar lining mucosa (Figures 2.1, 2.5–2.8, 2.10). The attached gingiva varies in width between individuals and between different areas of the same mouth (Grant et al., 1979; Lindhe and Karring, 1997). Moreover, the width of the attached gingiva is significantly modified by the eruption and exfoliation of teeth (Rose and App, 1973; Bimstein and Eidelman, 1988; Matsson, 1993; Peretz et al., 1996).

The dimensions of the marginal and attached gingiva are intimately related to each other. In fact, they may be considered as a gingival unit. In clinical situations, the width of the attached gingiva is calculated by subtracting the distance from the gingival margin to the CEJ (sulcus and crevice depth, which correspond to the marginal gingiva) from the distance from the gingival margin to the mucogingival junction (keratinized gingiva) (Rose and App, 1973; Hall, 1977).

The width of the attached gingiva is greater in adults than in children (Bowers, 1963). This widening is not linear since the attached gingiva in a newly erupted permanent tooth is significantly narrower than that of its deciduous predecessor (see Figures 2.5a, b, Table 2.1), as the result of a significantly deeper gingival crevice in the newly erupted permanent tooth (Rose and App, 1973; Bimstein and

Table 2.1 Width of attached gingiva (in mm) in central incisors in children

Age (yr)	Type of tooth	Maxilla		Mandible	
		Mean	SD	Mean	SD
3–5	Deciduous	3.31	0.70	2.16	0.48
5	Permanent	0.76	0.82	0.45	0.70
13–15	Permanent	2.59	0.87	1.54	0.63

Adapted from Tenenbaum and Tenenbaum (1986).
SD, standard deviation.

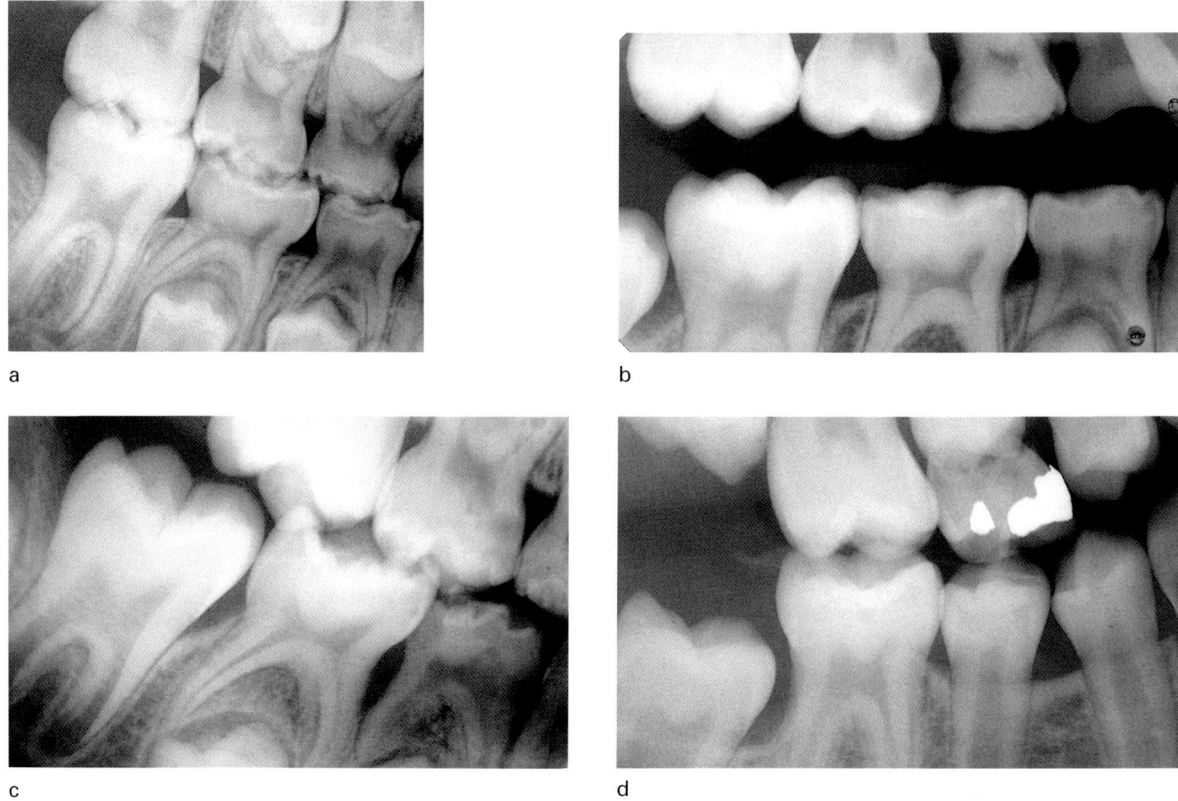

a   b

c   d

Figure 2.11

(a) Radiograph in which a normal alveolar bone height is evident in the deciduous and permanent teeth. (b) Radiograph in which a CEJ–ABC distance greater than 2 mm distal to the mandibular first deciduous molar is normal. (c) Radiograph in which a slope in the alveolar bone between the distal surface of the mandibular second primary molar and the mesial surface of the first permanent molar is normal. (d) Radiograph in which the angulation of the normal alveolar bone between the mandibular permanent teeth is dictated by the different height of each tooth, including the first permanent and the unerupted second permanent molars.

Eidelman, 1983, 1988; Bimstein et al., 1986; Tenenbaum and Tenenbaum, 1986; Peretz et al., 1996). It can be concluded that the width of the attached gingiva:

- changes concomitantly to changes in the sulcus and crevice depth during eruption and shedding
- increases with age in the primary dentition
- is significantly narrower in newly erupted permanent teeth than in their deciduous predecessors
- increases gradually with the eruption of the permanent teeth—however, in certain teeth it

may take many years until the width of the attached gingiva of the permanent tooth reaches the width of attached gingiva of its deciduous predecessor (Tenebaum and Tenenbaum, 1986)
- is normally minimal to none in newly erupted permanent teeth.

Alveolar bone

The alveolar bone in children has fewer trabeculae, larger marrow spaces, is less calcified, has a thinner lamina dura and wider periodontal membranes when compared with adults (Baer and Benjamin, 1974; Magnusson et al., 1981). In clinical situations the alveolar bone height, or presence of alveolar bone loss, is measured by the distance from the CEJ to the alveolar bone crest (ABC). In the primary dentition, a non-linear increase in the distance from the CEJ to the ABC takes place with age (Bimstein and Soskolne, 1988; Bimstein et al., 1990, 1993; Shapira et al., 1995; Needleman et al., 1997). This phenomenon is site-specific and has been related to attrition and facial growth (Bimstein et al., 1990, 1993) During facial growth, the maxilla and mandible are displaced in anterior and inferior directions (primary displacement), a "space" is created, and bone remodeling takes place with a consequent vertical drift of the teeth (Enlow, 1975a).

In the primary dentition, tooth eruption may take place at a faster rate than alveolar bone crest deposition, increasing the CEJ–ABC distance despite the claim by Enlow (1975b) that eruption brings the tooth to a definitive crown height above the gingiva and bone. In addition, exfoliation of primary teeth and/or eruption of adjacent permanent teeth can increase CEJ–ABC distances (Sjödin and Matsson, 1992).

Various CEJ–ABC distances for different deciduous teeth and jaws may be considered as cut-off values for the radiographic diagnosis of pathologic alveolar bone loss (Shapira et al., 1995). In most cases 2 mm is considered to be the borderline distance for a "healthy" alveolar bone height (Figure 2.11a). However, distances exceeding 2 mm may be normal in specific sites owing to approximation of exfoliation (Figure 2.11b) or adjacent erupting permanent teeth (Bimstein and Soskolne, 1988; Bimstein et al., 1990, 1993, 1994b; Sjödin and Matsson, 1992; Needleman et al., 1997). Distances of 2–3 mm have been considered as "questionable" and distances greater than 3 mm have been considered as "definitive" alveolar bone loss (Bimstein et al., 1994b). In any case, the quality of the crestal lamina dura must also be taken in consideration when diagnosing alveolar bone loss (Greenstein et al., 1981; Hausman et al., 1991; Bimstein, 1995).

In erupting permanent teeth, the alveolar bone crest is normally slightly apical to the CEJ. The discrepancy in the height of the CEJ of erupting teeth and their adjacent deciduous or permanent teeth gives the alveolar bone crest an angular appearance which should not erroneously be diagnosed as an angular bone defect (Figures 2.11c, d).

Conclusion

The clinician who treats children and adolescents must understand the influence of growth and development on the gingiva and the periodontium. Deep gingival crevices, minimal widths of attached gingiva (or none), red gingival color, lack of stippling, saddle-shaped interdental gingiva in spaced dentition, apical migration of the junctional epithelium, and CEJ–ABC distances greater than 2 mm may be normal findings in children and adolescents. Erroneous interpretation of these features may lead to inaccurate diagnosis of gingival or periodontal disease, resulting in unnecessary treatment and inaccurate disease prevalence values. Furthermore, comprehension of the potential developmental changes in the oral cavity allows the clinician to take advantage of these changes to benefit the young patient.

References

Baer PN, Benjamin SD (1974) The normal periodontium. In: *Periodontal Disease in Children and Adolescents*. Philadelphia: JB Lippincott, pp. 1–16.

Bernick S, Grant DA (1982) Development of the periodontal ligament. In: Berkovitz BKB, Moxham BJ, Newman HN (eds) *The Periodontal Ligament in Health and Disease*. Oxford: Pergamon, p. 197.

Bernick S, Rutherford RL, Rabinowitch BZ (1951) The role of the epithelial attachment in tooth resorption of primary teeth. *Oral Surg Oral Med Oral Path* **4**: 1444–50.

Bimstein E (1987) Periodontal considerations in the child dental patient. *Acta Odontol Pediatr* **8**: 13–19.

Bimstein E (1995) Radiographic diagnosis of the normal alveolar bone height in the primary dentition. *J Clin Pediatr Dent* **19**: 269–71.

Bimstein E, Eidelman E (1983) Dimensional differences in the attached gingiva and gingival sulcus in the mixed dentition. *ASDC J Dent Child* **50**: 264–7.

Bimstein E, Eidelman E (1988) Morphological changes in the attached and keratinized gingiva and gingival sulcus in the mixed dentition period. A 5-year longitudinal study. *J Clin Periodontol* **15**: 175–9.

Bimstein E, Matsson L (1999) Growth and development considerations in the diagnosis of gingivitis and periodontitis in children. *Pediatr Dent* **21**: 186–91.

Bimstein E, Soskolne WA (1988) A radiographic study of interproximal alveolar bone crest between the primary molars in children. *ASDC J Dent Child* **55**: 348–50.

Bimstein E, Lustmann J, Soskolne WA (1985) A clinical and histometric study of gingivitis associated with the human deciduous dentition. *J Periodontol* **56**: 293–6.

Bimstein E, Machtei E, Eidelman E (1986) Dimensional differences in the attached and keratinized gingiva and gingival sulcus in the early permanent dentition: a longitudinal study. *J Pedodont* **10**: 247–53.

Bimstein E, Soskolne WA, Lustmann J et al (1988) Gingivitis in the human deciduous dentition: a correlative clinical and block surface light microscopic (BSLM) study. *J Clin Periodontol* **15**: 575–80.

Bimstein E, Ranly DM, Skjonsby S (1990) Root exposure in the primary dentition studied in human skulls. *J Clin Periodontol* **17**: 317–20.

Bimstein E, Ranly DM, Skjonsby S, Soskolne AW (1993) The effect of facial growth, attrition, and age on the distance from the cementoenamel junction to the alveolar bone crest in the deciduous dentition. *Am J Orthod Dentofac Orthop* **103**: 521–5.

Bimstein E, Matsson L, Soskolne AW, Lustmann J (1994a) Histologic characteristics of the gingiva associated with the primary and permanent teeth of children. *Pediatr Dent* **16**: 206–10.

Bimstein E, Treasure ET, Williams SM, Dever JG (1994b) Alveolar bone loss in 5-year-old New Zealand children: its prevalence and relationship to caries prevalence, socio-economic status and ethnic origin. *J Clin Periodontol* **21**: 447–50.

Bowers GM (1963) A study of the width of attached gingiva. *J Periodontol* **34**: 201–9.

Enlow DE (1975a) Introductory concepts of the growth process. Part 2. In: Enlow DE (ed.) *Handbook of Facial Growth*. Philadelphia: WB Saunders, pp. 18–47.

Enlow DE (1975b) The facial growth process. Part 2. In: Enlow DE (ed.) *Handbook of Facial Growth*. Philadelphia: WB Saunders, pp. 76–146.

Gargiulo AW, Wentz FM, Orban B (1961) Dimensions and relations of the dentogingival junction in humans. *J Periodontol* **32**: 261–7.

Grant DA, Stern IB, Everett FG (1979) Periodontal health and disease. In: Grant DA, Stern IB, Everett FG (eds.) *Periodontics in the Tradition of Orban and Gottlieb*, 5th edn. St Louis: Mosby, pp. 3–19.

Greenstein G, Polson A, Iker H, Meitner S (1981) Associations between crestal lamina dura and periodontal status. *J Periodontol* **52**: 362–6.

Hall WB (1977) Present status of soft tissue grafting. *J Periodontol* **48**: 587–97.

Hausman E, Allen K, Clerehug V (1991) What alveolar crest level on a bite–wing radiograph represents bone loss? *J Periodontol* **62**: 570–2.

Jamison HC (1963) Prevalence of periodontal disease of the deciduous dentition. *J Am Dent Assoc* **66**: 208–15.

Keszthelyi G, Szabo I (1987) Attachment loss in primary molars. *J Clin Periodontol* **14**: 448–51.

Kleiner R, Garcia-Godoy F (1982) Gingival sulcus in the primary dentition. *J Pedodont* **6**: 288–93.

Levers BGH, Darling AI (1983) Continuous eruption of some adult human teeth of ancient population. *Arch Oral Biol* **28**: 401–8.

Lindhe J, Karring T (1989) The anatomy of the periodontum. In: Lindhe J (ed.) *Textbook of Clinical Periodontology*, 2nd edn. Copenhagen: Munksgaard, p. 19.

Lindhe J, Karring T (1997) Anatomy of the periodontum. In: Lindhe J, Karring T, Lang P (eds) *Clinical Periodontology and Implant Dentistry*, 3rd edn. Copenhagen: Munksgaard, pp. 19–68.

MacDonald RE, Avery DR, Weddell JA (1994) Gingivitis and periodontal disease. In: MacDonald RE, Avery DR (eds) *Dentistry for the Child and Adolescent*, 6th edn. St Louis: Mosby, p. 45.

Magnusson B, Matsson L, Modeer T (1981) Gingivitis and periodontal disease in children. In: Magnusson BO (ed.) *Pedodontics. A Systemic Approach*. Copenhagen: Munksgaard, p. 141–59.

Matsson L (1978) Development of gingivitis in preschool children and young adults. A comparative experimental study. *J Clin Periodontol* **5**: 24–34.

Matsson L (1993) Factors influencing the susceptibility to gingivitis during childhood—a review. *Int J Paed Dent* **3**: 119–27.

Matsson L, Goldberg P (1985) Gingival inflammatory reaction in children at different ages. *J Clin Periodontol* **12**: 98–103.

Needleman HL, Kue T-Ch, Nelson L et al (1997) Alveolar bone height of primary and first permanent molars in healthy seven-to-nine-year-old children. *ASDC J Dent Child* **64**: 188–96.

Newman HN, Levers BGH (1979) Tooth eruption and function in an early Anglo-Saxon population. *J Roy Soc Med* **72**: 341–50.

Parfitt GJ (1973) Periodontal diseases in children. The normal gingivae in childhood. In: Finn SB (ed.) *Clinical Pedodontics*, 4th edn. Philadelphia: WB Saunders, pp. 286–9.

Peretz B, Machtei EM, Bimstein E (1996) Periodontal status in childhood and early adolescence: three year follow up. *J Clin Pediatr Dent* **20**: 226–32.

Rose TR, App GR (1973) A clinical study of the development of attached gingiva along the facial aspect of the maxillary and mandibular anterior teeth in the deciduous, transitional and permanent dentitions. *J Periodontol* **44**: 131–9.

Rosenberg HM, Massler M (1967) Gingival stippling in young adult males. *J Periodontol* **38**: 473.

Rosenblum FN (1966) Clinical study of the depth of the gingival sulcus in the primary dentition. *ASDC J Dent Child* **33**: 289–97.

Shapira L, Tarazi E, Rosen L, Bimstein E (1995) The relationship between alveolar bone height and age in the primary dentition. *J Clin Periodontol* **22**: 408–12.

Sjödin B, Matsson L (1992) Marginal bone levels in the normal primary dentition. *J Clin Periodontol* **19**: 672–8.

Soskolne AW, Bimstein E (1977) Histomorphological study of the shedding process of human deciduous teeth at various chronological ages. *Arch Oral Biol* **22**: 331–5.

Tenenbaum H, Tenenbaum M (1986) A clinical study of the width of the attached gingiva in the deciduous, transitional and permanent dentition. *J Clin Periodontol* **13**: 270–5.

Wentz FM, Maier AW, Orban B (1952) Age changes and sex differences in the clinically "normal" gingiva. *J Periodontol* **23**: 13.

Zappler SE (1948) Periodontal disease in children. *JADA* **37**: 333 [quoted by Baer and Benjamin, 1974].

PART II

Gingival diseases and defects

3
Gingival diseases

Angelo J. Mariotti

There is growing acceptance that gingivitis is not a single disease, but an assortment of diseases that are the end result of a variety of different processes. Inflammation of the gingiva by bacteria is most common, but pathological changes in the gingiva can also result from systemic conditions (e.g., puberty), drugs (e.g., phenytoin) and neoplasms (e.g., leukemia). Hence, any disease that primarily affects gingival tissues should be broadly classified as a gingival disease.

The gingival diseases associated with children, adolescents, and young adults have several essential characteristics in common. Universal features include clinical signs of inflammation, signs and symptoms that are confined to the gingiva, reversibility of the disease on removal of the cause, and the presence of microbial-laden plaque to initiate or exacerbate the severity of the lesion. Although these features are common to all age groups, numerous studies have shown the severity and prevalence of gingival diseases will progressively intensify from the primary to the permanent dentition (Mackler and Crawford, 1973; Matsson, 1978; Hugoson and Koch, 1979; Matsson and Goldberg, 1985). The biological changes in periodontal structures (Zappler, 1948; Kelsten, 1955; Bradley, 1961; Ruben et al., 1971; Bimstein et al., 1994), the formation, organization, and maturation of dental plaque (Bailit et al., 1964; Socransky and Manganiello, 1971; Moore et al., 1984; Bimstein and Ebersole, 1989), and the development of the immune system (Longhurst et al., 1977, Seymour et al., 1977, 1982; Walsh et al., 1987; Bimstein and Ebersole, 1991) and endocrine system (Mariotti, 1994) account for the incidence and severity of many gingival diseases from infancy to adulthood.

Plaque-induced gingivitis

Plaque-induced gingivitis is an inflammation of the gingiva resulting from bacteria located at the gingival margin (Figure 3.1). The association of plaque with gingival inflammation made it a frequently postulated cause of gingivitis, but it was not until the elegant experimental human gingivitis studies of Löe and colleagues that a plaque bacterial etiology was confirmed (Löe et al., 1965). Epidemiological data have shown plaque-induced gingivitis to be prevalent at all ages of dentate populations (US Public Health Service, 1965, 1972, 1987; Stamm, 1986; Bhat, 1991) and this disease has been considered to be the most common form of periodontal disease (Page, 1985). In children, the prevalence of plaque-induced gingivitis increases with age until it reaches a zenith at puberty (Parfitt, 1957; Hugoson et al., 1981; Stamm, 1986). The initial histological changes from health to plaque-induced gingivitis may not be detectable clinically (Page and Schroeder, 1976; Bimstein et al., 1985; Bimstein et al., 1988), but as the gingivitis progresses, clinical signs become more obvious. Plaque-induced gingivitis begins at the gingival margin and can spread throughout the remaining gingival unit. Clinical signs of gingival inflammation involving changes to gingival contour, color, and consistency (Muhlemann and Son, 1971; Polson and Goodson, 1985) are associated with a stable periodontium which exhibits no loss of periodontal attachment or alveolar bone. In children, gingivitis is not as intense as that found in young adults with similar amounts of dental plaque (Matsson, 1978; Matsson and Goldberg, 1985). This age-related difference in

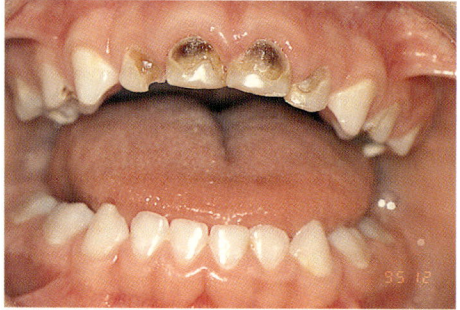

a

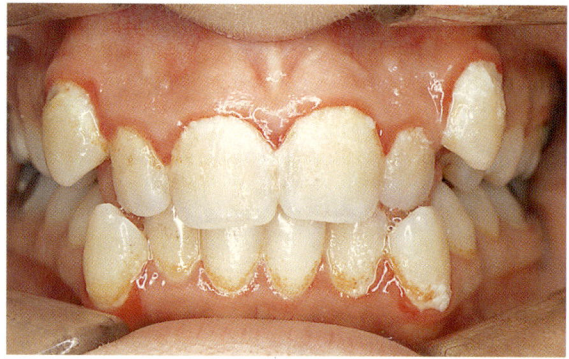

b

Figure 3.1

Plaque-induced gingivitis. (a) In the deciduous dentition (courtesy of Dr Enrique Bimstein). (b) In adolescence (courtesy of Dr Enrique Bimstein). (c) Severe gingivitis related to a long period without adequate oral hygiene (courtesy of Dr Howard L. Needleman).

c

the development and severity of gingivitis may be associated with the quantity or quality of dental plaque, the response of the immune system, or morphological differences in the periodontium between children and adults (Bimstein and Matsson, 1999). More specifically, the dental plaque of children usually contains lower concentrations of putative periodontal pathogens, and due to the presence of a thicker junctional epithelium coupled with increased vascularity in the gingival connective tissues and a developing immune system, the observable signs of inflammation in the child are usually more modest (Bimstein and Matsson, 1999).

The intensity of the clinical signs and symptoms of gingivitis will vary between individuals as well as between sites within a dentition. The common clinical findings of plaque-induced gingivitis include erythema, edema, bleeding, sensitivity, tenderness, and enlargement (Löe et al., 1965; Suzuki, 1988). Radiographic analysis or probing attachment levels of individuals with plaque-induced gingivitis will not indicate loss of supporting structures. Histopathologic changes include proliferation of basal junctional epithelium leading to apical and lateral cell migration, vasculitis of blood vessels adjacent to the junctional epithelium, progressive destruction of the collagen fiber network with changes in collagen types, cytopathologic alteration of resident fibroblasts, and a progressive inflammatory/immune cellular infiltrate (Page and Schroeder, 1976). Although the composition of bacterial flora associated with plaque-induced gingivitis differs from the flora associated with gingival health, no specific bacterial flora is pathognomonic for plaque-induced gingivitis (Ranney, 1993).

Gingival diseases associated with endogenous sex steroid hormones

Since the nineteenth century, evidence has accumulated to support the concept that tissues of the periodontium are modulated by androgens, estrogens, and progestins. Much of this evidence has come from observing the changes in gingival tissues during distinct endocrinological events (menstrual cycle, pregnancy, etc.). Although the gingiva can be a target for sex steroid hormones, the etiology of the changes has not been elucidated. The principal explanations for sex steroid hormone-induced changes in the gingiva have pointed to changes of microbiota in dental plaque, immune function, vascular properties, and cellular function in the gingiva (Mariotti, 1994). Certainly, the periodontal effects of sex steroid hormones are multifactorial in nature (Mariotti, 1994). Theoretically, sex steroid hormones will affect the host by influencing cellular function (in the blood vessels, the epithelium, and the connective tissue) and immune function, and together with hormone-selected bacterial populations occupying the gingival sulcus, induce specific observable changes in gingival tissues (Mariotti, 1994).

Puberty-associated gingivitis

Puberty is not a single episode but a complex process of endocrinological events that produce changes in the physical appearance and behavior of adolescents. Over the past two centuries the age of onset of puberty in both sexes has dramatically decreased (MacDonald et al., 1991): in the mid-nineteenth century the average age of menarche was 17.5 years, whereas today the average age of menarche is 12.5 years. The early onset of puberty, particularly for adolescent girls, increases the time of exposure of periodontal tissues to steroid hormones and the possibility of gingival disease.

The incidence and severity of gingivitis in adolescents are influenced by a variety of factors, including plaque levels, dental caries, mouth breathing, crowding of the teeth, and tooth eruption (Stamm, 1986); however, the dramatic rise in steroid hormone levels during puberty in both sexes has a transient effect on the inflammatory status of the gingiva (Mariotti, 1994). A number of studies have demonstrated an increase in gingival inflammation in circumpubertal individuals of both sexes without a concomitant increase in plaque levels (Parfitt, 1957; Sutcliffe, 1972; Hefti et al., 1981). Although puberty-associated gingivitis (Figure 3.2a, b) has many of the clinical features of plaque-induced gingivitis, this disease will develop frank signs of gingival inflammation in the presence of relatively small amounts of local irritants (plaque) during the circumpubertal period.

Menstrual cycle-associated gingivitis

Following menarche, there is a periodicity of sex steroid hormone secretion over a 25–30 day period—the menstrual cycle—during which clinically significant inflammatory changes in the gingiva have been observed (Muhlemann, 1948). However, the number of women who exhibit overt gingival changes fluctuating in conjunction with the menstrual cycle is small (Mariotti, 1994). The most common gingival changes involve minor signs of inflammation during ovulation. More specifically, gingival exudate has been shown to increase at least 20% during ovulation in over three-quarters of women tested (Hugoson, 1971). Since these changes in crevicular fluid flow are not observable unless measured electronically, most young women with gingival inflammation induced by the menstrual cycle will present with a very mild form of the disease.

Pregnancy-associated gingival disease

Some of the most remarkable endocrine and oral alterations accompany pregnancy as a result of the rise in plasma hormone levels over several months. During human gestation, pregnancy-associated gingivitis is characterized by an increase in the prevalence and severity of gingivitis during the second and third trimesters (Löe and Silness, 1963; Löe, 1965; Hugoson, 1971; Arafat, 1974b). Both longitudinal and

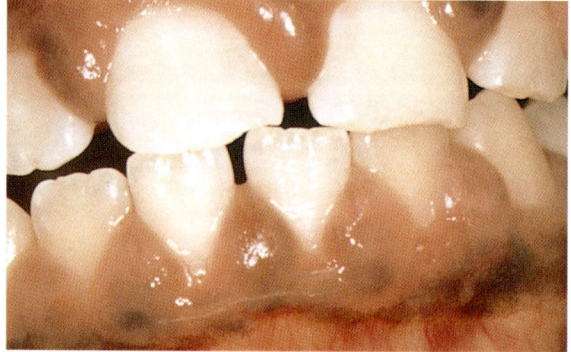

a

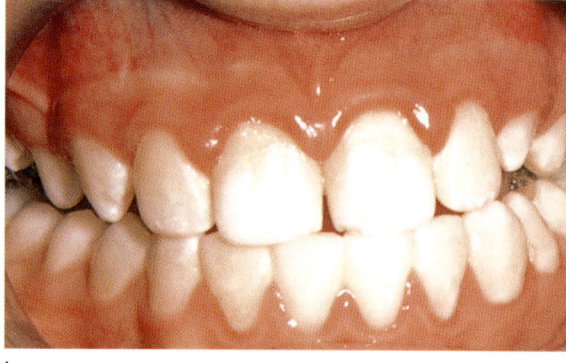

b

Figure 3.2

Gingival diseases associated with endogenous sex steroid hormones. (a, b) Puberty-associated gingivitis. (c) Pregnancy-associated pyogenic granuloma.

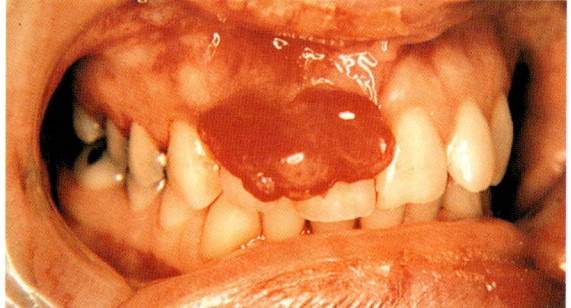

c

cross-sectional studies have found the prevalence and severity of gingival inflammation to be significantly higher during pregnancy than postpartum, even though plaque scores were the same in the two groups (Löe and Silness, 1963; Hugoson, 1971). In addition, gingival probing depths are deeper (Löe and Silness, 1963; Hugoson, 1971; Miyazaki et al., 1991), bleeding on probing or tooth brushing is increased (Arafat, 1974b; Miyazaki et al., 1991), and gingival crevicular fluid flow is elevated (Hugoson, 1971) in pregnant women. The features of pregnancy-associated gingivitis are similar to those of plaque-induced gingivitis, except for the propensity to develop frank signs of gingival inflammation in the presence of relatively little local irritation (i.e., plaque) during pregnancy.

Pregnancy-associated pyogenic granuloma or "pregnancy tumor" (Figure 3.2c) was described over a century ago (Coles, 1874). The pregnancy-associated pyogenic granuloma is not a tumor but an exaggerated inflammatory response during pregnancy to an irritation resulting in a solitary polyploid capillary hemangioma which can easily bleed upon mild provocation (Sills et al., 1996). These granulomas present clinically as a painless, protuberant, mushroom-like exophytic mass attached by a sessile or pedunculated base arising from the gingival margin or more commonly from an interproximal papilla (Sills et al., 1996). The pregnancy-associated pyogenic granuloma has been reported to occur in 0.5% to 5.0% of pregnant women (Ziskin and Nesse, 1946; Maier and Orban, 1949; Arafat, 1974a; Kristen, 1976). It is more common in the maxilla (Sills et al., 1996) and may develop as early as the first trimester (Sills et al., 1996), ultimately regressing or completely disappearing following parturition (Ziskin and Nesse, 1946).

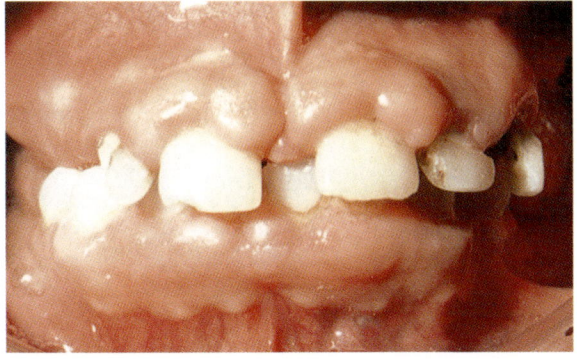

a

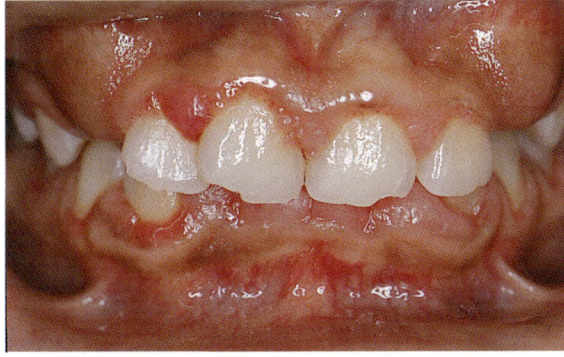

b

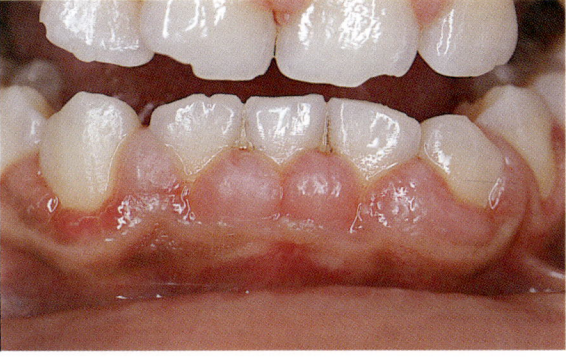

c

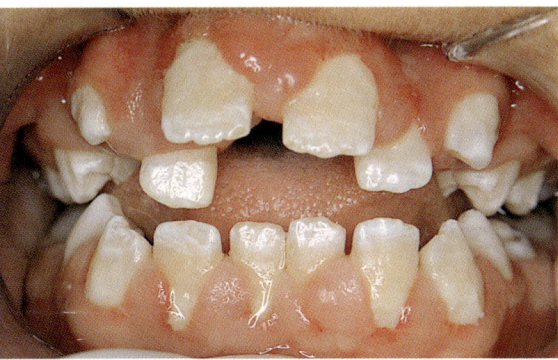

d

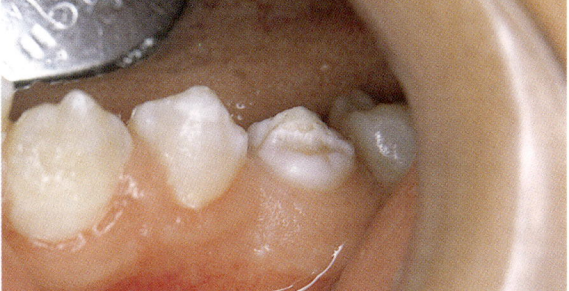

e

Figure 3.3

Drug-influenced gingival overgrowth. (a) Phenytoin associated overgrowth. (b) Cyclosporine-associated overgrowth in the permanent maxillary teeth of a child (courtesy of Dr Howard L. Needleman). (c) Cyclosporine-associated overgrowth in the permanent mandibular teeth of the same child as in (b) (courtesy of Dr Howard L. Needleman). (d) Cyclosporine-associated overgrowth in permanent anterior teeth in an adolescent (courtesy of Dr Enrique Bimstein). (e) Lateral view of the same adolescent as in (d). No gingival overgrowth is evident in the permanent mandibular cuspid and premolars (courtesy of Dr Enrique Bimstein).

Gingival diseases associated with medication

The use of chemicals for the benefit of humankind has led to an astonishing array of drugs for the alleviation of human afflictions as well as to the creation of new maladies that affect the gingiva.

Drug-influenced gingival enlargement

The disfiguring overgrowth of gingiva is a significant outcome principally associated with anticonvulsant drugs such as phenytoin (Figure 3.3a), immunosuppressors such as cyclosporine (Figure 3.3b–d), and calcium channel blockers such as nifedipine, verapamil, diltiazem and sodium valproate (Hassell and Hefti, 1991; Seymour et al., 1996). Common clinical characteristics of drug-influenced gingival enlargements include:

- patient variations in the pattern of enlargement, i.e., genetic predisposition (Hassell and Hefti, 1991; Seymour et al., 1996)
- a tendency to occur more often in anterior gingiva (Figure 3.3d, e) (Hassell and Hefti, 1991; Seymour et al., 1996)
- a higher prevalence in younger age groups (Esterberg and White, 1945; Rateitschak-Pluss et al., 1983; Hefti et al., 1994)
- onset within 3 months of use (Hassell and Hefti, 1991; Hassell, 1981; Seymour, 1991; Seymour and Jacobs, 1992) that is usually first observed in the papilla (Hassell and Hefti, 1991)
- although the condition can be found in a periodontium with or without bone loss, there is no association with attachment loss or tooth mortality (Hassell and Hefti, 1991; Seymour et al., 1996).

Furthermore, all of these drugs produce clinical lesions and histological characteristics that are indistinguishable from one another (Hassell and Hefti, 1991; Seymour et al., 1996). Finally, the influence of plaque on the induction of gingival enlargements by drugs in humans has not been fully elucidated (Hassell and Hefti, 1991); however, it does appear that the severity of the lesion is affected by the oral hygiene of the patient (Steinberg and Steinberg, 1982; Addy et al., 1983; Hassell et al., 1984; Tyldesley and Rotter, 1984; Daley et al., 1986; McGaw et al., 1987; Modeer and Dahllof, 1987; Yahia et al., 1988; Barclay et al., 1992).

Phenytoin

The first description of drug-induced enlargement of the gingiva involved phenytoin (Kimball, 1939). Used in a chronic regimen for the control of epileptic seizures, phenytoin induces gingival enlargements in approximately 50% of patients (Angelopoulous and Goaz, 1972). One prominent theory of the etiology of phenytoin-associated gingival enlargements suggests that the growth of genetically distinct populations of gingival fibroblasts results in the accumulation of connective tissues because of reduced catabolism of the collagen molecule (Hassell and Hefti, 1991).

Calcium channel blockers

Calcium channel blockers are a class of drugs that exert their effects principally at voltage-gated Ca^{2+} channels located in the plasma membrane, and are commonly prescribed as antihypertensive, antiarrhythmic, and antianginal agents. In 1984, calcium channel blockers were first linked to gingival enlargements (Ramon et al., 1984) and the prevalence of gingival lesions associated with these drugs has been estimated to be approximately 20% (Barclay et al., 1992). The mechanism of gingival enlargement is still under investigation, but these drugs may directly influence gingival connective tissues by stimulating an increase of gingival fibroblasts as well as an increase in the production of the connective tissue matrix (Fu et al., 1998).

Cyclosporine

Cyclosporine is a powerful immunoregulating drug used primarily in the prevention of organ transplant rejection (Seymour and Jacobs, 1992). The clinical features of cyclosporine-influenced gingival enlargement were first described in 1983 (Rateitschak-Pluss et al., 1983) and cyclosporine appears to affect 25–30% of the patients taking this medication (Hassell and Hefti, 1991; Seymour et al., 1987). Hypotheses explaining why cyclosporine affects the gingiva are diverse, but a leading theory suggests that the principal metabolite of cyclosporine, hydroxycyclosporine (M-17), in conjunction with the parent compound stimulates fibroblast proliferation (Mariotti et al., 1998). This increase in cell number coupled with a reduction in the breakdown of gingival connective tissues (Hassell and Hefti, 1991) has been postulated to be the cause of excessive extracellular matrix accumulation in cyclosporine-associated gingival enlargements.

Oral contraceptive-associated gingivitis

Oral contraceptive agents are one of the most widely used classes of drug in the world. The earlier onset of menarche, changing social mores, and increased emphasis on family planning have increased the use of oral contraceptives in adolescents and young adults. Case reports have described gingival enlargement induced by oral contraceptives in otherwise healthy women with no history of gingival overgrowth (Lynn, 1967; Kaufman, 1969; Sperber, 1969); in all cases, the increased gingival mass was reversed when oral contraceptive use was discontinued or the dosage reduced. Clinical studies have demonstrated that women using hormonal contraceptive drugs have a higher incidence of gingival inflammation than women who do not use these agents (Lindhe and Bjorn, 1967; El-Ashiry et al., 1970; Pankhurst et al., 1981) and that long-term use of oral contraceptives may affect periodontal attachment levels (Knight and Wade, 1974). All studies recording changes to gingival tissues by oral contraceptives were completed when dosage levels were much higher than today. A more recent clinical study in young women found that oral contraception had no effect on gingival tissues (Mariotti et al., 2000). It appears that current oral contraceptives are probably not as harmful to the periodontium as the early formulations.

Gingival diseases associated with systemic diseases

Leukemia-associated gingivitis

Leukemia is a progressive, malignant hematologic disorder characterized by an abnormal proliferation and development of leukocytes and precursors of leukocytes in the blood and bone marrow. Leukemia is classified according to its duration (acute or chronic) and the type of cell involved (myeloid or lymphoid) and the number of cells in the blood (leukemic or aleukemic). There are noticeable correlations of leukemias with age. For example, acute lymphoblastic leukemia constitutes 80% of all childhood leukemias, whereas acute myelogenous leukemia usually affects adults. Oral manifestations have primarily been described in acute leukemias; they consist of cervical adenopathy, petechiae, and mucosal ulcers, as well as gingival inflammation and enlargement (Lynch and

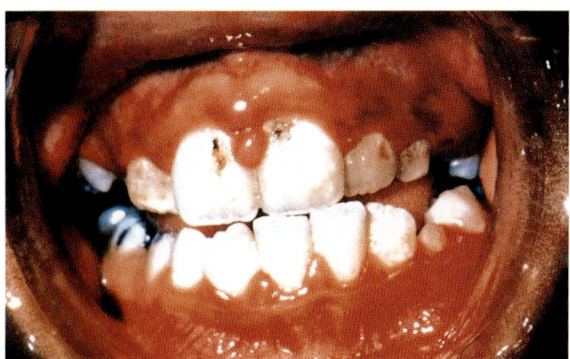

Figure 3.4

Leukemia-associated gingivitis.

Ship, 1967). Signs of inflammation in the gingiva include swollen, glazed, and spongy tissues which are red to deep purple in appearance (Figure 3.4) (Dreizen et al., 1984). Gingival bleeding is a common sign in patients with leukemia and is the initial oral sign or symptom in 17.7% and 4.4% of patients with acute and chronic leukemias, respectively (Lynch and Ship, 1967). Gingival enlargement has also been reported, initially beginning at the interdental papilla and followed by the marginal and attached gingiva (Dreizen et al., 1984). Although local irritants can predispose to and exacerbate the gingival response in leukemia, they are not prerequisites for lesions to form in the oral cavity (Dreizen et al., 1984).

Linear gingival erythema

Infection with the human immunodeficiency virus (HIV) produces an irreversible and progressive immunosuppression that renders the person infected susceptible to a variety of oral diseases. In humans, HIV depletes CD4+ lymphocytes (T helper cells), which leads to the development of a variety of fungal, viral, and bacterial oral infections (Connor and Ho, 1992).

Oral manifestations of HIV infection have been used to stage HIV disease (Justice et al., 1989; Royce et al., 1991; Prevention, 1992), to identify prophylactic treatment of other serious infections

(Force, 1993), and to indicate disease prognosis (Dodd et al., 1991; Katz et al., 1992). In the gingiva, manifestations of HIV infection were formerly known as HIV-associated gingivitis but are now known as linear gingival erythema (LGE). This condition is distinguished by a 2–3 mm marginal band of intense erythema in the free gingiva (Winkler et al., 1988), which may extend into the attached gingiva as a focal or diffuse erythema and/or extend beyond the mucogingival line into the alveolar mucosa (Winkler et al., 1988). The characteristics of LGE may be localized to one or two teeth but it is more commonly a generalized gingival condition.

The etiology of this gingival lesion is not well understood; however, research has begun to investigate the relationship of periodontal pathogens and the local host response in regard to how HIV infection affects the gingiva. Although LGE does not respond to conventional scaling, root planing, and plaque control (Winkler and Murray, 1987; Grassi et al., 1988; Winkler et al., 1988, 1989), the anaerobic microflora from subgingival sites of HIV-infected patients with gingivitis seems to be essentially the same as in non-infected patients (Moore et al., 1993). Despite the similarities in anaerobic microflora, organisms not generally associated with gingivitis in HIV-negative patients, such as *Candida* species, have been identified in LGE (Lamster et al., 1998). In addition, LGE lesions have been shown to have reduced proportions of T cells and macrophages and an increased number of immunoglobulin G plasma cells and polymorphonuclear leukocytes (Gomez et al., 1995). These host cell responses and unusual microbiota may be responsible for the refractory nature of this lesion to the conventional periodontal treatment of gingivitis.

Gingival diseases associated with malnutrition

Although some nutritional deficiencies can significantly exacerbate the response of the gingiva to plaque bacteria, the precise role of nutrition in the initiation or progression of periodontal diseases remains to be elucidated. Studies of the periodontal status of individuals in developed and in developing countries have failed to show any relationship between periodontal disease and general nutrition (Russell, 1962; Waerhaug, 1967; Wertheimer et al., 1967).

Severe vitamin C deficiency or scurvy was the earliest nutritional deficiency to be examined in the oral cavity (Lind, 1953). Even though scurvy is unusual in areas with an adequate food supply, certain populations on restricted diets (e.g., infants in families of low socioeconomic class) are at risk of developing this condition (Oeffinger, 1993). In scurvy the gingiva is typically bright red, swollen, ulcerated, and susceptible to hemorrhage (Carranza, 1996b; van Steenberghe, 1997). Although there is no dispute about the necessity of dietary ascorbic acid for periodontal health, in the absence of frank scurvy, the effect of declining ascorbic acid levels on the gingiva can be difficult to detect clinically (Woolfe et al., 1980) and when it is detected usually has characteristics that are similar to plaque-induced gingivitis.

Gingival diseases associated with heredity

Benign, non-inflammatory fibrotic enlargement of the maxillary and/or mandibular gingiva associated with a familial aggregation has been designated by such terms as gingivomatosis elephantiasis, familial elephantiasis, juvenile hyaline fibromatosis, congenital familial fibromatosis, idiopatic fibromatosis, idiopathic gingival fibromatosis, hereditary gingival hyperplasia, and hereditary gingival fibromatosis. Although there were almost a hundred published reports of hereditary associated gingival overgrowths in the twentieth century, information about the natural history of this rare disease is extremely limited and its etiology is unkown.

Hereditary gingival fibromatosis appears to be a slowly progressive gingival enlargement which develops upon eruption of the permanent dentition (Figure 3.5); however, gingival enlargement can also occur in the primary dentition (Emerson, 1965; Jorgenson and Cocker,1974; Lai et al., 1995; Miyake et al., 1995). The disease can be localized or generalized and may ultimately cover the occlusal surfaces of teeth. The enlarged gingiva is

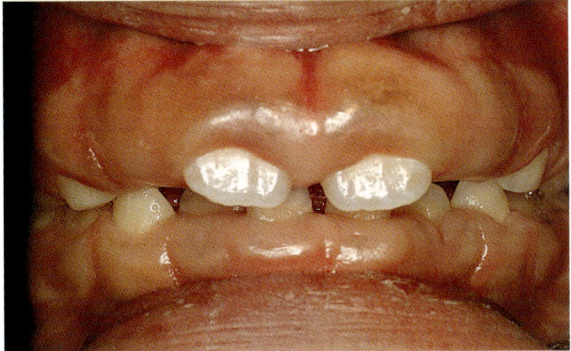

a

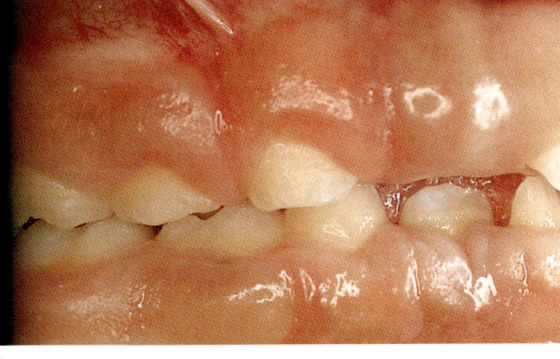

b

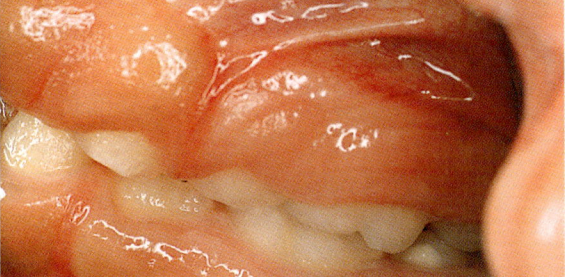

c

Figure 3.5

Hereditary gingival fibromatosis. (a) In erupting permanent anterior teeth (courtesy of Dr Orly Nir). (b) Lateral left view (mirror view) of the same child as in (a) (courtesy of Dr Orly Nir). (c) Lateral right view (mirror view) of the same child as in (a) (courtesy of Dr Orly Nir).

non-hemorrhagic and firm, but there can be an overlay of gingival inflammation which can augment the enlargement. The histologic features of hereditary gingival fibromatosis include dense fibrotic connective tissue as well as epithelial hyperplasia with elongated and increased rete pegs (Johnson et al., 1986; Clark, 1987).

Hereditary gingival fibromatosis can be inherited as a simple mendelian trait, in some chromosomal disorders and as a malformation syndrome (Witkop, 1971; Jones et al., 1977; Skrinjaric and Bacic, 1989; Takagi et al., 1991; Goldblatt and Singer, 1992; Hallet et al., 1995). Although the specific genes for this disease have not been identified, genetic analysis supports the presence of two different gene loci on chromosome 2p (Shashi et al., 1999). Research into the cellular responses of this disease suggests an accumulation of specific populations of gingival fibroblasts resulting in an abnormal accumula-

tion of connective tissues (Huang et al., 1997; Tipton et al., 1997).

Gingival diseases associated with ulcerative lesions

Necrotizing ulcerative gingivitis (NUG) has been known for centuries by numerous names including "trench mouth" and Vincent's infection. Acute necrotizing ulcerative gingivitis is a term used to describe the clinical onset of the disease and should not be used as a diagnostic classification, since some forms of NUG may be recurrent or possibly chronic.

Onset is usually sudden with intense gingival pain, which prompts the patient to seek professional care. Clinical signs include papillary necrosis, giving a "punched out" appearance of the

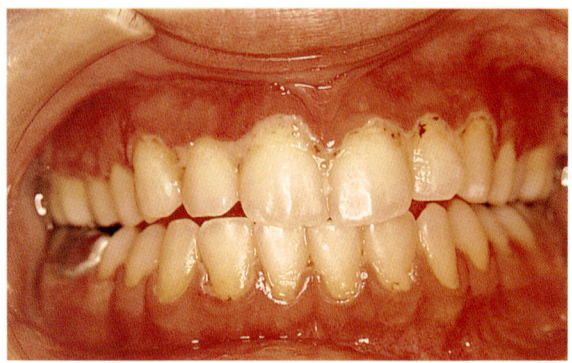

Figure 3.6

Necrotizing ulcerative gingivitis (courtesy of Dr Howard L. Needleman).

gingival papilla (Figure 3.6), and gingival bleeding that requires little or no provocation (Grupe and Wilder 1956; Goldhaber and Giddon, 1964; Johnson and Engel, 1986). Although these symptoms and signs must be present for a diagnosis of NUG, other features may occur such as fever, malaise, lymphadenopathy, metallic taste, and fetor ex ore (malodor) (Schluger, 1943; Wilson, 1952; Murayama et al., 1994). Systemic reactions of acute NUG are usually more severe in children (Carranza, 1996a). Significant destruction of the gingival connective tissue is possible with NUG but when attachment loss occurs this condition should be considered as a necrotizing ulcerative periodontitis.

The cause of NUG may be bacterial. The four zones of the NUG gingival lesion include the bacterial zone (the superficial area consisting of various bacteria and some spirochetes); the neutrophil-rich zone (follows the bacterial zone and contains leukocytes and bacteria including spirochetes); the necrotic zone (consisting of disintegrated cells and connective tissue elements with many large and intermediate spirochetes); and the spirochetal infiltration zone (the deepest zone that is infiltrated with no other bacteria but with intermediate and large spirochetes) (Listgarten, 1965). The cultivable flora of NUG that predominates includes *Prevotella intermedia* and *Fusobacterium* species, while microscopically, *Treponema* and *Selenomonas* species

are observed (Loesche et al., 1982; Rowland et al., 1993b). Additional factors such as smoking (AAP, 1996), psychological stress (Moulton et al., 1952; Cohen-Cole et al., 1983), malnutrition (Grupe and Wilder, 1956; Goldhaber and Giddon, 1964; Johnson and Engel, 1986) and immune suppression (Moulton et al., 1952; Rowland et al., 1993a) can predispose an individual to NUG.

Although NUG can affect any age group, it is considered to be a disease of young adults in industrialized countries (Melnick et al., 1988). In developing countries, NUG is a disease found in children from families with low socioeconomic status (Melnick et al., 1988). The onset of NUG in children is associated with inappropriate nutritional intake, especially low protein consumption (Sheiham, 1966; Taiwo, 1995). In addition, viral infections such as measles can induce NUG in malnourished children (Enwonwu, 1972; Osuji, 1990). Even though NUG has occurred in epidemic patterns, this disease is not considered communicable (Rosebury, 1942).

Gingival lesions associated with sexually transmitted bacterial diseases

Two common bacterial diseases that are transmitted by sexual contact are syphilis and gonorrhea. Syphilis is caused by *Treponema pallidum* and can affect all organ systems including the oral cavity. Although the majority of the lesions occur on the genitalia, the prevalence of extragenital lesions has risen owing to increased orogenital contact. The oral lesions are not limited to one area of the mouth and can affect the lips, tongue, palate, gingiva, and tonsils. Depending on the stage of syphilis, the lesions in the oral cavity can vary from an elevated and ulcerated nodule, to painless, gray-white patches covering ulcerated areas, to firm nodular masses that may in due course ulcerate.

Gonorrhea is caused by *Neisseria gonorrhoeae* and also non-specifically affects many areas of the oral cavity. Like syphilis, gonorrhea is increasing in prevalence in the oral cavity because of increased orogenital contact. The oral lesions of this disease may be similar to lesions produced by erythema multiforme, erosive lichen planus, and herpetic stomatitis (Schmidt et al., 1961). Although the gingiva may become erythematous and edematous, with papillary necrosis, the tonsils and the oropharynx are the oral sites most frequently affected by gonorrhea (Chue, 1975).

Gingival lesions manifested in childhood diseases

Acute herpetic gingivostomatitis

The herpes simplex virus produces some of the most common acute infections in humans. Of the two herpes simplex virus serotypes, type 1 is responsible for most oropharyngeal infections, including acute herpetic gingivostomatitis. This disease is observed in young adolescents and adults but has its highest incidence in infants and children younger than 6 years of age (Scott et al., 1941). There is no predilection for either sex with the primary infection. Following the primary infection, the virus moves through nerves to neuronal ganglia where it remains dormant until reactivated by various stimuli including trauma, exposure to sunlight or ultraviolet lamps, fever, stress, fatigue, menstruation, pregnancy, upper respiratory tract infection, allergy or gastrointestinal disturbances (Stevens, 1975; Shafer et al., 1974).

Although most cases of primary herpetic infection are asymptomatic (Gibson et al., 1990; McDonald et al., 1994), the primary infection in some cases may manifest as acute herpetic gingivostomatitis which is characterized by severe oral and systemic manifestations. The symptomatic infection is characterized by fever, malaise, headache, irritability, dysphagia, and lymphadenopathy. In the oral cavity, lesions can affect the lips, tongue, buccal mucosa, gingiva, palate, tonsils, and pharynx. Initially gingival inflammation characterized by a diffuse, erythematous, shiny appearance precedes the appearance of vesicles (White, 1998). The vesicles vary in size and are usually discrete, spherical sacs which rupture to form small, ragged, and painful ulcers that are covered by a gray membrane and surrounded by an erythematous, elevated halo (White, 1998). The ulcers persist for 7–10 days and heal spontaneously, leaving no scars (White, 1998).

The diagnosis for this infection is usually determined by the patient's history and clinical signs and symptoms, and confirmed by laboratory culture of the herpes simplex virus. Lesions of recurrent aphthous stomatitis have often been confused with acute herpetic gingivostomatitis, but can be distinguished clinically by the absence of diffuse erythema of the gingiva, acute toxic systemic symptoms, and herpes simplex virus culture.

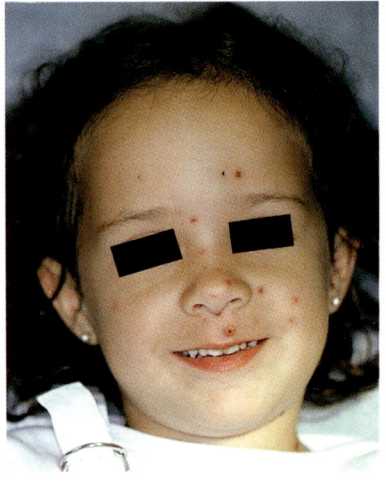

a

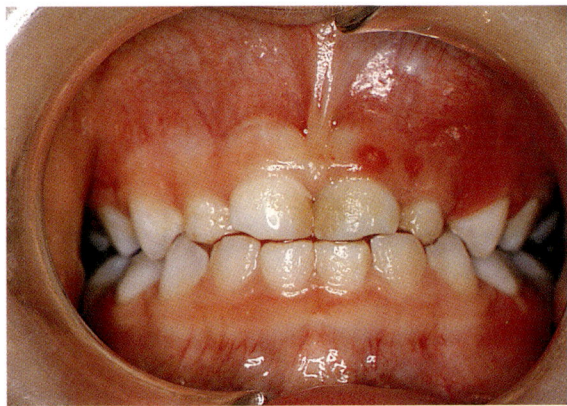

b

Figure 3.7

Chickenpox. (a) Facial view with skin lesions (courtesy of Dr Howard L. Needleman). (b) Intraoral view of the same child as in (a), showing ulcers (courtesy of Dr Howard L. Needleman).

Gingival lesions associated with chickenpox

Varicella is a herpesvirus infection that produces the clinical disease known as chickenpox. Varicella, which primarily affects individuals under the age of 15 years (Preblud, 1986), produces skin lesions characterized by vesicles and pustules that break and crust over (Figure 3.7a). In the oral cavity (Figure 3.7b) small ulcers may develop in any area of the mouth; however, lesions are found most often on the palate, gingiva, and buccal mucosa (Badger, 1980). The ulcers that appear during the course of the skin rash are usually not painful.

Gingival lesions associated with mononucleosis

Mononucleosis is produced by the Epstein–Barr virus and is primarily a disease of children and young adults. The clinical symptoms are most prominent in young adults, and common signs and symptoms include fatigue, malaise, headache, fever, sore throat, enlarged tonsils, and lymphadenopathy. Alterations in the oral cavity include gingival bleeding, petechiae of the soft palate, ulceration of the gingiva and buccal mucosa, and pericoronitis (White, 1998). Palatal petechiae are usually present before systemic symptoms become evident.

Soft tissue lesions associated with herpangina

The Coxsackie group A viruses are associated with herpangina. Although older children and adults can be affected, it is most commonly seen in young children. The clinical features are often of short duration and the manifestations are usually mild. The clinical presentation consists of numerous small vesicles which proceed to small ulcers contained on a gray base and inflamed periphery. The ulcers may appear on the anterior facial pillars, hard or soft palate, posterior pharyngeal wall, buccal mucosa, or tongue. The ulcers are generally not painful and usually heal within a few days to a week. This disease is frequently observed between May and October.

Soft tissue lesions associated with hand, foot, and mouth disease

The majority of cases of hand, foot, and mouth disease occur in children between 6 months and 5 years of age. The oral involvement of this disease has been reported to be caused by the Coxsackie group A viruses; however, Coxsackie group B viruses may also play a role in hand, foot, and mouth disease. As in herpangina, vesicular and ulcerative lesions form on the hard palate, tongue, and buccal mucosa, with a smaller percentage of lesions forming on the lips, gingiva, pharynx, and tongue. In the vast majority of patients, a sore mouth was reported which resulted in difficulty in eating. Unlike herpangina, additional vesicle formation can be found on the skin, particularly the hands, feet, legs, and arms, and sometimes the buttocks. This disease is generally self-limiting and will regress in 1–2 weeks.

Acute inflammatory gingival enlargement

A gingival abscess is an acute, painful, rapidly expanding lesion localized to the gingiva. Most gingival abscesses are detected on the marginal gingiva or the papilla. Gingival abscesses usually arise from an insult such as trauma caused by food which forces bacteria into the tissue. Within hours, a bright-red gingival swelling will convert to a lesion that is a pointed and fluctuant mass from which purulent exudate may be expressed. The lesion is generally self-limiting, ultimately rupturing if permitted to progress. The gingival abscess should not be confused with the periodontal abscess, which affects the supporting periodontal structures.

Gingival changes associated with tooth eruption

As the crown penetrates the oral mucosa, the marginal gingiva and sulcus form. During the physiologic process of eruption, the gingival margin becomes edematous and erythematous

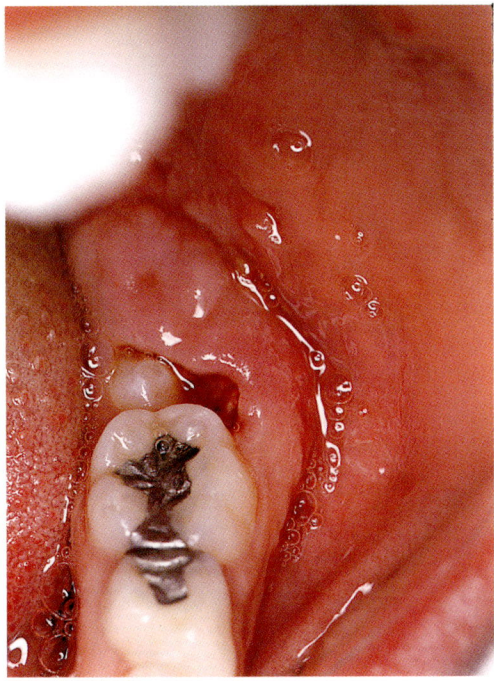

Figure 3.8

Gingival inflammation in the gingiva over an erupting permanent molar.

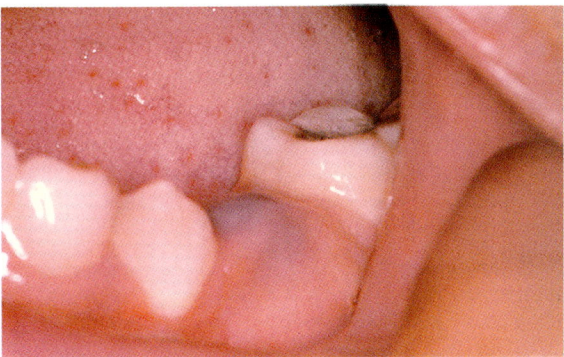

a

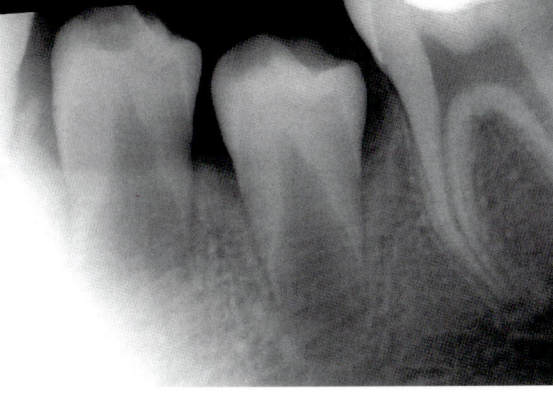

b

Figure 3.9

Eruption hematoma. (a) An eruption hematoma over a second premolar. (b) Radiograph of the area shown in (a). No alveolar bone disease is evident. The still undeveloped roots evidence the early eruption of both premolars. (Courtesy of Dr Enrique Bimstein.)

(Figure 3.8). It is not uncommon for erupting primary or permanent teeth to be associated with a form of dentigerous cyst called an eruption cyst or eruption hematoma. The eruption cyst usually appears as a site of translucent, fluctuant, circumscribed swelling over the erupting tooth. When the cystic cavity contains blood, the swelling appears as a purple or deep-blue fluctuant, circumscribed swelling termed an eruption hematoma (Figure 3.9). The occurrence of the eruption cyst has been reported to range from 11% to 30% depending on the teeth involved. Moreover, primary canines and molars appear to be more frequently involved than primary incisor teeth (Seward, 1973).

Conclusions

Gingival diseases are a diverse family of complex and distinct pathological entities which are the result of a variety of processes. While gingival diseases can affect infants or young adults, the phenotype and/or onset of the different gingival diseases are age-dependent. Although these periodontal diseases are limited to the gingiva, the inflammatory response initiated in gingival diseases appears to be a prerequisite for destruction of connective tissue attachment apical to the cementoenamel junction (Page et al., 1997; Sheiham, 1997). Therefore, the identification and treatment of gingival disease is an important first step in preventing more serious periodontal ailments in children, adolescents, and young adults.

References

[AAP] American Academy of Periodontology (1996) Tobacco use and the periodontal patient. *J Periodontol* **67**: 51–56.

Addy V, McElnay JC, Eyre DG et al (1983) Risk factors in phenytoin-induced gingival hyperplasia. *J Periodontol* **54**: 373–7.

Angelopoulous AP, Goaz PW (1972) Incidence of diphenylhydantoin gingival hyperplasia. *Oral Surg Oral Med Oral Path* **34**: 898–906.

Arafat A (1974a) The prevalence of pyogenic granuloma in pregnant women. *J Baltimore Coll Dent Surg* **29**: 64–70.

Arafat AH (1974b) Periodontal status during pregnancy. *J Periodontol* **45**: 641–3.

Badger GR (1980) Oral signs of chickenpox (varicella): report of two cases. *ASDC J Dent Child* **47**: 349–51.

Bailit HL, Baldwin DC, Hunt EE (1964) The increasing prevalence of gingival Bacteriodes melaninogenicus with age in children. *Arch Oral Biol* **9**: 435–8.

Barclay S, Thomason JM, Idle JR, Seymour RA (1992) The incidence and severity of nifedipine-induced gingival overgrowth. *J Clin Periodontol* **19**: 311–14.

Bhat M (1991) Periodontal health of 14–17-year-old US schoolchildren. *J Publ Health Dent* **51**: 5–11.

Bimstein E, Ebersole JL (1989) The age-dependent reaction of the periodontal tissues to dental plaque. *ASDC J Dent Child* **56**: 358–62.

Bimstein E, Ebersole JL (1991) Serum antibody levels to oral microorganisms in children and young adults with relation to severity of gingival disease. *Pediatr Dent* **13**: 267–72.

Bimstein E, Matsson L (1999) Growth and development considerations in the diagnosis of gingivitis and periodontitis in children. *Pediatr Dent* **21**: 186–91.

Bimstein E, Lustman, J, Soskolne WA (1985) A clinical and histometric study of gingivitis associated with the human deciduous dentition. *J Periodontol* **56**: 293–6.

Bimstein E, Soskolne WA, Lustman J et al. (1988) Gingivitis in the human deciduous dentition: a correlative clinical and block surface microscopical study. *J Clin Periodontol* **15**: 575–80.

Bimstein E, Matsson L, Soskolne A, Lustmann J (1994) Histologic characteristics of the gingiva associated with the primary and permanent teeth of children. *Pediatr Dent* **16**: 206–10.

Bradley RE (1961) Periodontal lesions of children: their recognition and treatment. *Dent Clin North Am* **5**: 671–85.

Carranza FA (1996a) Acute gingival infections. In: Carranza FA, Newman MG (eds) *Clinical Periodontology*, 8th edn. Philadelphia: WB Saunders, pp. 249–59.

Carranza Jr. FA (1996b) Influence of systemic diseases on the periodontium. In: Carranza FA, Newman MG (eds) *Clinical Periodontology*, 8th edn. Philadelphia: WB Saunders, pp. 185–205.

Chue PWY (1975) Gonorrhea—its natural history, oral manifestations, diagnosis, treatment and prevention. *J Am Dent Assoc* **90**: 1297–301.

Clark D (1987) Gingival fibromatosis and its related syndromes. A review. *J Can Dent Assoc* **2**: 137–40.

Cohen-Cole S, Cogen RB, Stevens AW et al. (1983) Psychiatric, pyschosocial, and endocrine correlates of acute and necrotizing ulcerative gingivitis (trench mouth): a preliminary report. *Psychiat Med* **1**: 215–25.

Coles O (1874) On the condition of the mouth and teeth during pregnancy. *Am J Dent Sci* **8**: 361–9.

Connor RJ, Ho DD (1992) Etiology of AIDS: biology of human retroviruses. In: DeVita T, Hellman S, Rosenberg SA (eds) *AIDS: Etiology, Diagnosis, Treatment and Prevention*. Philadelphia: JB Lippincott, pp. 13–38.

Daley TD, Wysocki GP, Day C (1986) Clinical and pharmacologic correlations in cyclosporine-induced gingival hyperplasia. *Oral Surg Oral Med Oral Path* **62**: 417–21.

Dodd CL, Greenspan D, Katz MH et al. (1991) Oral candidiasis in HIV infection: pesudomembranous and erythematous candidiasis show similar rates of progression to AIDS. *AIDS* **5**: 1339–43.

Dreizen S, McCredie KB, Keating MJ (1984) Chemotherapy-associated oral hemorrhages in adults with acute leukemia. *Oral Surg Oral Med Oral Path* **57**: 494–8.

El-Ashiry GM, El-Kafrawy AH, Nasr MF, Younis N (1970) Comparative study of the influence of pregnancy and oral contraceptives on the gingivae. *Oral Surg Oral Med Oral Path* **30**: 472–5.

Emerson T (1965) Hereditary gingival hyperplasia. A family pedigree of four generations. *Oral Surg Oral Med Oral Path* **19**: 1–9.

Enwonwu CO (1972) Epidemiological and biochemical studies of necrotizing ulcerative gingivitis and noma (cancrum oris) in Nigerian children. *Arch Oral Biol* **17**: 1357–71.

Esterberg HL, White PH (1945) Sodium dilantin gingival hyperplasia. *J Am Dent Assoc* **32**: 16–24.

Force USPHST (1993) Recommendations for prophylaxis against Pneumocystis carinii pneumonia for persons infected with human immunodeficiency virus. US Public Health Service Task Force on antipneumocystis prophylaxis in patients with human immunodeficiency virus infection. *J Acquir Immune Defic Syndr* **6**: 46–55.

Fu E, Nieh S, Hsiao CT et al. (1998) Nifedipine-induced gingival overgrowth in rats: brief review and experimental study. *J Periodontol* **69**: 765–71.

Gibson JJ, Hornung CA, Alexander GR et al. (1990) A cross-sectional study of herpes simplex virus types 1 and 2 in college students. Occurrence and determinants of infection. *J Infect Dis* **162**: 306–12.

Goldblatt J, Singer SL (1992) Autosomal recessive gingival fibromatosis with distinct facies. *Clin Genet* **42**: 306–8.

Goldhaber P, Giddon DB (1964) Present concepts concerning etiology and treatment of acute necrotizing ulcerative gingivitis. *Int Dent J* **14**: 468–96.

Gomez RS, Colsta JE, Loyola AM et al. (1995) Immunohistochemical study of linear gingival erythema from HIV-positive patients. *J Periodont Res* **30**: 355–9.

Grassi M, Williams CA, Winkler JR (1988) Management of HIV-associated periodontal diseases. In: Robertson PB, Greenspan JS (eds) *Perspectives of Oral Manifestations of AIDS. Proceedings of the First International Symposium on Oral Manifestations of AIDS.* Littleton: PSG Publishing, pp. 119–130.

Grupe HE, Wilder LS (1956) Observations of necrotizing gingivitis in 870 military trainees. *J Periodontol* **27**: 255–61.

Hallet KB, Bankier A, Chow CW et al. (1995) Gingival fibromatosis and Klippel-Trenaunay-Weber syndrome. Case report. *Oral Surg Oral Med Oral Path* **79**: 678–82.

Hassell TM (1981) Phenytoin: gingival overgrowth. In: Myers HM (ed.) *Epilepsy and the Oral Manifestations of Phenytoin Therapy.* Basel: Karger, 116–202.

Hassell TM, Hefti AF (1991) Drug-induced gingival overgrowth: old problem, new problem. *Crit Rev Oral Biol Med* **2**: 103–37.

Hassell T, O'Donnell J, Pearlman J et al. (1984) Phenytoin induced gingival overgrowth in institutionalized epileptics. *J Clin Periodontol* **11**: 242–53.

Hefti A, Engelberger T, Buttner M (1981) Gingivitis in Basel schoolchildren. *Helv Odontol Acta* **25**: 25–42.

Hefti A, Eshenaur AE, Hassell TM, Stone C (1994) Gingival overgrowth in cyclosporine A treated multiple sclerosis patients. *J Periodontol* **65**: 744–9.

Huang JS, Ho KY, Chen CC et al. (1997) Collagen synthesis in idiopathic and dilatin-induced gingival fibromatosis. *Kao Hsiung I Hsueh Tsa Chih* **13**: 141–8.

Hugoson A (1971) Gingivitis in pregnant women. A longitudinal clinical study. *Odontol Rev* **22**: 65–84.

Hugoson A, Koch G (1979) Oral health in 100 individuals aged 3–70 years in the community of Jonkoping. *Swed Dent J* **3**: 69–87.

Hugoson A, Koch G, Rylander H (1981) Prevalence and distribution of gingivitis-periodontitis in children and adolescents. Epidemiological data as a base for risk group selection. *Swed Dent J* **5**: 91–103.

Johnson BD, Engel D (1986) Acute necrotizing ulcerative gingivitis. A review of diagnosis, etiology and treatment. *J Periodontol* **57**: 141–50.

Johnson B, El-Guindy M, Ammons W et al. (1986) A defect in fibroblasts from an unidentified syndrome with gingival hyperplasia as the predominant feature. *J Periodont Res* **21**: 403–13.

Jones G, Wilroy RS, McHaney V (1977) Familial gingival fibromatosis associated with progressive deafness in five generations of a family. *Birth Def Orig Artic Ser* **13**: 195–201.

Jorgenson RJ, Cocker ME (1974) Variation in the inheritance and expression of gingival fibromatosis. *J Periodontol* **45**: 472–7.

Justice AC, Feinstein AR, Wells CK (1989) A new prognostic staging system for the acquired immunodeficiency syndrome. *New Engl J Med* **320**: 1388–93.

Katz MH, Greenspan D, Westenhouse J et al. (1992) Progression to AIDS in HIV-infected homosexual and bisexual men with hairy leukoplakia and oral candidiasis [see comments]. *AIDS* **6**: 95–100.

Kaufman AY (1969) An oral contraceptive as an etiologic factor in producing hyperplastic gingivitis and a neoplasm of the pregnancy tumor type. *Oral Surg Oral Med Oral Path* **28**: 666–70.

Kelsten LB (1955) Periodontal and soft tissue diseases in children. *Dent Med* **10**: 67–76.

Kimball O (1939) The treatment of epilepsy with sodium diphenyl-hydantoinate. *JAMA* **112**: 1244–5.

Knight GM, Wade AB (1974) The effects of hormonal contraceptives on the human periodontium. *J Periodont Res* **9**: 18–22.

Kristen VK (1976) Veranderungen der Mundschleimhaut wahrend Schwangerschaft und kontrazeptiver Hormonbehandlung. *Fortschr Med* **94**: 52–4.

Lai LL, Wang FL, Chan CP (1995) Hereditary gingival fibromatosis: a case report. *Chang Keng I Hsueh* **18**: 403–8.

Lamster IB, Grbic JT, Mitchell-Lewis DA et al. (1998) New concepts regarding the pathogenesis of periodontal disease in HIV infection. *Ann Periodontol* **3**: 62–75.

Lind (1953) The diagnostics, or signs. In: Stewart CP, Guthrie D (eds) *Lind's Treatise on Scurvy*. Edinburgh University Press, pp. 113–28.

Lindhe J, Bjorn AL (1967) Influence of hormonal contraceptives on the gingiva of women. *J Periodont Res* **2**: 1–6.

Listgarten MA (1965) Electron microscopic observations on the bacterial flora of acute necrotizing ulcerative gingivitis. *J Periodontol* **36**: 328–39.

Löe H (1965) Periodontal changes in pregnancy. *J Periodontol* **36**: 209–216.

Löe H, Silness J (1963) Periodontal disease in pregnancy. I. Prevalence and severity. *Acta Odontol Scand* **21**: 533–551.

Löe H, Theilade E, Jensen SB (1965) Experimental gingivitis in man. *J Periodontol* **36**: 177–87.

Loesche WJ, Syed SA, Laughon BE, Stall J (1982) The bacteriology of acute necrotizing ulcerative gingivitis. *J Periodontol* **53**: 223–30.

Longhurst P, Johnson NW, Hopps RM (1977) Differences in lymphocyte and plasma cell densities in inflamed gingiva in adults and young adults. *J Periodontol* **48**: 705–10.

Lynch MA, Ship II (1967) Initial oral manifestations of leukemia. *J Am Dent Assoc* **75**: 932–40.

Lynn BD (1967) "The pill" as an etiologic agent in hypertrophic gingivitis. *Oral Surg Oral Med Oral Path* **24**: 333–4.

MacDonald PC, Dombroski RA, Casey ML (1991) Recurrent secretion of progesterone in large amounts: an endocrine/metabolic disorder unique to young women? *Endocrin Rev* **12**: 372–401.

Mackler SB, Crawford JJ (1973) Plaque development and gingivitis in the primary dentition. *J Periodontol* **44**: 18–24.

Maier AW, Orban B (1949) Gingivitis in pregnancy. *Oral Surg Oral Med Oral Path* **2**: 334–73.

Mariotti A (1994) Sex steroid hormones and cell dynamics in the periodontium. *Crit Rev Oral Biol Med* **5**: 27–53.

Mariotti A, Hassell T, Jacobs D et al (1998) Cyclosporin A and hydroxycyclosporine (M-17) affect the secretory phenotype of human gingival fibroblasts. *J Oral Pathol Med* **27**: 260–1.

Mariotti A, Knutson M, Preshaw P (2000) The effects of oral contraceptives on gingival inflammation. *J Periodont Res* **79**: (in press).

Matsson L (1978) Development of gingivitis in preschool children and young adults. A comparative experimental study. *J Clin Periodontol* **5**: 24–34.

Matsson L, Goldberg P (1985) Gingival inflammatory reaction in children at different ages. *J Clin Periodontol* **12**: 98–103.

McDonald RE, Avery DR, Weddell JA (1994) Gingivitis and periodontal disease. Acute gingival disease. Herpes simplex virus infection. In: McDonald RE, Avery DR (eds) *Dentistry for the Child and Adolescent* (6th edn) St Louis: Mosby, pp. 458–9.

McGaw T, Lam S, Coates J (1987) Cyclosporin-induced gingival overgrowth: correlation with dental plaque scores, gingivitis scores, and cyclosporine levels in serum and saliva. *Oral Surg Oral Med Oral Path* **64**: 293–7.

Melnick SL, Roseman JM, Engel D, Cogen RB (1988) Epidemiology of acute necrotizing ulcerative gingivitis. *Epidemiol Rev* **10**: 191–211.

Miyake I, Tokumaru H, Sugino H et al. (1995) Juvenile hyaline fibromatosis. Case report with five years' follow up. *Am J Dermatopathol* **17**: 584–90.

Miyazaki H, Yamashita Y, Shirahama R et al. (1991) Periodontal condition of pregnant women assessed by CPITN. *J Clin Periodontol* **18**: 751–4.

Modeer T, Dahllof G (1987) Development of phenytoin-induced gingival overgrowth in non-institutionalized epileptic children subjected to different plaque control programs. *Acta Odontol Scand* **45**: 81–5.

Moore WEC, Holdeman LV, Smibert RM et al. (1984) Bacteriology of experimental gingivitis in children. *Infect Immun* **46**: 1–6.

Moore LVH, Moore WEC, Riley C et al. (1993) Periodontal microflora of HIV positive subjects with gingivitis or adult periodontitis. *J Periodontol* **64**: 48–56.

Moulton R, Ewwn S, Thieman W (1952) Emotional factors in periodontal disease. *Oral Surg Oral Med Oral Path* **5**: 833–60.

Muhlemann HR (1948) Eine Gingivitis intermenstrualis. *Schweiz Monatsschr Zahnheilk* **58**: 865–85.

Muhlemann HR, Son S (1971) Gingival sulcus bleeding—a leading symptom in initial gingivitis. *Helv Odontol Acta* **15**: 107–13.

Murayama Y, Kurihara H, Nagai A et al. (1994) Acute necrotizing ulcerative gingivitis: risk factors involving host defense mechanisms. *Periodontol 2000* **6**: 116–124.

Oeffinger KC (1993) Scurvy: more than historical relevance. *Am Fam Phys* **48**: 609–13.

Osuji OO (1990) Necrotizing ulcerative gingivitis and cancrum oris (noma) in Ibadan, Nigeria. *J Periodontol* **61**: 769–72.

Page RC (1985) Oral health status in the United States: prevalence of inflammatory periodontal diseases. *J Dent Educ* **49**: 354–64.

Page RC, Schroeder HE (1976) Pathogenesis of inflammatory periodontal disease. *Lab Invest* **33**: 235–49.

Page RC, Offenbacher S, Schroeder HE et al. (1997) Advances in the pathogenesis of periodontitis: summary of developments, clinical implications and future directions. *Periodontol 2000* **14**: 216–48.

Pankhurst CL, Waite IM, Hicks KA et al. (1981) The influence of oral contraceptive therapy on the periodontium—duration of drug therapy. *J Periodontol* **52**: 617–20.

Parfitt GJ (1957) A five year longitudinal study of the gingival condition of a group of children in England. *J Periodontol* **28**: 26–32.

Polson AM, Goodson JM (1985) Periodontal diagnosis. Current status and future needs. *J Periodontol* **56**: 25–34.

Preblud SR (1986) Varicella: complications and costs. *Pediatrics* **78**: 728–35.

Prevention CDC (1992) 1993 revised classification system for HIV infection and expanded surveillance case definition for AIDS among adolescents and adults. *MMWR* **41**: 1–19.

Ramon Y, Behar S, Kishon Y, Engelberg IS (1984) Gingival hyperplasia caused by nifedipine—a preliminary report. *Int J Cardiol* **5**: 195–204.

Ranney RR (1993) Classification of periodontal diseases. *Periodontol 2000* **2**: 13–25.

Rateitschak-Pluss EM, Hefti A, Lortscher R, Thiel G (1983) Initial observation that cyclosporin-A induces gingival enlargement in man. *J Clin Periodontol* **10**: 237–46.

Rosebury T (1942) Is Vincent's infection a communicable disease? *J Am Dent Assoc* **29**: 823–34.

Rowland RW, Escobar MR, Friedman RB, Kaplowiz LG (1993a) Painful gingivitis may be an early sign of infection with the human immunodeficiency virus. *Clin Infect Dis* **16**: 233–6.

Rowland RW, Mestecky J, Gunsolley JC, Cogen RB (1993b) Serum IgG and IgM levels to bacterial antigens in necrotizing ulcerative gingivitis. *J Periodontol* **64**: 195–201.

Royce RA, Luckman RS, Fusaro RE, Winkelstein W (1991) The natural history of HIV-1 infection: staging classification of disease. *AIDS* **5**: 355–64.

Ruben M, Frankl SN, Wallace S (1971) The histopathology of periodontal disease in children. *J Periodontol* **42**: 473–84.

Russell AL (1962) Periodontal disease in well- and malnourished populations. A preliminary report. *Arch Environ Health* **5**: 153–7.

Schluger S (1943) The etiology and treatment of Vincent's infection. *J Am Dent Assoc* **39**: 524–32.

Schmidt H, Hjorting-Hansen E, Philipsen HP (1961) Gonococcal stomatitis. *Acta Derm Venereol* **41**: 324–7.

Scott TFM, Steigman AS, Convey JH (1941) Acute infectious gingivostomatitis: etiology, epidemiology, and clinical picture of common disorders caused by virus of herpes simplex. *JAMA* **117**: 999–1005.

Seward MH (1973) Eruption cyst: an analysis of its clinical features. *J Oral Surg* **31**: 31–5

Seymour RA (1991) Calcium channel blockers and gingival overgrowth. *Br Dent J* **170**: 376–9.

Seymour RA, Jacobs DJ (1992) Cyclosporin and the gingival tissues. *J Clin Periodontol* **19**: 1–11.

Seymour GJ, Crouch MS, Powell RN (1977) The phenotypic characterization of lymphoid cell subpopulations in gingivitis in children. *J Periodont Res* **16**: 582–92.

Seymour GJ, Crouch MS, Powell RN et al. (1982) The identification of lymphoid subpopulations in sections of human lymphoid tissue and gingivitis in children using monoclonal antibodies. *J Periodont Res* **17**: 247–56.

Seymour RA, Smith DG, Rogers SR (1987) The comparative effects of azathioprine and cyclosporin on some gingival health parameters of renal transplant patients. A longitudinal study. *J Clin Periodontol* **14**: 610–13.

Seymour RA, Thomason JM, Ellis JS (1996) The pathogenesis of drug-induced gingival overgrowth. *J Clin Periodontol* **23**: 165–75.

Shafer WG, Hine MK, Levy BM (1974) Diseases of microbial origin. Recurrent, or secondary, herpetic stomatitis. In: Saunders WB (ed) *A Textbook of Oral Pathology*, 3rd edn. Phil;adelphia, pp. 328–31.

Shashi V, Pallos D, Pettenati MJ et al. (1999) Genetic homogeneity of gingival fibromatosis on chromosome 2p. *J Med Genet* **36**: 683–6.

Sheiham A (1966) An epidemiological survey of acute ulcerative gingivitis in Nigerians. *Arch Oral Biol* **11**: 937–42.

Sheiham A (1997) Is the chemical prevention of gingivitis necessary to prevent severe periodontitis? *Periodontol 2000* **15**: 15–24.

Sills ES, Zegarelli DJ, Hoschander MM, Strider WE (1996) Clinical diagnosis and management of hormonally responsive oral pregnancy tumor (pyogenic granuloma). *J Reprod Med* **41**: 467–70.

Skrinjaric I, Bacic M (1989) Hereditary gingival fibromatosis: report on three families and dermatoglyphic analysis. *J Periodontol* **24**: 303–9.

Socransky SS, Manganiello SD (1971) The oral microbiota of man from birth to senility. *J Periodontol* **42**: 485–96.

Sperber GH (1969) Oral contraceptive hypertrophic gingivitis. *J Dent Assoc S Africa* **24**: 37–40.

Stamm JW (1986) Epidemiology of gingivitis. *J Clin Periodontol* **13**: 360–6.

Steinberg SC, Steinberg AD (1982) Phenytoin-induced gingival overgrowth control in severely retarded children. *J Periodontol* **53**: 429–33.

Stevens JG (1975) Latent herpes simplex virus and the nervous system. *Curr Top Microbiol Immunol* **70**: 31–50.

Sutcliffe P (1972) A longitudinal study of gingivitis and puberty. *J Periodont Res* **7**: 52–8.

Suzuki JB (1988) Diagnosis and classification of the periodontal diseases. *Dent Clin North Am* **32**: 195–216.

Taiwo JO (1995) Severity of necrotizing ulcerative gingivitis in Nigerian children. *Periodont Clin Investig* **17**: 24–7.

Takagi M, Yamamoto H, Mega H et al. (1991) Heterogeneity in the gingival fibromatoses. *Cancer* **68**: 2202–12.

Tipton DA, Howell KJ, Dabbous MK (1997) Increased proliferation, collagen, and fibronectin production by hereditary gingival fibromatosis fibroblasts. *J Periodontol* **68**: 524–30.

Tyldesley WR, Rotter E (1984) Gingival hyperplasia induced by cyclosporin-A. *Br Dent J* **157**: 305–9.

US Public Health Service NCHS (1965) *Periodontal Disease in Adults, United States 1960–1962*. Washington, DC: Government Printing Office.

US Public Health Service NCHS (1972) *Periodontal Diseases and Oral Hygiene Among Children, United States*. Washington, DC: Government Printing Office.

US Public Health Service NIDR (1987) *Oral Health of United States Adults; National Findings*. Bethesda, MD: NIDR.

Van Steenberghe D (1997) Systemic disorders and the periodontium. In: Lindhe J, Karring T, Lang NP (eds) *Clinical Periodontology and Implant Dentistry*, 3rd edn. Copenhagen: Munksgaard, pp. 332–55.

Waerhaug J (1967) Prevalence of periodontal disease in Ceylon. Association with age, sex, oral hygiene, socio-economic factors, vitamin deficiencies, malnutrition, betel and tobacco consumption and ethnic group. Final report. *Acta Odontol Scand* **25**: 205–31.

Walsh LJ, Armitt KL, Seymour GJ, Powell RM (1987) The immunohistology of chronic gingivitis in children. *Pediatr Dent* **9**: 26–32.

Wertheimer FW, Brewster RH, White CL (1967) Periodontal disease and nutrition in Thailand. *J Periodontol* **38**: 100–4.

White DK (1998) Acute viral infections of the oral cavity and parotid gland. *Oral Maxillofac Surg Clin North Am* **10**: 75–94.

Wilson JR (1952) Etiology and diagnosis of bacterial gingivitis including Vincent's disease. *J Am Dent Assoc* **44**: 671–9.

Winkler JR, Murray PA (1987) Periodontal disease. A potential intraoral expression of AIDS may be rapidly progressive periodontitis. *Can Dent Assoc J* **15**: 20–4.

Winkler JR, Grassi M, Murray PA (1988) Clinical description and etiology of HIV-associated periodontal diseases. In: Robertson PB, Greenspan JS (eds) *Perspectives of Oral Manifestations of AIDS*. Proceedings of the First International Symposium on Oral Manifestations of AIDS. Littleton: PSG Publishing, pp. 49–70.

Winkler JR, Murray PA, Grassi M, Hammerle C (1989) Diagnosis and management of HIV-associated periodontal lesions. *J Am Dent Assoc* (suppl): 25S–34S.

Witkop CJ (1971) Heterogeneity in gingival fibromatosis. *Birth Def Orig Artic Ser* **7**: 210–21.

Woolfe SN, Hume WR, Kenney EB (1980) Ascorbic acid and periodontal disease: a review of the literature. *J West Soc Periodontol Periodont Abstr* **28**: 44–56.

Yahia N, Seibel W, McCleary L et al. (1988) Effect of toothbrushing on cyclosporine-induced gingival overgrowth in beagles. *J Dent Res* **67**: 332.

Zappler SE (1948) Periodontal disease in children. *J Am Dent Assoc* **37**: 333–45.

Ziskin DE, Nesse GJ (1946) Pregnancy gingivitis: history, classification, etiology. *Am J Orthod Oral Surg* **32**: 390–432.

4
Mucogingival defects and their treatment

Nadeem Karimbux and Narawat Wara-aswapati

Mucogingival defects involve the morphology, position, and/or amount of gingiva supporting the teeth. The most common defect is gingival recession, which has been defined as the location of the gingival marginal tissue apical to the cementoenamel junction (CEJ).

Recession of the gingiva can occur in children and adolescents (Gorman, 1967; O'Leary, 1967) and its early diagnosis is important in both prevention and treatment. Early treatment of gingival recession in children and adolescents is simple, its prognosis is good, and irreversible complications impairing the quality of life are prevented. Recession can be due to the buccal eruption patterns of a tooth or to displacement of a tooth after orthodontic treatment. In some cases, habits such as nail picking (Figure 4.1) or inadequate tooth brushing can cause recession. Recession can also be the result of progressive periodontitis, caused by the inflammatory response to microbiological plaque. The essence of the problem is the loss of the attached gingiva, a keratinized band of tissue that protects the neck of the teeth from the everyday trauma of eating and brushing. Loss of attached gingiva beyond the mucogingival line results in the exposure of the alveolar mucosa (a non-keratinized, highly elastic tissue prone to inflammatory breakdown) to the advancing plaque front present on the root surface. Following exposure to the oral environment, root sensitivity is a common complaint and the roots of teeth are at a higher risk of developing caries.

The treatment of gingival recession may be either conservative (meticulous oral hygiene and follow-up) or surgical. In children, the transition from a deciduous tooth to its permanent successor is accompanied by a significant reduction in the width of attached gingiva, which will subsequently increase with the eruption of the permanent tooth (Tenenbaum and Tenenbaum, 1986; Bimstein and Eidelman, 1988a, b; Peretz et al., 1996), allowing potential self-repair of minimal widths of attached gingiva (Bimstein et al., 1988, Bimstein, 1989). Furthermore, since most studies of mucogingival defects have been completed in adults, their principles can be applied to children or adolescents only after taking into consideration the morphological changes caused by the growth and development in the primary, mixed, and young permanent dentitions.

Mucogingival surgery is used to correct defects in the morphology, position, and amount of gingiva supporting the teeth (Nevins et al., 1992). The development of techniques to correct alveolar ridge form and soft tissue esthetics has led to use of the term "periodontal plastic surgery" instead. Defects in the gingiva more commonly occur in the form of gingival recession on the

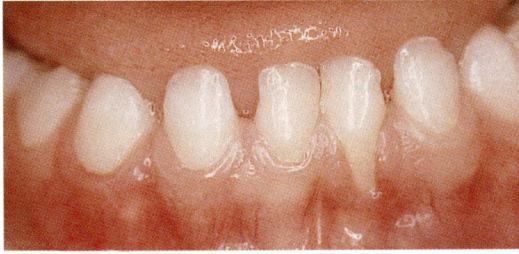

Figure 4.1

Gingival recession due to fingernail picking in a mandibular deciduous central incisor (courtesy of Dr Enrique Bimstein).

buccal surfaces of the teeth. The two main objectives of mucogingival surgery are to cover previously exposed root surfaces, and to augment the band of attached tissue.

Mucogingival defects in children occur commonly on the mandibular central incisors: the prevalence of such problems was 12–19% in a sample of 100 patients examined (Maynard and Ochsenbein, 1975). However, a complete absence of attached gingiva was observed in only 1% of 1302 teeth randomly studied (Gliksberg et al., 1989).

The concept of "adequate" width of keratinized tissue

Prior to the 1980s it was generally accepted that a certain apicocoronal width of keratinized tissue and attached gingiva was required for periodontal health and for the prevention of soft tissue recession. A study by Lang and Löe (1972) demonstrated that over 80% of the areas with at least 2 mm of keratinized tissue corresponding to 1 mm of attached gingiva was clinically healthy, while all areas with less than 2 mm of keratinized tissue and with less than 1 mm of attached gingiva showed some degree of clinical inflammation. At that time, it was recommended that 2 mm of keratinized tissue with at least 1 mm of attached gingiva was adequate to maintain gingival health. Subsequent studies, however, failed to support the concept of minimal width; for example, Miyasato et al. (1977) reported that there were no differences in gingival health observed between surfaces with appreciable widths (2 mm or more) and those with minimal widths (1 mm or less) of keratinized tissue. This study also revealed that sites with appreciable keratinized tissue were no more resistant to developing plaque-induced inflammation than sites with minimal or no keratinized gingiva. Subsequent experimental studies (Wennstrom and Lindhe, 1983) indicated that a free gingival unit supported by loosely attached alveolar mucosa is no more susceptible to inflammation than a free gingival unit supported by a wide zone of attached gingiva.

Several studies (Kennedy et al., 1985; Schoo and van der Velden, 1985; Salkin et al., 1987; Wennstrom, 1987; Freedman et al., 1992) demonstrated that in patients maintaining good oral hygiene the incidence of soft tissue recession was no greater at sites with minimal or no attached gingiva than at sites with wide zones of attached gingiva. In addition, areas with minimal bands of gingiva and even mucosal margins can be maintained without progressive soft tissue recession if traumatic tooth brushing and inflammation are controlled (Dorfman et al., 1980). It is interesting, however, to note that in a longitudinal study by Kennedy et al. (1985) the sites with little or no attached gingiva in the unmaintained patients had a 20% higher frequency of further recession when compared with the free soft tissue grafted sites in the same patient group.

Early detection of mucogingival defects in children allows for simple treatment and prevention of complications in adulthood. The dimensional differences of the attached gingiva during development of dentitions—primary, mixed, and permanent—should be taken into consideration. The width of attached gingiva is greater in adults than in children at the primary dentition stage (Bowers, 1963; Rose and App, 1973); the decrease in width in the mixed dentition results from deeper crevices in the permanent teeth compared with their deciduous predecessors (Bimstein and Eidelman, 1988a, b; Peretz et al. 1996; Srivastava et al., 1990). Tenenbaum and Tenenbaum (1986) reported that the attached gingiva increases with age in both the primary and permanent dentitions. A series of studies (Ainamo and Talari, 1976; Ainamo et al., 1981) have shown that, in adults aged 23 years old and over, the band of attached gingiva continues to increase unless there is concurrent reduction in height of marginal tissue due to periodontal breakdown. The decision to postpone mucogingival surgery in all cases should be tempered by the patient's home care and the other treatment that is planned for the patient (e.g., preorthodontic, preprosthetic, and preorthognathic treatments).

The dimensional changes in the attached gingiva may allow spontaneous improvement of recession defects in young children during growth and development (Figure 4.2), if adequate oral hygiene is maintained. Therefore, it has been suggested that mucogingival surgery to correct soft tissue recession or increase the amount of attached gingiva in children should be postponed until possible spontaneous improvement has been allowed to take place (Bimstein and Eidelman, 1988a, b; Bimstein et al., 1988; Andlin-Sobocki et al., 1991; Saario et al., 1994, 1995).

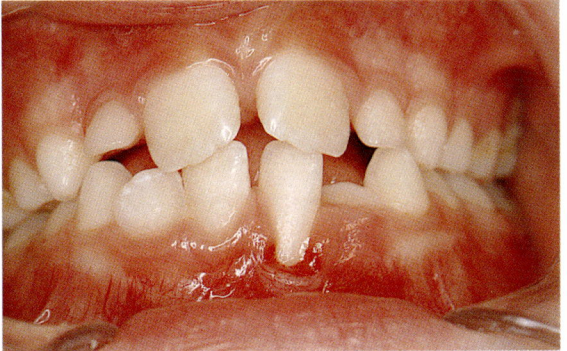

a

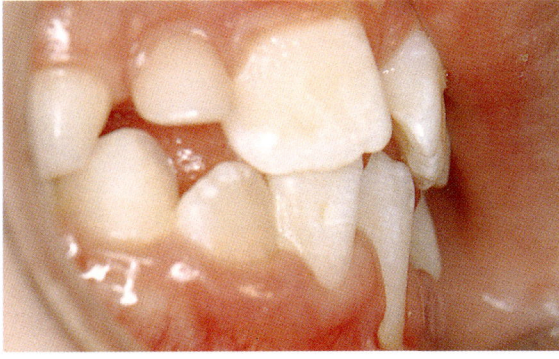

b

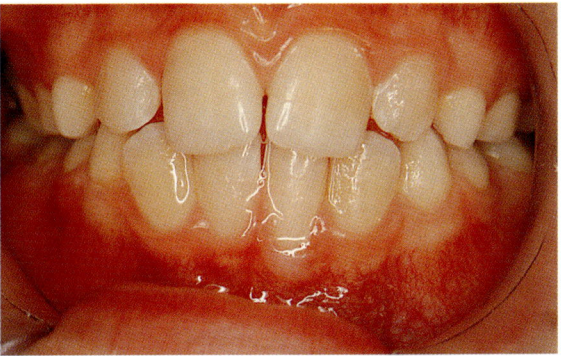

c

Figure 4.2

Non-surgical repair of gingival pseudorecession (courtesy of Dr Enrique Bimstein). (a) Buccal view at baseline. Gingival recession is evident at the mandibular left central incisor. (b) Lateral view at baseline. (c) Buccal view after 21 months with adequate oral hygiene. No recession is evident, the gingival height of both mandibular incisors is normal. Note the developmental change in tooth position that contributed to resolution of the recession.

If recession of the marginal tissue is progressive and inflammation is present despite good oral hygiene, a gingival graft should be performed. However, the question of how long the clinician should monitor the patient before making a recommendation for soft tissue grafting has not been clearly addressed. As a preventive measure and prior to orthodontic or prosthetic treatment, a free gingival graft has been prescribed to prevent incipient mucogingival defects from progressing in young children (Maynard, 1998). The placement of a graft over a properly prepared bed when the involved tooth has had no root exposure is a far more predictable procedure than that of covering up the root surface once the recession has occurred (Maynard and Ochsenbein, 1975). The conservative approach advocates watching areas of recession, because in the absence of bacterial plaque, little or no keratinized tissue is required to maintain periodontal health. However, a plaque-free mouth may be difficult to attain. Therefore, it has been recommended that in a child or young adult, once the marginal tissue recedes apical to the CEJ, and if there is no attached gingiva or minimal keratinized tissue (1 mm or less of keratinized tissue) and if a frenulum pull is present, a frenectomy alone or combined with a gingival graft should be performed. In all treatment plans, the relationships of the existing attached gingival margin, alveolar mucosa margin, and width of the bone to the CEJ should be the dictating factors, not the monitoring of attachment levels over long periods (Maynard and Wilson, 1980).

Influence of tooth position on gingival and alveolar height

Tooth eruption patterns and the thickness of the periodontium have a significant effect on mucogingival defects (Maynard and Wilson, 1980). Teeth that erupt in labioversion or are

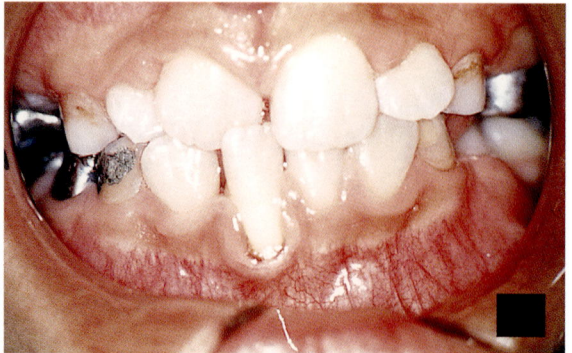

a

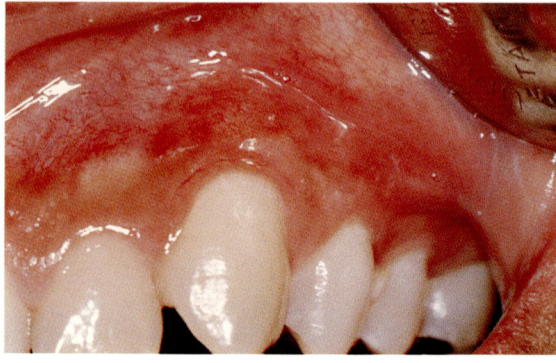

b

Figure 4.3

Influence of tooth position on the gingiva. A minimal width of keratinized gingiva is evident in the following examples. (a) A mandibular permanent central incisor displaced in a labial direction. Note the crossbite with its antagonist tooth (courtesy of Dr Enrique Bimstein). (b) A bulky, buccally displaced maxillary permanent canine. (c) A bulky, buccally displaced mandibular permanent canine.

c

forced in a labial direction are likely to exhibit minimal keratinized tissue and reduced osseous support at the facial aspect (Figure 4.3); in addition, a wide zone of keratinized tissue and a thick alveolar plate would be present at the lingual aspect of the tooth, with the soft tissue margin more coronal on the lingual aspect than on the labial aspect. Patients with thin keratinized tissue (less than 2 mm) and a thin labiolingual width of the alveolar process should be a cause for concern (Maynard and Wilson, 1980); however, clinicians must take into consideration that minimal or no attached gingiva in newly erupted permanent teeth is a normal feature (Figure 4.4).

Figure 4.4

A mixed dentition in which the width of the attached gingiva in the recently erupted permanent incisors is minimal or absent. The adjacent deciduous teeth have a significantly wider band of attached gingiva (courtesy of Dr Enrique Bimstein, with permission of *Acta Odontologica Pediatrica*, from Bimstein, 1987).

Recession: diagnosis and classification

Gingival recession is defined as the "location of the marginal tissue apical to the cementoenamel

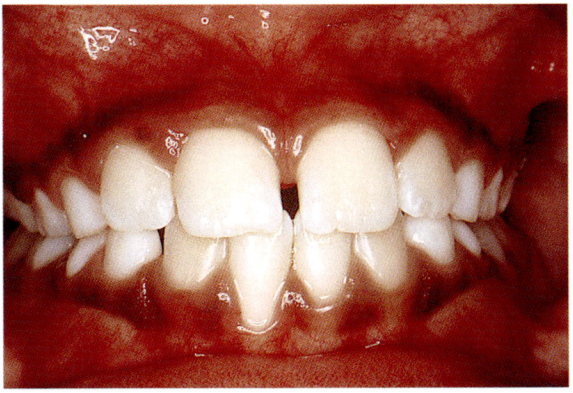
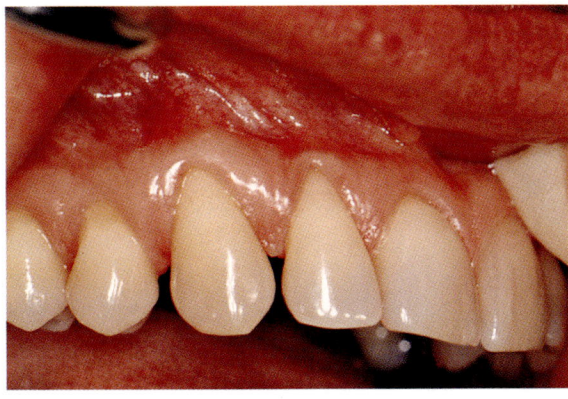

a   b

Figure 4.5

Pseudorecession. The marginal gingiva is located apical to that of the adjacent teeth but coronal to the cementoenamel junction. (a) Mandibular permanent central incisor (courtesy of Dr Enrique Bimstein). (b) Maxillary permanent canine.

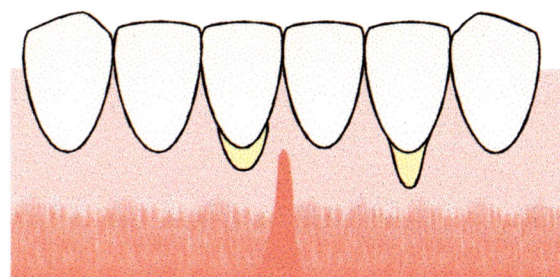

Class I

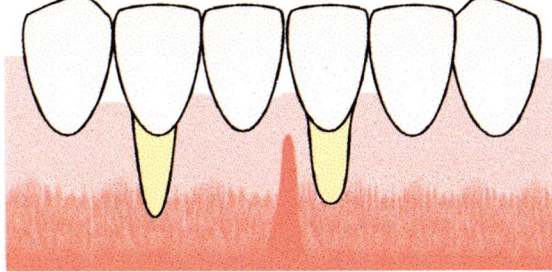

Class III

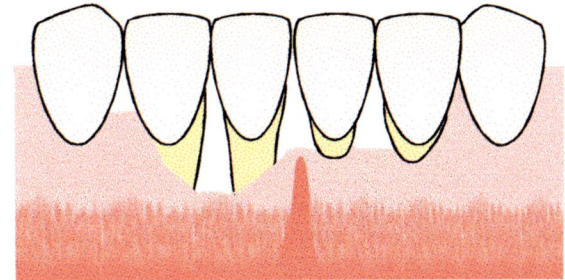

Class II

Class IV

Figure 4.6

Miller's classification of marginal tissue recession.

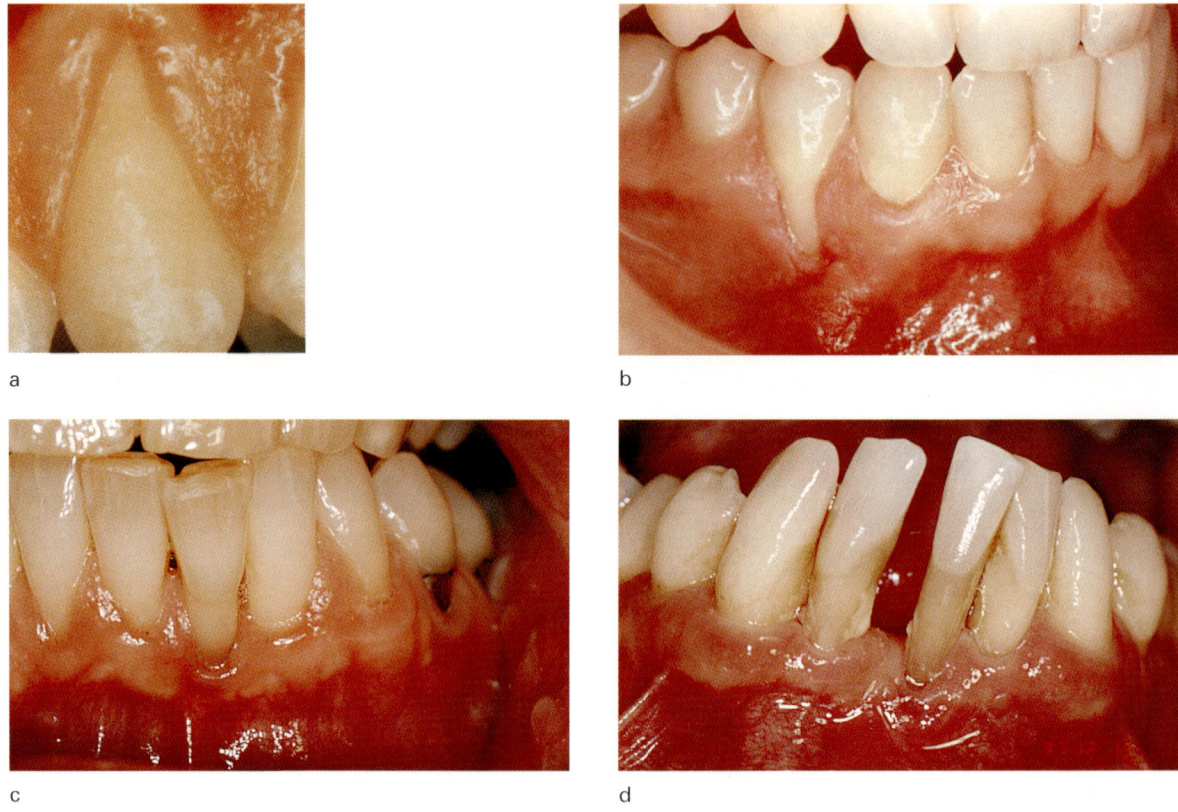

a   b

c   d

Figure 4.7

Clinical examples of Miller's classification of marginal tissue recession. True recession: the marginal tissue is apical to the cementoenamel junction. (a) Class I. (b) Class II. (c) Class III. (d) Class IV.

junction" (Nevins et al., 1992). The terms "soft tissue recession" and "marginal tissue recession" may be preferred on the grounds that the soft tissue margin may not always be composed of gingiva (it may be alveolar mucosa, if all the keratinized tissue has been lost). The soft tissue recession on a particular tooth may be readily determined by comparing the marginal tissue level to that of the adjacent teeth. However, this method may give a false interpretation. Clinicians should be aware that not every case of marginal tissue discrepancy is indicative of true recession: the soft tissue margin of one tooth may be more apical than that of the adjacent teeth, but it may not be apical to the CEJ. Using the CEJ as a reference point, clinicians can clearly differentiate between

"pseudorecession" (Figures 4.5a, b) and "true recession" (Figures 4.6, 4.7), as pseudorecession exhibits marginal tissue at the level coronal to the CEJ (Stoner and Mazdyasna, 1980; Bimstein, 1989).

Conditions implicated as predisposing factors to soft tissue recession include minimal attached gingiva (buccolingual and/or apicocoronal dimension), prominence of the tooth in the arch, frenum pull, inflammation related to plaque, improper brushing, and iatrogenesis (Wilson, 1983; Miller, 1993; Wennstrom, 1996). Miller (1985a) described four types of marginal tissue recession (Table 4.1, Figures 4.6, 4.7). He stated that the amount of root coverage that can be anticipated is dependent on the height of the adjacent papilla.

Table 4.1 Miller's classification of marginal tissue recession

Class	Description
I	Marginal tissue recession that does not extend to the mucogingival junction. There is no loss of interdental bone or soft tissue, and 100% root coverage can be anticipated
II	Marginal tissue recession that extends to or beyond the mucogingival junction. There is no loss of interdental bone or soft tissue, and 100% root coverage can be anticipated
III	Marginal tissue recession that extends to or beyond the mucogingival junction. Interdental bone or soft tissue loss is present or there is malpositioning of the teeth, which prevents the attempting of 100% root coverage. Partial root coverage can be anticipated
IV	Marginal tissue recession that extends to or beyond the mucogingival junction. The interdental bone or soft tissue loss and/or malpositioning of teeth is so severe that root coverage cannot be anticipated

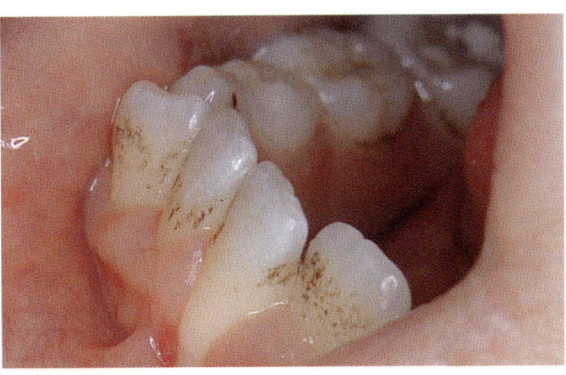

Figure 4.8

High frenum attachment. The mandibular central incisors exhibit a high labial frenum attachment, marginal tissue recession, and minimal keratinized tissue. The vestibulum is shallow and causes difficulties in tooth brushing. A frenectomy is recommended in this case (courtesy of Dr Enrique Bimstein, with permission of the *ASDC J Dent Child*, from Bimstein et al., 1988).

High frenum attachments: diagnosis

Hirschfeld (1939) associated the frenum inserting close to the gingival margin with gingival recession and pocket formation (Nevins and Cappetta, 1998a). He also discussed it as a possible etiologic factor in periodontal disease. Ochsenbein and Maynard (1974) suggested that when the width of attached gingiva is inadequate, a high frenum attachment may cause excessive tension on the marginal tissue (Figure 4.8). In the presence of inflammation, this condition may result in gingival recession. Therefore, a procedure to increase the band of attached gingiva such as a frenectomy or a free autogenous gingival graft combined with a frenectomy may be recommended (Ochsenbein and Maynard, 1974).

Treatment considerations

Oral hygiene and improvement due to growth and development

Periodontal inflammation should be controlled before a mucogingival defect is diagnosed or

mucogingival surgery is recommended (Figure 4.9). Mucogingival surgery should be considered if the recession is progressing. It is important to keep in mind that absence (or minimal thickness) of keratinized tissue alone is not an absolute indication for mucogingival surgery. However, when an inadequate width of keratinized tissue is associated with circumstances that either compromise the patient's ability to control plaque or by themselves stimulate inflammatory response of the periodontal tissues, mucogingival surgery is generally recommended. In addition, the stage of growth and development and its impact on changes in the width of attached gingiva should also be taken into account prior to mucogingival surgery (see Figure 4.2).

Mucogingival considerations for orthodontic patients

Tooth position significantly influences the width of the attached gingiva (Maynard, 1998). In addition, orthodontic appliances may compromise oral hygiene, and plaque-induced inflammation combined with excessive orthodontic

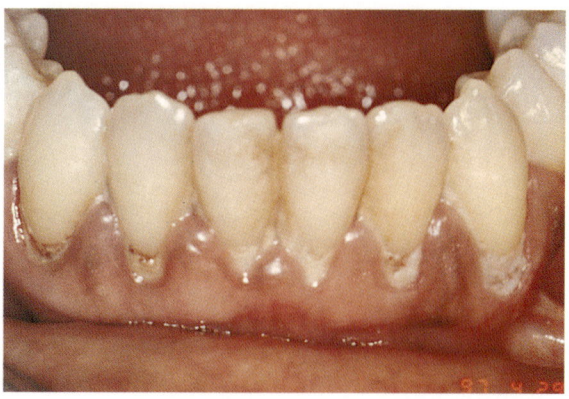

a

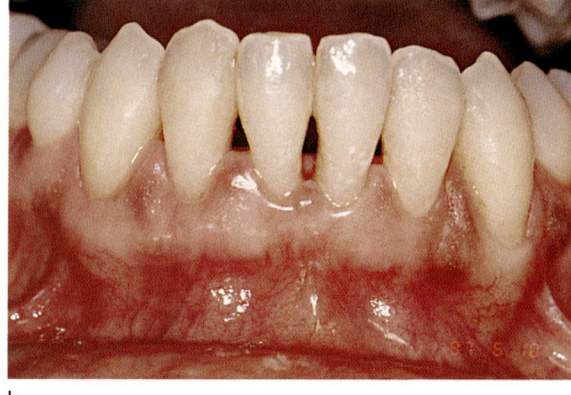

b

Figure 4.9

Treatment to reduce periodontal inflammation is recommended prior to the diagnosis and treatment for a mucogingival defect. (a) Before initial debridement and plaque control. (b) After initial debridement and plaque control.

forces may result in attachment loss and marginal tissue recession (Coatoam et al., 1981; Figure 4.10).

A review of mucogingival surgery and gingival augmentation was included in the World Workshop in Clinical Periodontics sponsored by the American Academy of Periodontology in 1989 (Hall, 1989). It was recommended that in the absence of an adequate thickness of keratinized gingiva, the probability of marginal tissue recession during the orthodontic tooth movement is sufficiently high to justify augmentation of the gingiva. Grafting prior to orthodontic therapy in a patient with a thin periodontium should be advised. This procedure is highly predictable with assured connective tissue attachment to the tooth, and will reduce the risk of soft tissue recession during orthodontic therapy. This gingival augmentation should be considered therapeutic.

Mucogingival considerations following the orthodontic alignment of impacted maxillary cuspids have been discussed in several studies. The location of the impacted cuspid (whether it is in a palatal or a labial position), the timing and technique for hard and soft tissue surgical management to expose the cuspid, and the mechanics of tooth movement are factors that have a significant effect on the periodontal status of the cuspid after alignment (Wise, 1981). The palatally impacted cuspid shows no loss of attached gingiva, but can exhibit bone loss after the orthodontic therapy

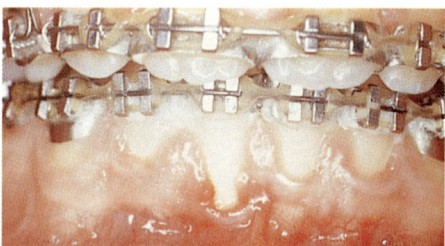

Figure 4.10

Orthodontic appliances can compromise the patient's plaque control. A free soft tissue graft is recommended in areas of marginal tissue recession during orthodontics where an "inadequate" width of keratinized tissue is observed.

(Becker et al., 1983). In contrast, the alignment of labially displaced cuspids is usually accompanied by the loss of attached gingiva (Kohavi et al., 1984). A study conducted by Adrian Becker and colleagues has reported that there is approximately 0.8 mm of attached gingiva remaining on the orthodontically treated cuspids whereas there is 2.44 mm of attached gingiva left on the untreated controls (normal cuspids) (Becker et al., 1983).

Clinicians should be alert to the possibility of mucogingival defects both prior to and following orthodontic therapy, and all cases should be assessed periodontally before and after treatment. The relation between malocclusion, orthodontic treatment, and gingival health is discussed in Chapter 13.

Mucogingival considerations for restorative dentistry

Soft tissue recession may facilitate the development of root caries and dentine hypersensitivity. For the treatment of root caries, placement of the restorative margin intracrevicularly can induce gingival inflammation and compromise the ability to control plaque. Although it is generally accepted that no keratinized tissue is required to maintain periodontal health of an intact tooth, this rule is changed when a restoration is planned. The unintentional irritation and insults associated with restorative procedures such as tooth preparation, impression taking, and casting try-ins call for a more secure periodontium (Wilson and Maynard, 1981; Nevins and Cappetta, 1998a). Therefore, gingival augmentation should be considered in order to minimize the risk of marginal tissue recession.

In the pediatric permanent dentition, the pulp chamber and root canals are larger than in the adult tooth. Root exposure in children frequently results in more drastic sensitivity to mechanical and thermal stimuli than that observed in adults with similar root exposure (Maynard, 1998). As a result, the child avoids brushing the sensitive sites, leading to plaque accumulation and gingival inflammation. Soft tissue grafting is one of several procedures that should be considered as a treatment alternative in cases of root exposure (Maynard, 1998). This procedure is recommended for the treatment of root sensitivity or shallow carious lesions, particularly when appearance is important.

Mucogingival surgery

The 1989 World Workshop on Clinical Periodontics recognized eight procedures of mucogingival surgery: the pedicle graft, the lateral sliding flap, the free gingival graft, the coronally positioned graft, the double papilla flap, the semilunar positioned flap, the connective tissue graft, and the edentulous ridge augmentation. Guided tissue regeneration procedures have been shown to be a predictable treatment in specific cases for the treatment of soft tissue recession. In addition, an acellular dermal matrix graft offering unlimited grafting material has been demonstrated as an acceptable treatment for root coverage. Each mucogingival procedure has different indications, strengths, and weaknesses. Clinicians need to select a treatment suitable for each individual patient. The nature of the attachment of the grafted gingiva to the root in various mucogingival procedures appears to be the most significant area of research. For both guided tissue regeneration and the traditional free gingival graft procedures, there is human biopsy evidence of a connective tissue attachment to new cementum on the exposed root surface (Cortellini et al., 1993; Pasquinelli, 1995).

Indications for mucogingival surgery

- To establish an adequate zone of attached gingiva prior to coronal positioning of a graft and/or for restorative considerations, particularly if the restorative margins will be placed subgingivally.
- To facilitate proper plaque control. This may be the case in the presence of a high frenum and muscle attachments, a deep and narrow recession defect, and where a recession extends to the level of the vestibular fornix.
- To eliminate the pull of frena and muscle attachments on the gingival margin.
- To increase vestibular depth.
- To correct soft tissue recession by root coverage techniques or to cover gingival clefts.
- To modify the edentulous ridges prior to prosthetics.
- To assist in orthodontic therapy, e.g., uncovering an impacted canine, and when facial tooth movement results in alveolar bone dehiscence.
- To cover exposed roots for esthetic reasons (Figure 4.11), root sensitivity, or to prevent root caries.

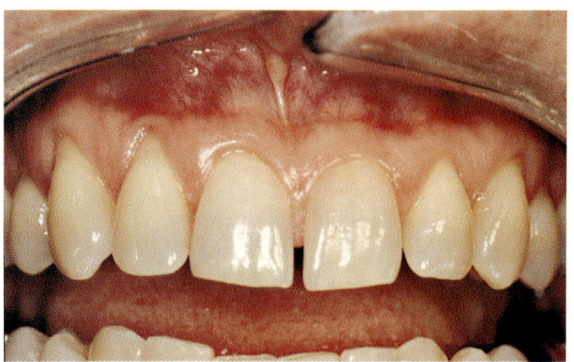

Figure 4.11

Marginal tissue recession presenting in unesthetic zone (maxillary right lateral incisor and canine). Mucogingival surgery for esthetic purposes is indicated, regardless of the amount of attached gingiva.

Techniques

Lateral sliding flap

The lateral sliding flap procedure was first described by Grupe and Warren (1956) and has been modified by several clinicians over the years. It can be used to increase the amount of attached gingiva and to cover a root with localized recession (Figure 4.12). Utilizing gingiva from an adjacent donor source and a pedicle design that retains its blood supply, the lateral sliding flap has a success rate of approximately 70% with excellent color and texture match (Nevins and Cappetta, 1998b).

The lateral sliding flap may be prepared as a full thickness or partial thickness flap to avoid recession at the donor site. It is recommended that the width of the pedicle be three times the width of the root area to be covered, at least 3 mm of gingiva in an apicocoronal direction,

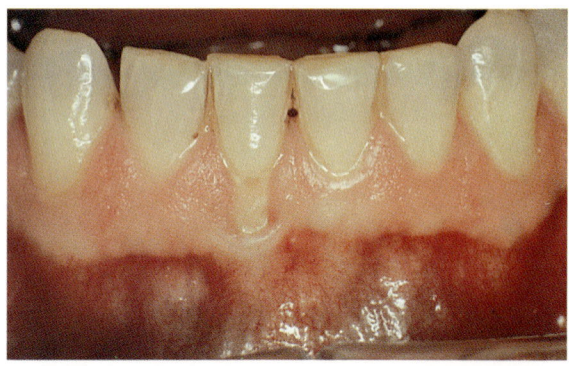

a

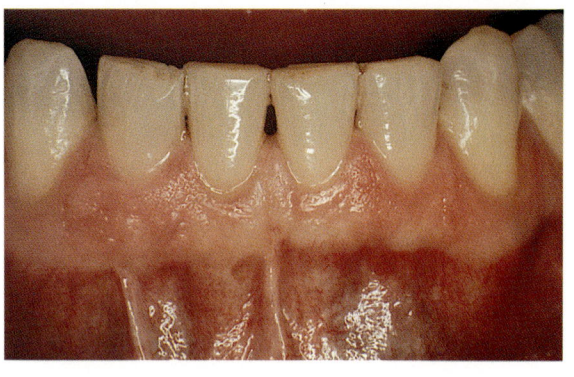

c

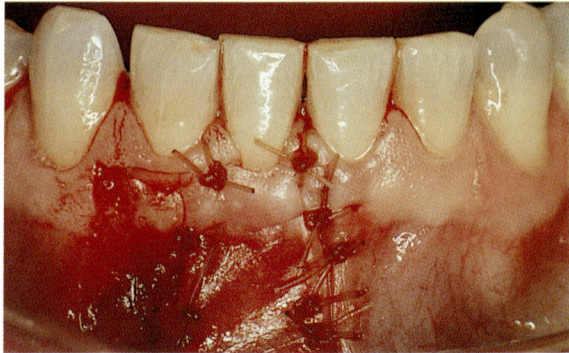

b

Figure 4.12

The lateral sliding flap (courtesy of Dr David Greenfield). (a) Marginal tissue recession presented at the mandibular permanent right central incisor. (b) Gingiva from the adjacent teeth was utilized as a donor source for the lateral sliding flap procedure. The pedicle flap design provided good blood supply. (c) Ten-month postoperative view showed complete root coverage and a significant increase in the width of attached gingiva.

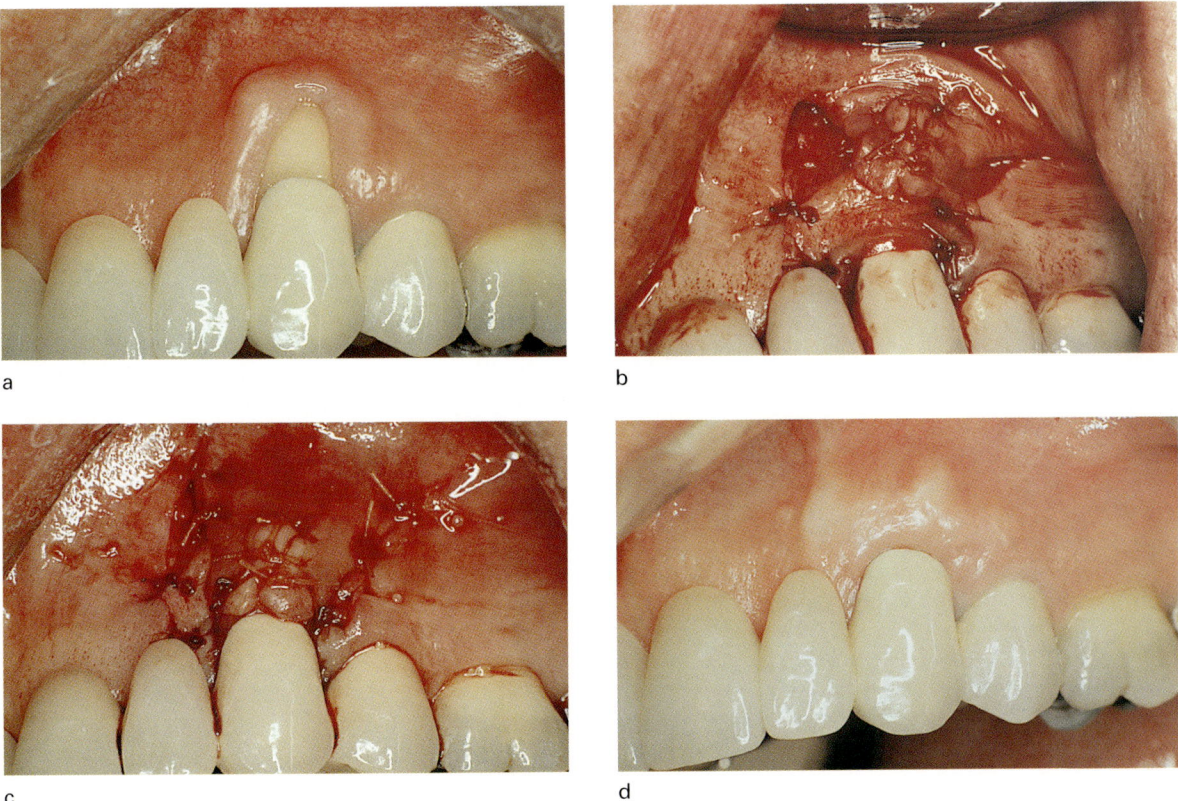

a

b

c

d

Figure 4.13

The double papilla flap combined with a connective tissue graft (courtesy of Dr David Greenfield). (a) Marginal tissue recession presented at the maxillary permanent left canine. (b) The double papilla flap procedure combined with a connective tissue graft was performed. (c) The double papilla flap is placed coronally and sutured in situ over the connective tissue graft. (d) One-year postoperative view shows esthetic results. Complete root coverage and a significant increase in the width of attached gingiva were accomplished.

with sufficient thickness in the donor site (Allen and Miller, 1989). Tension on the flap should be eliminated prior to suturing to facilitate wound healing. The narrower and shorter the area to be covered, the more likely is the procedure to be successful. Several modifications of this procedure include treatment of the root surface with citric acid and covering connective tissue grafts in a bilaminar procedure (Nelson, 1987; Harris, 1992).

If a lateral sliding flap is planned in a young patient, the clinician needs to be aware of anatomical and developmental circumstances at this particular stage (Ochsenbein and Maynard, 1974). The keratinized tissue at the donor site

may be over the enamel surface, since the tooth is not fully erupted. In the lateral sliding flap procedure, most of the keratinized gingiva that has only enamel beneath it may be removed. There will then be no replacement of the tissue during healing, resulting in no attached gingiva in the area of the donor site.

Double papilla flap

The double papilla pedicle graft was introduced by Cohen and Ross (1968). In this procedure, interdental papillae on either side of a tooth with recession are joined to create a band of gingiva sufficient to cover the exposed root surface (Figure 4.13). Its use is limited to cases where gingival color matching cannot be achieved by a free gingival graft, partly due to its poor predictability. The donor papillae must have sufficient width and height when joined together to cover the recession, and deep gingival grooves should not be present.

Coronally positioned flap (coronally positioned pedicle graft)

The coronally positioned flap was first described as a treatment for root coverage. It provides the advantages of an excellent match of color, texture, and contour, as well as a single surgical site. This flap is recommended as a treatment for shallow areas of recession (class I of Miller's classification) where 3 mm of keratinized gingiva is present. The predictability and efficacy of this procedure in covering exposed roots have been questioned. Several modifications designed to improve its predictability have been reported, including the use of citric acid root preparation and a combined technique using a free gingival graft with a coronally positioned flap. The coronally positioned flap is more predictable when combined with the prior placement of a free gingival graft than when used alone (Bernimoulin et al., 1975). The free gingival graft is first placed apical to the area of localized recession with inadequate attached gingiva. Two months later, the coronally positioned flap procedure is performed to obtain the gingival margin at the CEJ level. Although the combined procedure significantly increases the predictability, there are esthetic concerns. The free gingival graft as the first step in this technique results in color and texture mismatches. Because there is no significant difference in root coverage between the two-stage combined procedure and the free gingival graft alone (Laney et al., 1992), the use of the combined procedure has decreased in recent years.

In a series of studies by Caffesse and Guinard (Caffesse and Guinard, 1978, 1980; Guinard and Caffesse, 1978), both the lateral sliding flap and the combined technique of free gingival graft with the coronally positioned flap were shown to be more predictable than the double papilla approach. They reported an approximate 65% coverage of study sites at 6 months. The height of the interdental papillae adjacent to the recession determines how much root coverage can be obtained.

Epithelialized free gingival graft

The free gingival graft procedure was first described by Bjorn (1963). Subsequently, Nabers (1966a, b) reported the use of this treatment to increase the amount of attached gingiva and to cover exposed roots; in this study only partial root coverage was achieved. The inability of the free gingival graft to predictably cover exposed roots in the early years led clinicians to advocate limiting its use to increasing the dimension of attached gingiva.

Miller (1985b) demonstrated that the free gingival graft was a predictable treatment for root coverage. Others reported similar results (Corn and Mark, 1983; Holbrook and Ochsenbein, 1983). Miller (1985b) reported 100% root coverage by the free gingival graft in 87% (incidence) of deep–wide recession defects and 100% root coverage in 100% of the shallow–narrow recession defects. Citric acid root preparation was used in Miller's technique. In addition, a thick graft (approximately 1.5–2.0 mm) was recommended in order to achieve root coverage. The amount of root coverage that can be obtained is limited by the height of the interproximal bone of adjacent interdental papillae.

Although it is generally accepted that the free gingival graft is the most versatile, most widely used, and most predictable pure mucogingival surgical procedure, it has a major weakness of which the clinician should be aware. The free gingival graft is not recommended where esthetic considerations are important. Color mismatches of the palatal donor gingiva and gingiva adjacent to the recipient site, and keloid formation in the grafted site, appear to be the most serious concerns (Figure 4.14).

The free gingival graft technique described below (Figure 4.15) is suitable for gingival augmentation. For root coverage, the technique requires modification (Miller, 1987). In addition, a phenomenon known as "creeping attachment"

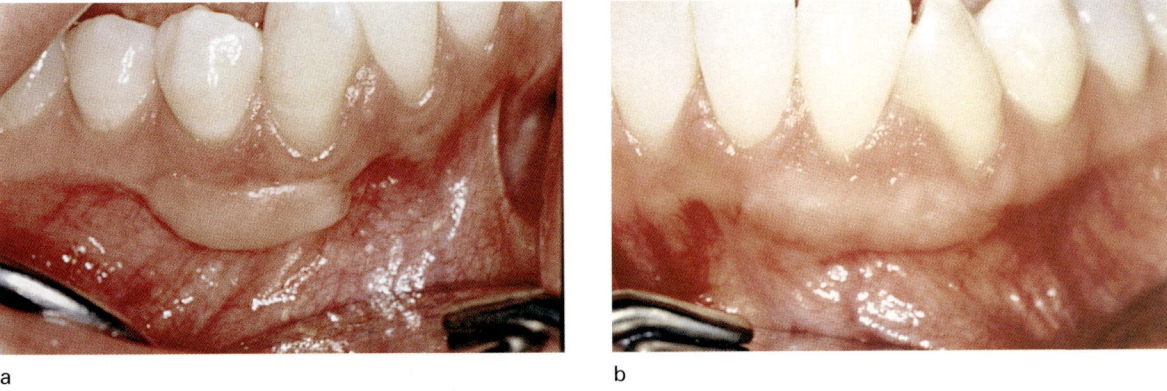

a   b

Figure 4.14

Free gingival graft procedures completed on the mandibular right (a) and left (b) premolar areas. A compromised esthetic result is a weakness of this procedure (a).

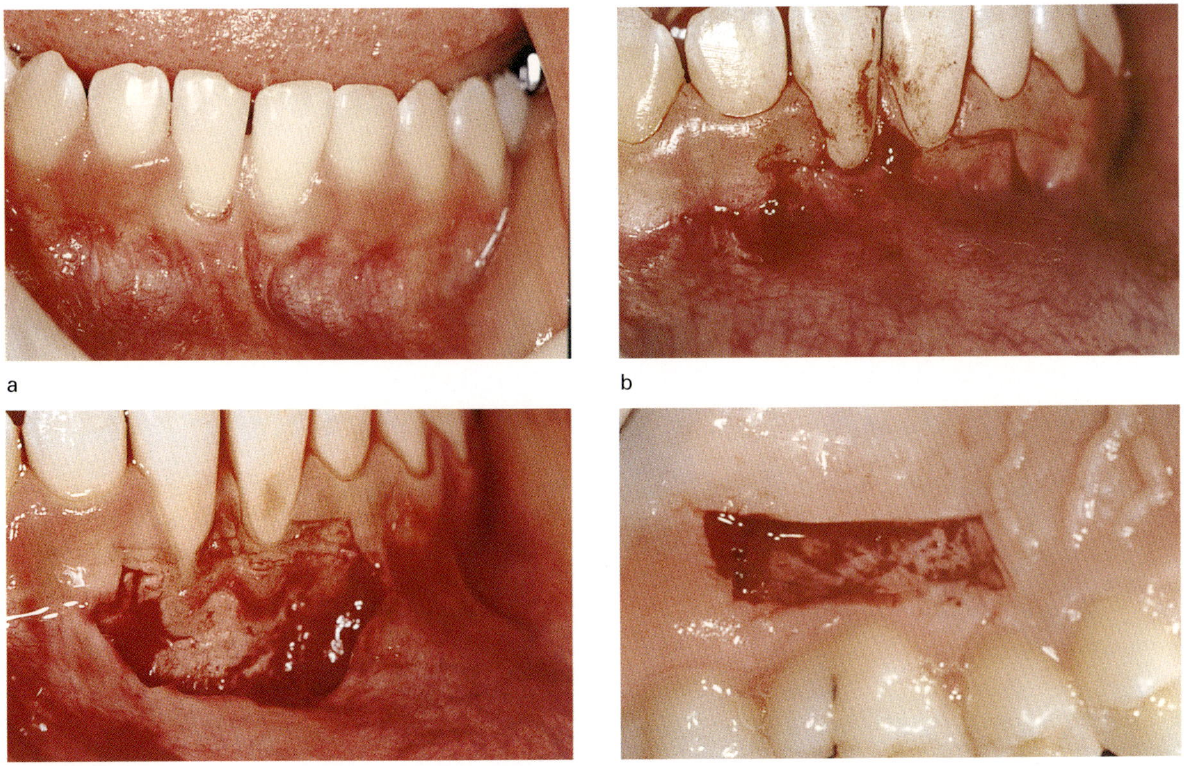

a   b

c   d

Figure 4.15

Free gingival graft for gingival augmentation. (a) Inadequate width of keratinized tissue with chronic inflammation and a high frenum attachment were observed in the mandibular central incisor area. After initial phase therapy, a free gingival graft was recommended. (b) A horizontal incision with two vertical releasing incisions was made. (c) The periosteal recipient bed was prepared by partial thickness dissection. (d) Shown is the donor surgical site after the free gingival graft was removed.

Continued overleaf

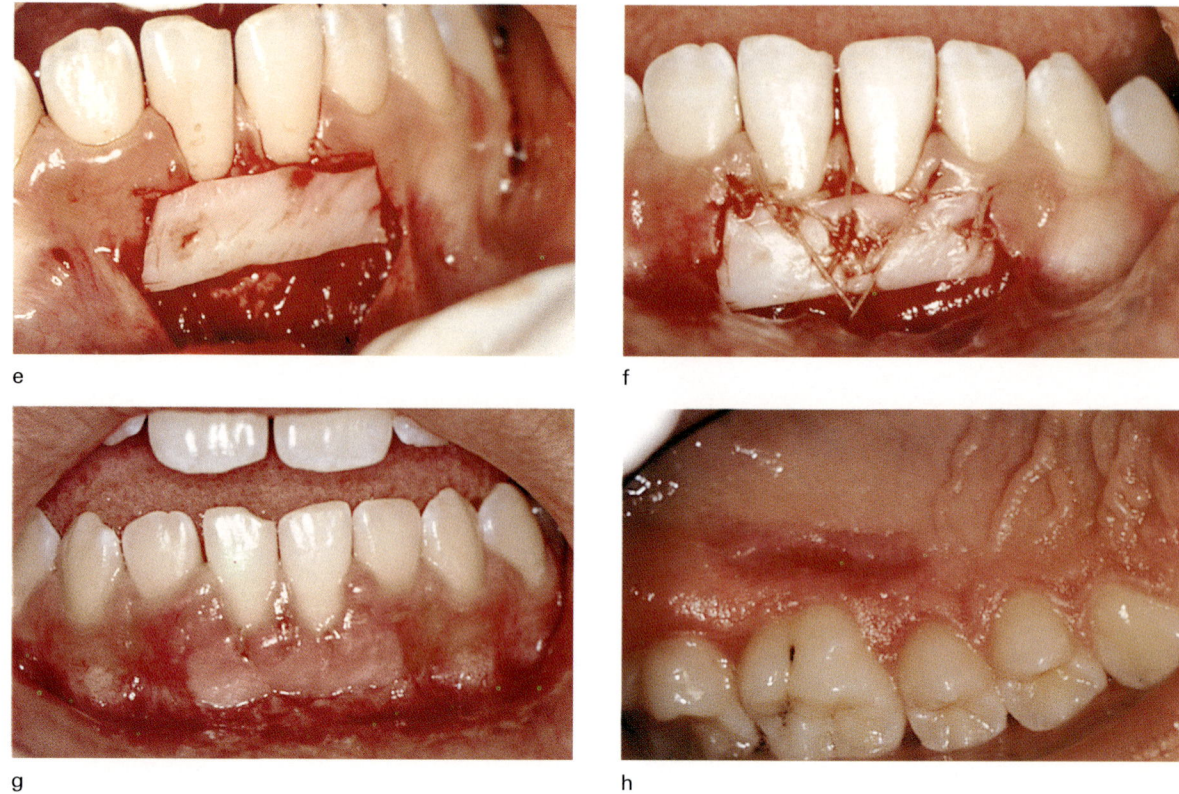

e

f

g

h

Figure 4.15 *continued*

(e) The donor tissue was placed on the prepared recipient bed and pressure was applied with a damp gauze to prevent a dead space between the graft and prepared bed. (f) The graft was stabilized by interrupted and suspensory sutures. (g) Two-week postoperative view of the grafted sites. (h) Two-week postoperative view of the donor sites.

may occur in some cases during healing, resulting in some minor root coverage.

Recipient site preparation (bed preparation)

Local infiltration or blockade with local anesthetic solution is delivered at the recipient site. A no. 15 surgical blade held at 90° to the gingival surface is used to make a superficial incision at a level just coronal to the mucogingival junction (Figure 4.15b). The periosteal recipient bed is then prepared by partial thickness dissection in an apical direction with the no. 15 blade held parallel to the alveolar process. The flap is apically positioned. The periosteal bed should extend approximately 6–8 mm apical to the mucogingival junction, and should be trimmed free of any irregular connective tissue tags and muscle attachments (Figure 4.15c). The dimensions of the prepared bed are determined with a periodontal probe or by preparing an adhesive tinfoil template.

Donor site

The most common donor site is the palatal gingiva which should be posterior to the rugae, coronal to the vessels and nerves exiting the anterior palatine foramen, and at least 1 mm apical to the gingival margins of adjacent teeth to avoid recession at the donor site. The selected donor area should be palpated to ascertain the thickness and the presence of exostoses. Local anesthetic infiltration is administered around the donor area. The measured dimensions are outlined with the no. 15 surgical blade or a prefabricated template. A 1.5–2.0 mm thickness of palatal gingiva is removed gently and smoothly from the hard palate (Figure 4.15d). The donor material should be uniform in thickness and smoothness of the underlying surface, and free of adipose tissue.

Graft suturing

The donor tissue is placed on the prepared recipient bed and pressure is applied with damp gauze (Figure 4.15e). The choice of suture material varies among clinicians; in most cases a more delicate needle is preferred. A suture is placed at each end of the graft and at the papillary areas. Suspensory sutures may be necessary if additional graft stabilization is needed (Figure 4.15f).

Postoperative care and instructions

Placement of a periodontal dressing is recommended for both the donor and the grafted sites. Care should be taken not to disturb the graft during its placement. The patient should be advised to refrain from retracting the lips and cheeks, to keep the tongue away from the surgical sites, and to avoid brushing or flossing in the grafted area. An ice pack can be applied to the grafted area externally during the postoperative period to minimize swelling. Chlorhexidine mouthwash may be prescribed. Postoperative discomfort is most often associated with the palatal donor site and can be managed with an over-the-counter pain medication. The dressing and sutures are removed 7 days postoperatively (Figures 4.15g, h). The patient is advised to continue use of the chlorhexidine mouth rinse for an additional 1–2 weeks.

Subepithelial connective tissue graft

There are few reports on the use of subepithelial connective tissue grafts in children and adolescents. This may in part be due to the anatomy of the hard palate during development. A study by Studer et al. (1997) using bone sounding techniques demonstrated that in adults the keratinized tissue in the canine–premolar region and the tuberosity was significantly thicker than in other areas of the hard palate.

The subepithelial connective tissue graft was introduced by Langer and Langer (1985). The procedure has high predictability for root coverage with good gingival color and texture matches and minimal keloid formation. Long-term benefits in both increasing the amount of attached gingiva and obtaining root coverage have been demonstrated (Jahnke et al., 1993; Paolantonio et al., 1997). Double blood supply— that of the gingival flap covering the graft, and that of the recipient connective tissue bed including the adjacent papilla—appears to be a factor that increases its success rate. In addition, this procedure is more comfortable postoperatively for the patient than the free gingival graft, because the palatal donor site can be completely closed.

Several modifications of this procedure have been reported. In the technique described by Langer and Langer (1985), the grafted connective tissue is left exposed at the portion placed over the previously denuded root surface. In addition, a 2 mm band of epithelium is retained at the graft margin to facilitate the handling quality. Raetzke (1985) proposed the "envelope" technique; the epithelium was retained on the connective tissue graft only where it would cover the exposed root (Figure 4.16). Nelson used a laterally positioned full thickness flap or a double papilla flap to cover the connective tissue graft to provide the double blood supply (Nelson, 1987). Harris covered the graft with partial thickness pedicle flaps (Harris, 1992).

Recipient site preparation

In order to avoid compromising the blood supply, a mandibular or dental block is given in the mandible. In the maxilla, an injection into the immediate graft site should be avoided. Interpapillary injections are kept to a minimum. A horizontal right-angle incision is carried out with a no. 15 surgical blade at or slightly coronal

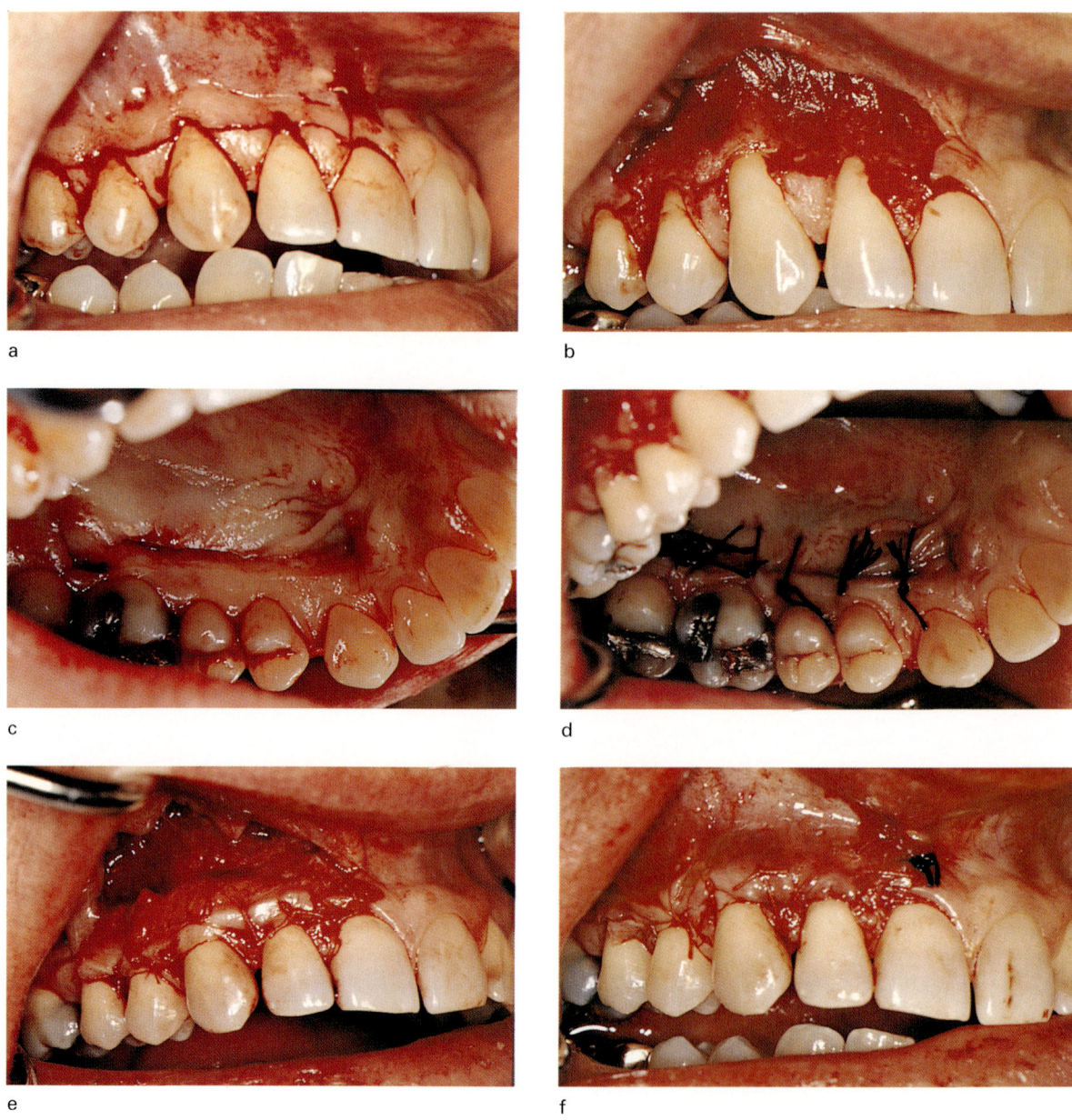

Figure 4.16

The subepithelial connective tissue graft. (a) Initial incision at the cementoenamel junction level. (b) The recipient site was prepared by a partial thickness dissection. (c) Appearance of the donor surgical site after the subepithelial connective tissue graft was removed. (d) The donor surgical site was sutured. Note the complete closure of the donor surgical site was obtained. (e) Donor connective tissue was placed and stabilizes at the prepared recipient site. (f) The overlying partial thickness flap is replaced by interrupted sutures into the papillae.

to the CEJ of the tooth with recession. The inter-proximal papillae are left intact (Figure 4.16a). A partial thickness flap is created with or without two vertical incisions by sharp dissection (Figure 4.16b). If the vertical incisions are not made, the mesiodistal length of the horizontal incision should be extended to provide easy access to the denuded root. The dissection should be extended apically, well beyond the mucogingival junction, without perforations. The flap should have no tension when pulled coronally beyond the CEJ. The roots are planed thoroughly. If the root is overly convex, it may be planed to lie within the bony housing. Following root planing, the root may be treated with citric acid or tetracycline depending on the clinician's preference. The dimensions of the prepared bed are determined with a periodontal probe or by preparing an adhesive tinfoil template.

Donor site preparation

After local anesthesia is obtained, the thickness of the donor palatal tissue can be determined by bone sounding. The first horizontal incision is made on the palate perpendicularly to the long axis of the teeth, approximately 2–3 mm apical to the gingival margin of the maxillary teeth. The second incision is made parallel and approximately 1–2 mm apical to the first incision. This is continued far enough apically to obtain a sufficient height of connective tissue to cover the exposed root and the prepared periosteal bed. The more coronal incision is likewise carried apically. The palatal bone is scored apically, mesially, and distally, to enable the operator to remove the connective tissue graft. Alternatively, a small periosteal elevator may be used to raise a full thickness periosteal connective tissue graft. Vertical incisions can be made mesially and distally through the flap and the connective tissue graft to facilitate the removal of the graft (Figure 4.16c). The graft thickness is ideally 1.5 mm. The band of epithelium at the coronal part of the graft is retained in order to facilitate tissue handling. A crossed horizontal suspensory suture or interrupted sutures with 4-0 silk is used to approximate the palatal wound (Figure 4.16d).

Graft suturing

The length and thickness of the graft can be modified by a surgical blade, while the graft is placed on a moist, sterile gauze pad. Excess adipose and glandular tissues should be removed. The connective tissue graft is secured to the interdental papillae with interrupted sutures using 6-0 monofilament pliabilized nylon or 5-0 chromic gut with an atraumatic needle. It is important that the graft be closely adapted to the recipient site, avoiding blood clot formation between the graft tissue and the periosteal recipient bed (Figure 4.16e). The recipient overlying flap is positioned coronally to cover as much of the graft as possible (Figure 4.16f). Tension on the flap when sutured over the graft should be eliminated.

Postoperative care and instructions

A periodontal dressing is placed over the recipient site. For the palatal donor site, a dressing is optional. Chlorhexidine mouthwash, oral non-steroidal anti-inflammatory drugs, and narcotic or non-narcotic analgesics are prescribed. Patients should be advised to refrain from retracting the lips and cheeks, to keep the tongue away from the surgical sites, and to avoid brushing or flossing in the grafted area. Intermittent ice pack application is recommended for the first 12 hours. The dressing and sutures are removed 7 days postoperatively. The patient is advised to continue use of the chlorhexidine mouth rinse for an additional 1–2 weeks.

Semilunar coronally positioned flap

The semilunar coronally positioned flap was described in the adult by Tarnow (1986). An incision with a semilunar form is made at the mucogingival junction or apical to it, and a partial thickness flap is raised by inserting a blade into the sulcus and filleting a flap free over the root. The flap, still attached at both lateral borders to the adjacent papilla, is moved coronally to cover the exposed root surface and held in place with or without suture. In the semilunar coronally positioned flap procedure a free gingival graft is not performed first, so the esthetic result is good. It was reported that clinically successful root coverage (approximately 2–3 mm) can be obtained in over 20 teeth by a single session of the semilunar coronally positioned flap procedure.

Guided tissue regeneration

As the ultimate goal of periodontal therapy is periodontal regeneration, guided tissue regeneration (GTR) appears to be the treatment of choice. Tinti and Vincenzi (1990) described the use of expanded polytetrafluoroethylene (e-PTFE) membranes for the treatment of recession. In later years, the use of bioabsorbable membranes combined with various flap designs was reported as a treatment of gingival recession (Genon et al., 1994; Pini Prato et al., 1995). It has been shown that GTR is an effective and predictable procedure to obtain root coverage for deep–wide (larger than 5 mm) isolated facial recessions, resulting in improved appearance and gains in clinical attachment (Pini Prato et al., 1992, 1996). The technique does not require a secondary donor surgical site, eliminating postoperative discomfort.

A comparison was made of two root coverage techniques: GTR with a bioabsorbable membrane, and a connective tissue graft combined with a coronally positioned pedicle flap without vertical incisions (Harris, 1998a). Both procedures resulted in statistically similar amounts of mean root coverage. However, the connective tissue graft combined with a coronally positioned flap produced a significant increase in the amount of keratinized tissue, while the GTR did not.

Acellular dermal allograft

An acellular dermal allograft has been used to increase the amount of keratinized gingiva and to cover the exposed root surface. This procedure offers unlimited grafting material and does not require a secondary donor site, eliminating postoperative discomfort. An acellular dermal matrix graft (Alloderm, Lifecore Biomedical Inc., Chaske, Minn., USA) is commercially available.

This material is aseptically processed from donated human skin, removing cells that would be targets for immune response without altering the collagen and extracellular matrix proteins. Its use results in clinical and histologic outcomes comparable with the connective tissue graft with partial thickness double pedicle (Harris, 1998b) and the free gingival (Silverstein et al., 1999), but the esthetic result is better than an autogenous palatal graft. Additional studies are needed to determine the predictability and longevity of root coverage obtained from this allograft.

Frenectomy

The frenum position changes with age (Geiger, 1980), and the clinician treating a child with a high frenum attachment should take this into consideration. Evaluation of the patient's oral hygiene is particularly important for a treatment decision. A frenectomy is indicated if the frenum is located apical to an area of recession associated with an inability to adequately cleanse or debride the area.

Nevins (1986) stated that a shallow vestibule impedes oral cleansing and that the frenum must be carefully considered as a threat to long-term periodontal health when superimposed on a shallow vestibule (Nevins and Cappetta, 1998a).

Frenectomy can result in scar formation which could prevent the mesial movement of the central incisors (West, 1968). Thus, it is suggested that frenectomy is performed after orthodontic therapy. Relapse separation of the teeth has been reported in the case of orthodontic closure of diastema without excision of associated frena (Edwards, 1977).

Technique

Local infiltration or blockade with local anesthetic solution is delivered at the recipient site. The frenum can be grasped with a hemostat and retracted, or if it is broad, simply retracting the lip will suffice. Starting at the apex, a no. 15 scalpel blade is used to release each side individually. The incisions at the base are extended to allow proper tapering of the flap. The wound can either be left to heal with a periodontal dressing

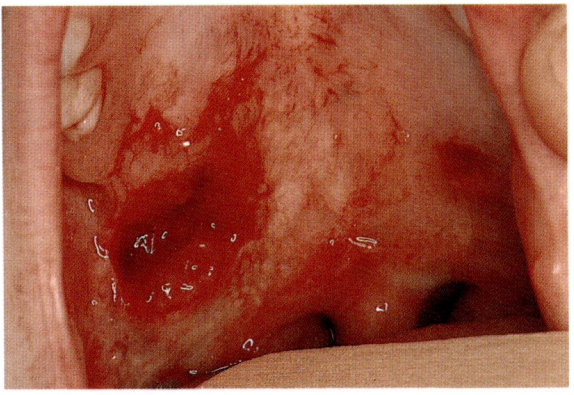
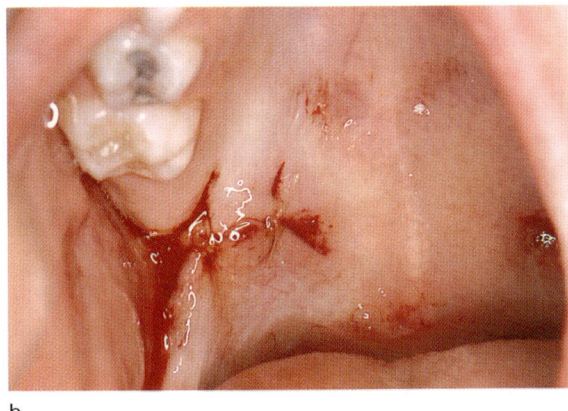

a   b

Figure 4.17

Treatment of gingival abrasion and contusion. (a) Cleansing of the wound with saline and removal of foreign bodies. (b) Suturing of the wound to try to achieve primary closure.

in place, or several resorbable sutures can be placed; this depends on how the tissue "falls" after the incisions have been made.

Management of gingival injuries in children and adolescents

Children treated in hospital emergency departments often present with dental and oral soft tissue trauma (Andreasen, 1970; Galea, 1984; O'Neil et al., 1989). The soft tissues usually involved are the lip, alveolar mucosa, and gingiva. The recommended treatment approach includes a diagnostic phase, an evaluation of antibiotic coverage, initial treatments of dental injuries prior to soft tissue management, wound debridement, and repositioning and suturing of displaced tissues (Andreasen, 1994). In the diagnostic phase, the nature, extent, and contamination of the lesion should be thoroughly examined after administration of local anesthesia.

Gingival injuries can involve abrasion, contusion, laceration, or avulsion (tissue loss). Improper management of gingival wounds in children may lead to mucogingival defects in adulthood. Treatment of gingival abrasion and contusion (Figure 4.17) is limited to cleansing of

the wound with saline and removal of foreign bodies. Complete healing is anticipated owing to the high degree of vascularity of the gingival tissue. It is essential that optimal oral hygiene is maintained during the healing period; this may include daily mouth rinsing with 0.12% chlorhexidine. In cases of gingival laceration (Figure 4.18), it is recommended that after wound debridement and removal of foreign bodies (Figure 4.18a) the displaced teeth should be repositioned (Figure 4.18b) before the lacerated gingiva is brought back into a normal position (Figure 4.18c). A minimal number of fine sutures such as 5-0 or 6-0 silk may be placed to immobilize the repositioned gingival tissue (Figure 4.18d). The sutures are removed 4–5 days afterwards (Figure 4.18e).

Gingival tissue loss can result in the exposure of alveolar bone. In such cases, a gingival flap should be raised and elongated by the placement of periosteal incisions to achieve a complete coverage of the exposed bone. If the gingival avulsion or displacement occurs in the area of erupting teeth, an assessment in relation to the CEJ is required. It has been suggested that if the gingival wound does not extend beyond the CEJ of the erupting tooth, further eruption and physiologic gingival retraction will normalize the clinical appearance with time (Andreasen, 1994).

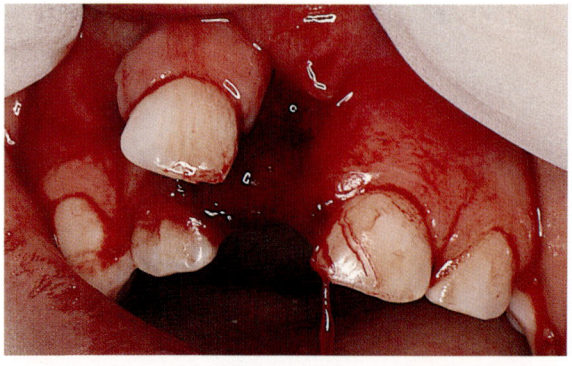

a

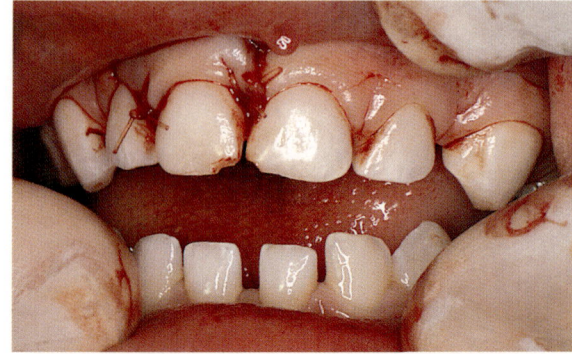

b

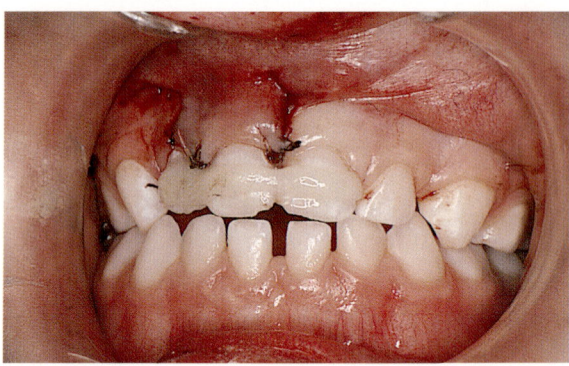

d

c

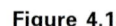

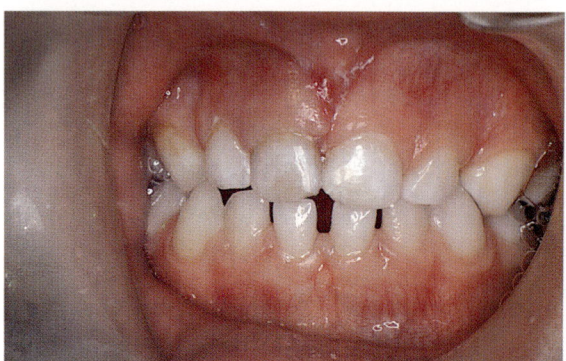

e

Figure 4.18

Treatment of gingival laceration (courtesy of Dr Howard L. Needleman). (a) Wound debridement and removal of foreign bodies. (b) Reposition of displaced teeth. (c) Lacerated gingiva brought back into a normal position. (d) A minimal number of fine sutures such as 5-0 or 6-0 silk may be placed to immobilize the repositioned gingival tissue. (e) The sutures are removed 4–5 days later.

Acknowledgments

The authors express their deepest appreciation to Dr Paul Levi and Dr David S. Greenfield for their instructive illustrations.

References

Ainamo J, Talari A (1976) The increase with age of the width of attached gingiva. *J Periodont Res* **11**: 182–8.

Ainamo A, Ainamo J, Poikkeus R (1981) Continuous widening of the band of attached gingiva from 23 to 65 years of age. *J Periodont Res* **16**: 595–9.

Allen EP, Miller PD (1989) Coronal positioning of existing gingiva: short term results in the treatment of shallow marginal tissue recession. *J Periodontol* **60**: 316–19.

Andlin-Sobocki A, Marcusson A, Persson M (1991) 3-year observations on gingival recession in mandibular incisors in children. *J Clin Periodontol* **18**: 155–9.

Andreasen JO (1970) Etiology and pathogenesis of traumatic dental injuries. A clinical study of 1298 cases. *Scand J Dent Res* **78**: 329–42.

Andreasen JO (1994) Soft tissue injuries. In: Andreasen JO, Andreasen FM (eds) *Textbook and Color Atlas of Traumatic Injuries to the Teeth*, 3rd edn. Copenhagen: Munksgaard, pp. 495–516.

Becker A, Kohavi D, Zilberman Y (1983) Periodontal status following the alignment of palatally impacted canine teeth. *Am J Orthodont* **84**: 332–6.

Bernimoulin JP, Luscher B, Muhlemann HR (1975) Coronally repositioned periodontal flap. Clinical evaluation after one year. *J Clin Periodontol* **2**: 1–13.

Bimstein E (1989) Non-surgical treatment of pseudo-recession in children and adolescents. *Am J Dent* **2**: 25–7.

Bimstein E, Eidelman E (1988a) Longitudinal changes in the width of attached gingiva in children. *Pediatr Dent* **10**: 22–4.

Bimstein E, Eidelman E (1988b) Morphological changes in the attached and keratinized gingiva and gingival sulcus in the mixed dentition period. A 5-year longitudinal study. *J Clin Periodontol* **15**: 175–9.

Bimstein E, Machtei E, Becker A (1988) The attached gingiva in children: diagnostic, developmental and orthodontic considerations for its treatment. *ASDC J Dent Child* **55**: 351–6.

Bjorn H (1963) Free transplantation of gingiva propria. *Sven Tandlak Tidskr* **22**: 684.

Bowers G (1963) A study of the width of attached gingiva. *J Periodontol* **34**: 201–9.

Caffesse RG, Guinard EA (1978) Treatment of localized gingival recessions. Part II. Coronally repositioned flap with a free gingival graft. *J Periodontol* **49**: 357–61.

Caffesse RG, Guinard EA (1980) Treatment of localized gingival recessions. Part IV. Results after three years. *J Periodontol* **51**: 167–70.

Coatoam GW, Behrents RG, Bissada NF (1981) The width of keratinized gingiva during orthodontic treatment: its significance and impact on periodontal status. *J Periodontol* **52**: 307–13.

Cohen DW, Ross SE (1968) The double papillae repositioned flap in periodontal therapy. *J Periodontol* **39**: 65–70.

Corn H, Mark MH (1983) Gingival grafting for deep-wide recession. *Compend Contin Educ Dent* **4**: 167.

Cortellini P, Clauser C, Prato GP (1993) Histologic assessment of new attachment following the treatment of a human buccal recession by means of a guided tissue regeneration procedure. *J Periodontol* **64**: 387–91.

Dorfman HS, Kennedy JE, Bird WC (1980) Longitudinal evaluation of free autogenous gingival grafts. *J Clin Periodontol* **7**: 316–24.

Edwards JG (1977) The diastema, the frenum, the frenectomy: a clinical study. *Am J Orthod* **71**: 489–508.

Freedman AL, Salkin LM, Stein MD, Green K (1992) A 10-year longitudinal study of untreated mucogingival defects. *J Periodontol* **63**: 71–2.

Galea H (1984) An investigation of dental injuries treated in an acute care general hospital. *J Am Dent Assoc* **109**: 434–8.

Geiger AM (1980) Mucogingival problems and the movement of mandibular incisors: a clinical review. *Am J Orthod* **78**: 511–27.

Genon P, Genon-Romagna C, Gottlow J (1994) Treatment of gingival recessions with guided tissue regeneration: a bioresorbable barrier. *J Parodontol Implantol* **13**: 289–96.

Gliksberg JH, Mintz A, Hochberg MS, Sher MR (1989) The incidence of mucogingival defects: report of case. *J Am Dent Assoc* **119**: 625–6.

Gorman WJ (1967) Prevalence and etiology of gingival recession. *J Periodontol* **38**: 316–22.

Grupe HE, Warren RF (1956) Repair of gingival defects by a sliding flap operation. *J Periodontol* **27**: 92–5.

Guinard EA, Caffesse RG (1978) Treatment of localized gingival recessions. Part III. Comparison of results obtained with lateral sliding and coronally repositioned flaps. *J Periodontol* **49**: 457–61.

Hall WB (1989) Gingival augmentation/mucogingival surgery. In: Nevins M, Becker W, Kornman K (eds) *Proceedings of the World Workshop in Clinical Periodontics*. Chicago: American Academy of Periodontology, VII1–21.

Harris RJ (1992) The connective tissue and partial thickness double pedicle graft: a predictable method of obtaining root coverage. *J Periodontol* **63**: 477–86.

Harris RJ (1998a) A comparison of 2 root coverage techniques: guided tissue regeneration with a bioabsorbable matrix style membrane versus a connective tissue graft combined with a coronally positioned pedicle graft without vertical incisions. Results of a series of consecutive cases. *J Periodontol* **69**: 1426–34.

Harris RJ (1998b) Root coverage with a connective tissue with partial thickness double pedicle graft and an acellular dermal matrix graft: a clinical and histological evaluation of a case report. *J Periodontol* **69**: 1305–11.

Hirschfeld I (1939) The toothbrush; its use and abuse. *J Am Dent Assoc* **26**: 1237–40.

Holbrook T, Ochsenbein C (1983) Complete coverage of the denuded root surface with a one-stage gingival graft. *Int J Periodont Rest Dent* **3**: 9–27.

Jahnke PV, Sandifer JB, Gher ME et al. (1993) Thick free gingival and connective tissue autografts for root coverage. *J Periodontol* **64**: 315–22.

Kennedy JE, Bird WC, Palcanis KG, Dorfman HS (1985) A longitudinal evaluation of varying widths of attached gingiva. *J Clin Periodontol* **12**: 667–75.

Kohavi D, Zilberman Y, Becker A (1984) Periodontal status following the alignment of buccally ectopic maxillary canine teeth. *Am J Orthod* **85**: 78–82.

Laney JB, Saunders VG, Garnick JJ (1992) A comparison of two techniques for attaining root coverage. *J Periodontol* **63**: 19–23.

Lang NP, Löe H (1972) The relationship between the width of keratinized gingiva and gingival health. *J Periodontol* **43**: 623–7.

Langer B, Langer L (1985) Subepithelial connective tissue graft technique for root coverage. *J Periodontol* **56**: 715–20.

Maynard JG (1998) Mucogingival considerations for the adolescent patient. In: Nevins M, Mellonig JT (eds) *Periodontal Therapy: Clinical Approaches and Evidence of Success*. Carol Stream, IL: Quintessence, pp. 291–304.

Maynard JG, Ochsenbein C (1975) Mucogingival problems, prevalence and therapy in children. *J Periodontol* **46**: 543–52.

Maynard JG, Wilson RD (1980) Diagnosis and management of mucogingival problems in children. *Dent Clin North Am* **24**: 683–703.

Miller PD (1985a) A classification of marginal tissue recession. *Int J Periodont Rest Dent* **5**: 8–13.

Miller PD (1985b) Root coverage using the free soft tissue autograft following citric acid application. III. A successful and predictable procedure in areas of deep-wide recession. *Int J Periodont Rest Dent* **5**: 14–37.

Miller PD (1987) Root coverage with the free gingival graft. Factors associated with incomplete coverage. *J Periodontol* **58**: 674–81.

Miller PD (1993) Root coverage grafting for regeneration and aesthetics. *Periodontol 2000* **1**: 118–27.

Miyasato M, Crigger M, Egelberg J (1977) Gingival condition in areas of minimal and appreciable width of keratinized gingiva. *J Clin Periodontol* **4**: 200–9.

Nabers JM (1966a) Extension of the vestibular fornix utilizing a gingival graft—case history. *Periodontics* **4**: 77–9.

Nabers JM (1966b) Free gingival grafts. *Periodontics* **4**: 243–5.

Nelson SW (1987) The subpedicle connective tissue graft. A bilaminar reconstructive procedure for the coverage of denuded root surfaces. *J Periodontol* **58**: 95–102.

Nevins M (1986) Attached gingiva—mucogingival therapy and restorative dentistry. *Int J Periodont Rest Dent* **6**: 9–27.

Nevins M, Cappetta EG (1998a) Mucogingival surgery: the rationale and long-term results. In: Nevins M, Mellonig JT (eds) *Periodontal Therapy: Clinical Approaches and Evidence of Success*. Carol Stream, IL: Quintessence, pp. 279–90.

Nevins M, Cappetta EG (1998b) An overview of surgery to cover the exposed root surface. In: Nevins M, Mellonig JT (eds) *Periodontal Therapy: Clinical Approaches and Evidence of Success*. Carol Stream, IL: Quintessence, pp. 339–54.

Nevins M, Becker W, Kornman K, (eds.) (1992) *Glossary of Periodontal Terms*. Chicago: American Academy of Periodontology.

Ochsenbein C, Maynard JG (1974) The problem of attached gingiva in children. *ASDC J Dent Child* **41**: 263–72.

O'Leary T (1967) The periodontal screening examination. *J Periodontol* **38** (suppl): 617–24.

O'Neil DW, Clark MV, Lowe JW, Harrington MS (1989) Oral trauma in children: a hospital survey. *Oral Surg Oral Med Oral Path* **68**: 691–6.

Paolantonio M, di Murro C, Cattabriga A, Cattabriga M (1997) Subpedicle connective tissue graft versus free gingival graft in the coverage of exposed root surfaces. A 5-year clinical study. *J Clin Periodontol* **24**: 51–6.

Pasquinelli KL (1995) The histology of new attachment utilizing a thick autogenous soft tissue graft in an area of deep recession: a case report. *Int J Periodont Rest Dent* **15**: 248–57.

Peretz B, Machtei E, Bimstein E (1996) Periodontal status in children and early adolescence: a three-year follow up. *J Clinic Pediatr Dent* **20**: 229–32.

Pini Prato G, Tinti C, Vincenzi G et al. (1992) Guided tissue regeneration versus mucogingival surgery in the treatment of human buccal gingival recession. *J Periodontol* **63**: 919–28.

Pini Prato G, Clauser C, Magnani C, Cortellini P (1995) Resorbable membranes in the treatment of human buccal recession: a nine case report. *Int J Periodont Rest Dent* **15**: 258–67.

Pini Prato G, Clauser C, Cortellini P et al. (1996) Guided tissue regeneration versus mucogingival surgery in the treatment of human buccal recessions. A 4-year follow-up study. *J Periodontol* **67**: 1216–23.

Raetzke PB (1985) Covering localized areas of root exposure employing the "envelope" technique. *J Periodontol* **56**: 397–402.

Rose ST, App GR (1973) A clinical study of the development of the attached gingiva along the facial aspects of the maxillary and mandibular anterior teeth in the deciduous, transitional and permanent dentitions. *J Periodontol* **44**: 131–9.

Saario M, Ainamo A, Mattila K, Ainamo J (1994) The width of radiologically-defined attached gingiva over permanent teeth in children. *J Clin Periodontol* **21**: 666–9.

Saario M, Ainamo A, Mattila K et al. (1995) The width of radiologically-defined attached gingiva over deciduous teeth. *J Clin Periodontol* **22**: 895–8.

Salkin LM, Freedman AL, Stein MD, Bassiouny MA (1987) A longitudinal study of untreated mucogingival defects. *J Periodontol* **58**: 164–6.

Schoo WH, van der Velden U (1985) Marginal soft tissue recessions with and without attached gingiva. A five year longitudinal study. *J Periodont Res* **20**: 209–11.

Silverstein LH, Gornstein RA, Callan DP, Singh B (1999) Similarities between a cellular dermal allograft and a palatal graft, for tissue augmentation: clinical report. *Periodont Insights* **6**: 3–6.

Srivastava B, Chandra S, Jaiswal JN et al. (1990) Cross-sectional study to evaluate variations in attached gingiva and gingival sulcus in the three periods of dentition. *J Clin Ped Dent* **15**: 17–24.

Stoner JE, Mazdyasna S (1980) Gingival recession in the lower incisor region of 15-year-old subjects. *J Periodontol* **51**: 74–6.

Studer SP, Allen EP, Rees TC, Kouba A (1997) The thickness of masticatory mucosa in the human hard palate and tuberosity as potential donor sites for ridge augmentation procedures. *J Periodontol* **68**: 145–51.

Tarnow DP (1986) Semilunar coronally repositioned flap. *J Clin Periodontol* **13**: 182–5.

Tenenbaum H, Tenenbaum M (1986) A clinical study of the width of the attached gingiva in the deciduous, transitional and permanent dentitions. *J Clin Periodontol* **13**: 270–5.

Tinti C, Vincenzi G (1990) La rigenerazione guidata dei tessuti con Gore-Tex: nuove prospettive? *Quintess Int* [Italian edn], **6**: 45–9.

Wennstrom JL (1987) Lack of association between width of attached gingiva and development of soft tissue recession. A 5-year longitudinal study. *J Clin Periodontol* **14**: 181–4.

Wennstrom JL (1996) Mucogingival therapy. *Ann Periodontol* **1**: 671–701.

Wennstrom JL, Lindhe H (1983) Plaque-induced gingival inflammation in the absence of attached gingiva in dog. *J Clin Periodontol* **10**: 266–76.

West EE (1968) Diastema—a cause for concern. *Dent Clin North Am (July)*: 425–34.

Wilson RD (1983) Marginal tissue recession in general dental practice: a preliminary study. *Int J Periodont Rest Dent* **3**: 40–53.

Wilson RD, Maynard G (1981) Intracrevicular restorative dentistry. *Int J Periodont Rest Dent* **1**: 34–49.

Wise RJ (1981) Periodontal diagnosis and management of the impacted maxillary cuspid. *Int J Periodont Rest Dent* **1**: 56–73.

PART III

Periodontal diseases

5

Periodontal diseases in children, adolescents, and young adults

Andrew J. Delima, Bengt E. Sjödin, Maurizio S. Tonetti, Enrique Bimstein, Hubert N. Newman, and Thomas E. Van Dyke

Periodontal diseases represent a spectrum of pathologic entities. It has been known since antiquity that the periodontium is susceptible to a wide range of destructive conditions (Löe, 1993). It has also been recognized that gingival lesions can be demonstrated in children and young adults. McCall, as early as 1938, demonstrated that gingivitis can be observed in children as young as 4–5 years old (McCall, 1938). A review of the periodontal literature affirms that children are not immune to gingival and periodontal pathology. In fact, gingivitis is a common finding in children of different geographic regions and countries, cultures, and socioeconomic groups (Ramfjord, 1961; Basu and Dutta, 1963; Russell, 1971; Lennon and Davies, 1974; Blankenstein et al., 1978; Stamm, 1986; Pilot et al., 1987; Wolfe and Carlos, 1987; Bimstein et al., 1989). From this brief survey, it is evident that during the past few decades there has been an increasing interest in the manifestation and progression of gingival and periodontal diseases in young individuals.

The early occurrence and apparent rapid course of these diseases and their similar clinical characteristics have given a false impression of a homogeneous disease entity in afflicted children and young adults. However, microbiological and immunological research has revealed a number of disease processes with different etiologies, distinct degrees of severity, and contrasting clinical courses and outcomes. The focus of this chapter is the periodontopathologies that affect the deeper periodontal tissues and manifest themselves as alterations in cementum, periodontal ligament, and/or alveolar bone, and can lead to premature exfoliation of the deciduous or permanent dentition (or both).

Historical perspective

In 1923, Gottlieb described a disease that he called "diffuse atrophy of the alveolar bone". He believed that extraoral or systemic factors played a major role in the pathogenesis of this lesion and later in 1928 attempted to prove that metabolic alterations in cementum were responsible for the disease (Gottlieb, 1923, 1928). Subsequently, Wannenmacher (1938) was the first to distinguish this disease entity as a rapidly progressing form of periodontitis found predominantly in young adults. The disease, which he called *paradontosis*, was characterized by alveolar bone loss around the incisors and first molars. Further reports of the same disease by Thoma and Goldman (1940), Orban and Weinmann (1942) and later by Miller (1948) led to the introduction of the term *periodontosis*, subsequently replaced by the term *juvenile periodontitis* (Butler, 1969).

Baer (1971) defined periodontosis as "a disease of the periodontium occurring in an otherwise healthy adolescent which is characterized by a rapid loss of alveolar bone about more than one tooth of the permanent dentition." He described a localized form, in which only the permanent first molars and incisors were affected, and a generalized form, in which most of the dentition was affected. He also noted that the tissue destruction seen in both forms of this disease entity was "not commensurate with the amount of local irritants present." The discovery of periodontosis/juvenile periodontitis was important in that it was considered the only form of periodontitis affecting children and adolescents that did not have a specific systemic etiologic origin. For example, in 1977 the only two forms of periodontitis that were recognized by the American Academy of Periodontology were juvenile periodontitis and chronic marginal periodontitis.

During the 1980s, reports of variations of destructive periodontitis (Page et al., 1983a, b; Spektor et al., 1985) led to a re-evaluation of the classification of periodontal disease. In 1982, Page and Schroeder in their publication *Periodontitis in Man and Other Animals* described four major forms of periodontitis: adult periodontitis (AP), rapidly progressive periodontitis (RPP), juvenile periodontitis (JP), and prepubertal periodontitis (PP), with the last three forms manifesting themselves in children and adolescents. This work represented a marked departure from previous groupings of periodontal disease since it was becoming evident that periodontitis in children was a far more heterogeneous entity than previously thought (Page and Schroeder, 1982).

Rapidly progressive periodontitis (Page et al., 1983a) was described as severe gingival inflammation and rapid destruction of the periodontal tissues. The disease may have periods of remission where the gingiva is free of inflammation but with deep pockets and significant loss of alveolar bone. Lesions are generalized throughout the dentition but without any consistent pattern of distribution. It was thought to occur in young adults with an onset between puberty and 30 years of age. The finding that 75% of the patients had functional defects in neutrophils or monocytes suggested a genetic factor in the pathogenesis of this form of disease.

Juvenile periodontitis has its onset at puberty, but it is often diagnosed later. Severe bony defects are found confined to the first permanent molar and sometimes the incisors, with a symmetrical distribution. The rates and severity of periodontal destruction are not consistent with the sparse plaque accumulation and lack of clinical inflammation, which often leads to its delayed diagnosis.

Prepubertal periodontitis (Page et al., 1983b) at this time had not been well characterized, and

was considered to be a rare occurrence with an onset subsequent to the eruption of the deciduous dentition. The disease was thought to manifest itself in localized or generalized forms: localized prepubertal periodontitis (LPP) and generalized prepubertal periodontitis (GPP). However, no clear demarcation between the localized and generalized forms was reported, nor was a maximum number of involved deciduous teeth specified for the localized form. Most data on prepubertal periodontitis originated from case presentations, and it seems that most (though not all) cases of GPP were medically compromised individuals, while most case reports on LPP included otherwise healthy children.

Localized prepubertal periodontitis affects only a few teeth in the deciduous dentition, with little gingival inflammation and a milder form of tissue destruction (see Figure 1.2c–f). Leukocyte defects are found in polymorphonuclear cells or monocytic cells, but not both. Page et al. (1983b) considered the localized form to be treatable with antibiotics and gingival curettage. Generalized prepubertal periodontitis was characterized by intense acute inflammation, severe gingivitis, spontaneous gingival bleeding, gingival recession concurrent with rapid destruction of marginal alveolar bone, and premature loss of deciduous teeth (see Figure 1.2g–h). The generalized form affects both the deciduous and permanent dentition and was thought to be caused by functional defects in both peripheral neutrophils and monocytic cells. Neutrophils are completely absent from the gingival tissues, yet the numbers of peripheral white cells are elevated. This form of the disease was considered refractory to treatment with antibiotics, consequently Waldrop et al. (1987) found this form of periodontitis to be a manifestation of the systemic disease *leukocyte adhesion deficiency* (LAD). In 1990, Watanabe sought to further characterize prepubertal periodontitis. He excluded patients with blood dyscrasias and other forms of systemic disease, and proposed that the disease was caused by common periodontopathogens: *Prevotella intermedia, Porphyromonas gingivalis, Capnocytophaga,* and *Eikenella corrodens* (Watanabe, 1990).

In response to the overwhelming evidence that the term "periodontitis" represented a diverse family of related but distinct diseases, the

American Academy of Periodontology (AAP) adopted a new disease classification in 1986. It recognized four major forms of periodontitis: adult, juvenile, necrotizing ulcerative gingivoperiodontitis, and refractory. The juvenile category was further subdivided into prepubertal periodontitis, localized juvenile periodontitis, and generalized juvenile periodontitis.

Later, Suzuki (1988) classified periodontal disease into categories that described the clinical features pathognomonic for gingivitis and for adult, rapidly progressive, juvenile, post-juvenile, and prepubertal forms of periodontitis. Little information was added to the original description of adult, juvenile, and prepubertal periodontitis of Page and Schroeder (1982). Suzuki further subdivided the rapidly progressive disease into types A and B, based primarily on the age of onset. The A form followed Page and Schroeder's earlier description of rapidly progressive periodontitis with an onset at 14–26 years of age and a predilection for females (2:1 to 3:1). In type B the patients are usually older (at least 26 years) and there is no predetermined sex predilection. Suzuki (1988) also added to his classification of periodontal diseases the category of post-juvenile periodontitis, originally described by Van Dyke et al. (1980). This disease entity resembled juvenile periodontitis except that the patients were generally older (26–35 years), and the rate of destruction of the periodontal tissues was markedly slower than in juvenile periodontitis; it was therefore thought to be an arrested or "burnt out" form of juvenile periodontitis (Baer and Benjamin, 1974). Although this grouping of destructive periodontal diseases was far more descriptive than previous classifications, a major flaw is that all groups described by Suzuki except for adult periodontitis could be a manifestation of a rapidly progressing disease.

In 1989, the World Workshop in Clinical Periodontics called for a reclassification of periodontal disease (Caton, 1989). The consensus report proposed eight distinct forms of periodontal disease, based on criteria including age of disease onset, rate of tissue destruction, and the intraoral distribution of the disease (localized or generalized). This classification also took into account the superimposition of systemic complications and specific microbial and host etiologic factors, as well as the response to periodontal therapy. This classification specified five primary forms of periodontitis, one containing three subdivisions:

I   Adult periodontitis
II Early onset periodontitis
    a. prepubertal (generalized and localized)
    b. juvenile (generalized and localized)
    c. rapidly progressive periodontitis
III Periodontitis associated with systemic disease
IV Necrotizing ulcerative periodontitis
V Refractory periodontitis

For the first time, in an attempt to differentiate between periodontal diseases in juvenile patients and the disease entity "juvenile periodontitis", the term "early onset periodontitis" (EOP) was introduced. This term is used to describe periodontal diseases with an onset at less than 35 years of age, typically demonstrating a rapid rate of tissue destruction, various manifestations of a defective host response, and a pathogenic bacterial flora that differs significantly from adult periodontitis. Early onset periodontitis was further subdivided into three disease entities, depending on the age of onset: prepubertal periodontitis (onset before puberty), juvenile periodontitis (initiated during the circumpubertal to late teenage years), and rapidly progressive periodontitis (onset in the early to late 20s). Both prepubertal and juvenile periodontitis were further divided into localized and generalized forms. This division was supposed to divide early onset periodontal disease into a variety of clinically distinct entities in order to help clinicians make a differential diagnosis.

However, this system of classification has not met with universal acceptance and several flaws have been acknowledged (Schenkein and Van Dyke, 1994; Novak and Novak, 1996). One criticism is that the disease categories overlap and there are potential cases that do not fit neatly into any one category. Another target of criticism is that the division of disease entities is based on the age of onset, but these age restrictions are not sensitive enough to differentiate between disease subtypes such as generalized juvenile periodontitis and rapidly progressive periodontitis. There are aspects of EOP that can occur later in a patient's life past the arbitrarily established age of 35 years, and it is also evident that there are features of "adult" periodontitis that can be demonstrated in even young children. Yet another problem is that the classification is based too heavily on clinical presentation and radiographic signs, while the importance of disease etiology and host and other risk factors in the manifestation of disease is basically ignored.

Prepubertal periodontitis associated with systemic disorders had constituted a specific group within the AAP's 1989 classification system (AAP, 1989). However, otherwise healthy children with prepubertal periodontitis have sometimes, but not always, been included in the group of EOP. Though a classification of disease

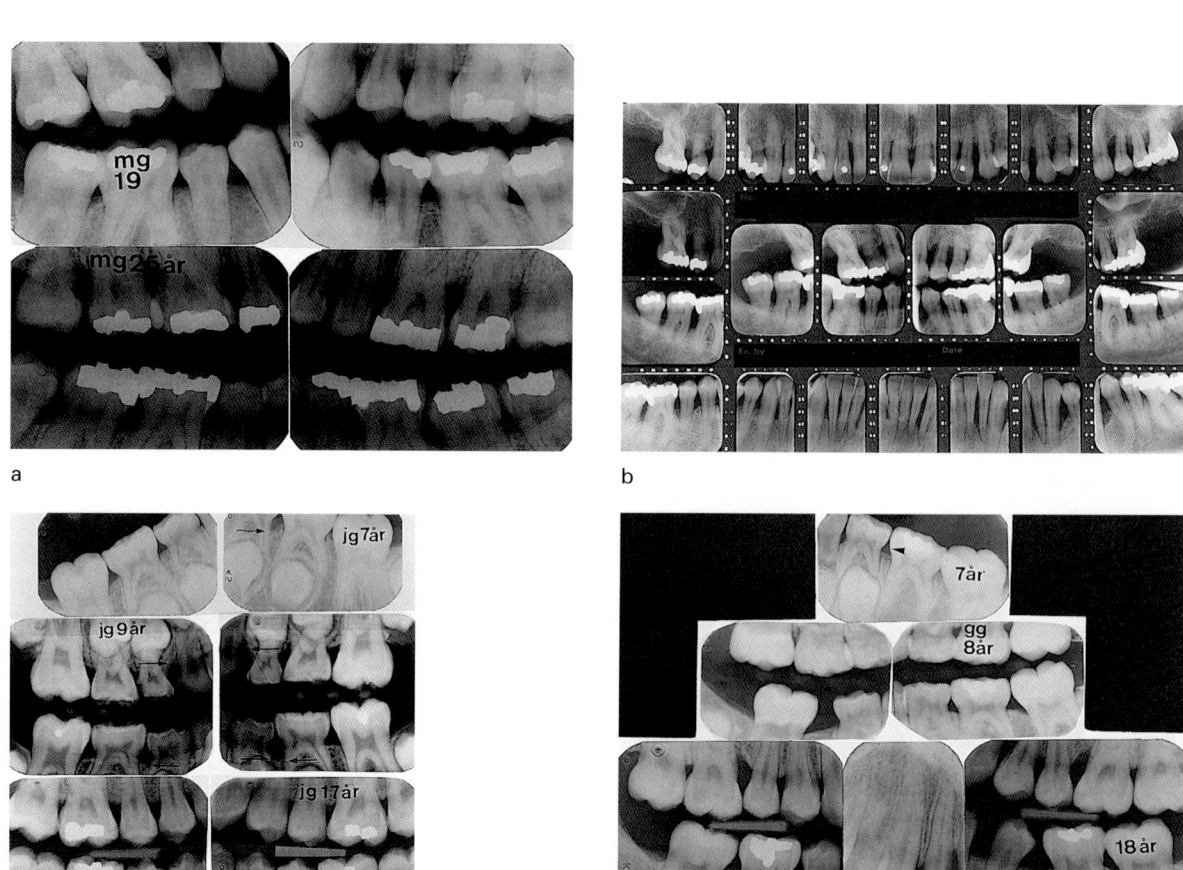

a

b

c

d

Figure 5.1

Dental radiographs of a family in which the mother had aggressive periodontitis in the permanent dentition, and the son and daughter had localized childhood periodontitis in the deciduous teeth and developed localized aggressive periodontitis in the permanent dentition. (a) The mother at age 19 years (upper radiographs) and 26 years (lower radiographs) with aggressive periodontitis. (b) The mother at age 33 years with further deterioration of the periodontium due to aggressive periodontitis. (c) The son at age 7 years (upper radiographs) and age 9 years (center radiographs) with signs of localized childhood periodontitis in the deciduous teeth, and at age 17 years (lower radiographs) with localized aggressive periodontitis in the permanent dentition. (d) The daughter at age 7 years (upper radiograph) and 8 years (center radiographs) with signs of localized childhood periodontitis affecting the deciduous teeth, and at age 18 years (lower radiographs) with localized aggressive periodontitis affecting the permanent dentition. Arrows indicate the presence of alveolar bone loss.

entities implies a mutual and specific etiologic background, the classification of periodontal diseases is primarily determined by the age of the patient and the number of teeth involved. Several family studies, which reported the occurrence of severe periodontal disease in siblings and relatives irrespective of dentition or age, indicated that disease classification may be a matter of a point in time rather than actual different disease entities (Butler, 1969; Sakamoto et al., 1984; Boughman et al., 1986; Mandel and Gaffar, 1986; López, 1992; Marazita et al., 1994; Brown et al., 1996; Bimstein et al., 1997) (Figure 5.1). A sequential occurrence of prepubertal and juvenile periodontitis in longitudinally monitored patients further supports this concept (Ngan et al., 1984; Shapira et al., 1994). In retrospective radiographic studies it has been shown that a substantial proportion of JP patients exhibit signs of bone loss in deciduous dentition in childhood (Figures 5.1c, d, 5.2 and 5.3) (Sjödin et al., 1989; Cogen et al., 1992; Sjödin and Matsson, 1992).

In an attempt to make a more acceptable classification of periodontal diseases, Ranney in 1991 and again in 1993 proposed a new organization. He divided periodontitis into four categories: adult periodontitis, EOP, necrotizing

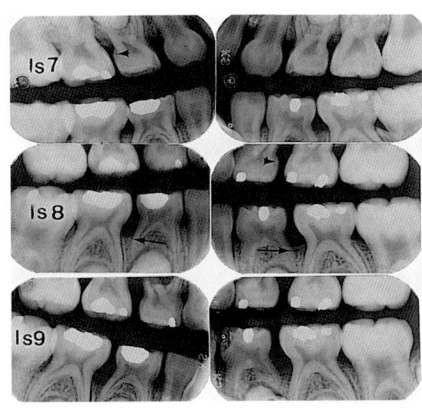

a

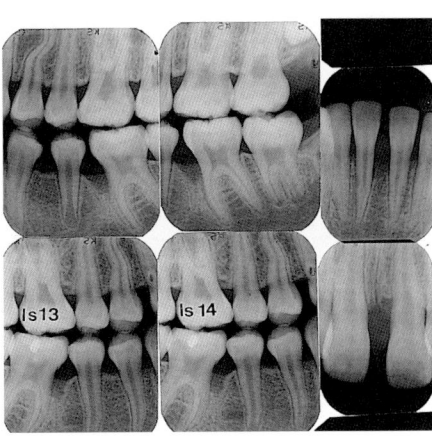

c

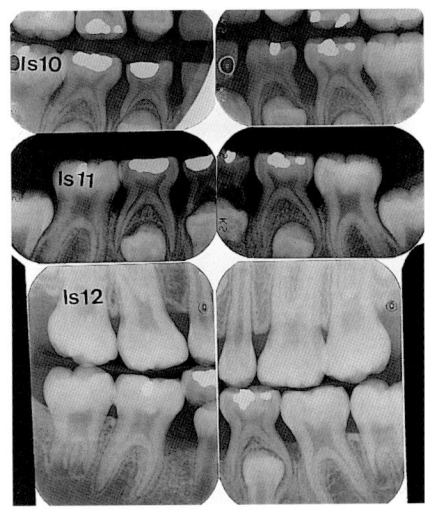

b

Figure 5.2

Radiographs of a girl with localized childhood periodontitis in the primary teeth and localized aggressive periodontitis in adolescence. (a) From age 7 years (upper radiographs), to 8 years (center radiographs) and 9 years (lower radiographs) childhood periodontitis deteriorated from localized to generalized. (b) From age 10 years (upper radiographs), to 11 years (center radiographs) and 12 years (lower radiographs) the childhood periodontitis facilitated the appearance of localized aggressive periodontitis in permanent teeth. (c) At age 13 years with localized aggressive periodontitis affecting several anterior and posterior permanent teeth. Arrows indicate the presence of alveolar bone loss; arrowheads indicate the presence of calculus.

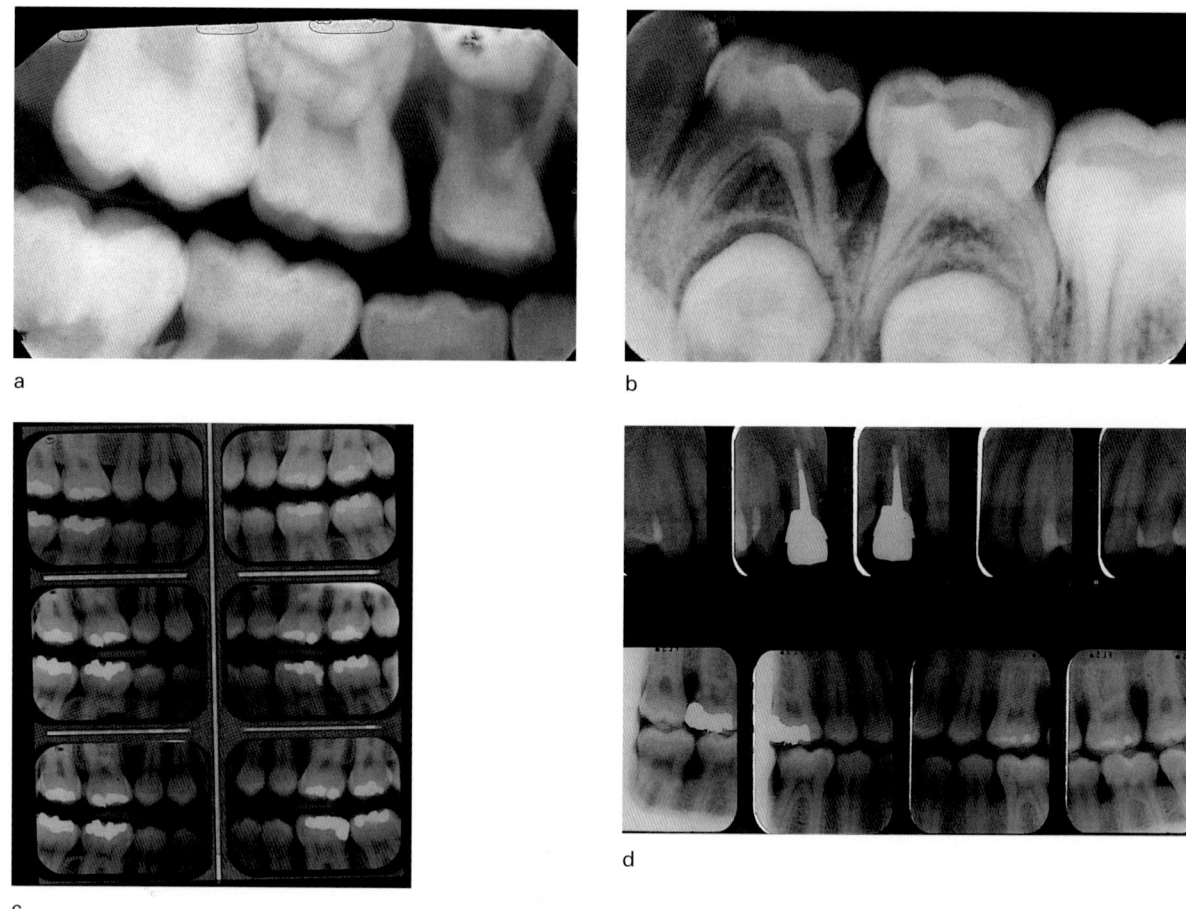

Figure 5.3

Radiographs of a boy with localized childhood periodontitis in the primary teeth and localized aggressive periodontitis in adolescence and early adulthood. (a, b) At age 8 years localized childhood periodontitis is evident in the deciduous teeth. (c) At ages 14 years, 16 years, and 19 years. (d) At age 22 years with signs of aggressive periodontitis affecting the permanent dentition.

ulcerative periodontitis, and periodontal abscesses. He further subdivided his early onset category into localized EOP, generalized EOP, EOP related to systemic disease, and EOP with unknown systemic determinants (Ranney, 1991, 1993). This was done to recognize the importance of systemic health on the manifestation of early onset disease. Ranney also accepted the influence of host factors in the pathogenesis of early onset disease by identifying the importance

of neutrophil abnormalities in subsets of both localized and generalized EOP patients.

Newman (1992) offered a more descriptive and comprehensive classification. He noted that, "While most periodontal diseases are infectious inflammatory in type, the periodontium, in fact, is subjected to a range of pathology as wide as that of any other body tissue or system." The basis for his classification was not only chronicity (acute versus chronic) and specificity (non-specific versus specific) but also the etiology and pathology of the disease process. The major groupings of his system comprise developmental, traumatic, inflammatory, cystic, neoplastic, blood, and lymphoreticular forms of disease, as well as hormonal, nutritional/metabolic, immunological, soft connective tissue, bone and cementum disorders, and epulides. Like Ranney's classifications in 1991 and 1993, this grouping not only takes into account the effects of systemic disease and host abnormalities in the pathogenesis of periodontal diseases, but also recognizes the role of biologic processes such as neoplasias and heredity in the development of periodontal disease.

In 1991, the Research, Science and Therapy Committee of the AAP published a position paper entitled "Periodontal Diseases of Children and Adolescents" (AAP, 1996). This work recognized the following distinct disease entities in young individuals: chronic gingivitis; EOP; necrotizing ulcerative gingivitis/ periodontitis; and periodontitis associated with systemic diseases. This new classification also took into account systemic and microbiologic factors that might influence periodontal disease. The early onset group was once again subdivided into localized and generalized forms.

At a symposium in 1996 on the pathogenesis of EOP, participants called for the revision of the classification of EOP into two broad categories: localized and generalized (Van Dyke and Schenkein, 1996). It was also concluded that there was no evidence to support the notion that generalized juvenile periodontitis and rapidly progressing periodontitis were two separate disease processes, and suggested that the two should be combined and redesignated as generalized juvenile periodontitis to distinguish them from the localized form. The group also called for research into host, microbiologic, and other risk factors for early onset disease in order to gain further insight of the nature and classification of the disease.

Epidemiology

It used to be thought that periodontal disease in children was limited to gingivitis, but epidemio-

logical studies have shown that children are vulnerable to periodontal afflictions similar to those seen in adults, albeit at a lower prevalence. Destructive periodontal diseases (periodontitis) are reported to have prevalence rates of 1–9% in children aged 5–11 years and 1–46% in those aged 12–15 years (Delaney, 1986; Wei et al., 1986; Wolfe and Carlos, 1987; Pilot et al., 1987; Bimstein et al., 1988a, 1994; Durward and Wright, 1989; Miyazaki et al., 1989; Löe and Brown, 1991; Papapanou, 1996). These studies demonstrate a wide variability in the expression of periodontitis in children and young adults that may represent differences between some populations. However, the disparate findings are more probably due to different epidemiological techniques, including differences in the cohorts studied and the criteria and clinical methods used for diagnosis. Nevertheless, epidemiological data clearly support the notion that children and adolescents are susceptible to destructive forms of periodontal disease. It should also be noted that most frequency studies of periodontal destruction in children investigated populations attending dental clinics and the samples are potentially biased. It seems that such populations regularly show higher frequencies of loss of periodontal support than randomly selected samples.

Epidemiological methodology

The methods used in epidemiological studies of young individuals have ranged from clinical measurements to radiographic assessments (Tables 5.1–5.3). Irrespective of the method used, there is debate about the correct criteria to use for recognition of the early signs of periodontal disease.

Clinical attachment loss

The measurement used in many epidemiological studies is the clinical attachment loss (CAL), usually assessed by probing the gingival tissues. Measurement of small amounts of loss of attachment in adolescents using a periodontal probe has been shown to be valid (Clerehugh and Lennon, 1984), but no reproducibility study has

Table 5.1 Epidemiological surveys of periodontal conditions in children.

Author(s)	Age (years)	N	Country	Measurements	Threshold	Prevalence (%)	Dentition Primary	Dentition Permanent
Jamison, 1963	5–14	159	USA	Clinical attachment loss	(Ramfjord PDI >3)	25	+	
Russell, 1971	5–9	?		Pocket formation		0.1	?	+
Buckley, 1986	7–12	1 492	Ireland	ABL		1.7		+
Schlossman et al., 1986	5–9	?	USA (Native American)	Clinical attachment loss ≥ 2 mm		7.7	+	+
Keszthelyi and Szabó, 1987			Hungary	Extracted teeth		94	+	
Sweeney et al., 1987	5–11	2 264	USA	ABL	Reduced bone level	0.8	+	
Bimstein et al., 1988a	4–11	752	USA	ABL	CEJ–ABC >2 mm	11	+	+*
Bimstein et al., 1993	3–12	500	Israel	ABL	CEJ–ABC >3 mm plus absence of lamina dura	0–17.4	+	+*
Sjödin and Matsson, 1994	7–9	4 545	Sweden	ABL	CEJ–ABC >2 mm	2–4.5	+	
Bimstein et al., 1994	5	317	New Zealand	ABL	CEJ–ABC >2 mm plus absence of lamina dura	2.1	+	
Drummond and Bimstein 1995	4–14	187	New Zealand	ABL	CEJ–ABC >2 mm plus absence of lamina dura	20.8 (children) 4.7 (surfaces)	+	+*
Bimstein et al., 1996a	6–9	354	Israel	ABL	CEJ–ABC >2 mm plus absence of lamina dura	26.8 (children) 4 (surfaces)	+	
Carranza et al., 1998	3–10	115	Mexico	ABL	CEJ–ABC >2 mm plus absence of lamina dura	7.8	+	

Some studies have included both children and adolescents and primary and/or permanent teeth; in some instances the prevalence for the primary dentition has been calculated from data presented in the studies.
*Mesial surfaces of first permanent molars. ABC, alveolar bone crest; ABL, alveolar bone loss; CEJ, cementoenamel junction; PDI, periodontal disease index.

Table 5.2 Epidemiological surveys of periodontal conditions in adolescents.

Author(s)	Year	Age (years)	N	Country	Criteria	Prevalence (%)
Clerehugh and Lennon	1986	14, 16	229	Great Britain	CAL ≥ 1 mm	4.4
Wolfe and Carlos	1987	14–19	618	USA	CAL >2 mm	88.7
Aass et al.	1988	14	2 767	Norway	Radiographic bone loss	4.5
Albandar et al.	1989	14	1 318	Denmark, Iraq, Norway	Radiographic bone loss	1.7–6
Van der Velden et al.	1989	14–17	4 465	Netherlands	CAL ≥ 1 mm	5
Källestål and Matsson	1990	16, 18	570	Sweden	CAL (proximal measurements)	2.8, 4.9
					Radiographic bone loss >2 mm	1
Perry and Newman	1990	12–15	307	USA	CAL ≥ 2 mm and ≥ 5 mm ppd	12.7
Bhat	1991	14–17	11 111	USA	CAL ≥ 2 mm	21.7
Källestål and Matsson	1991	16	400	Sweden	Radiographic bone loss	3.5
Löe and Brown	1991	14–17	40 694	USA	CAL ≥ 3 mm	2.3
Neely	1992	10–12	1 872	USA	Radiographic bone loss ≥ 2 mm	11.7
Hansen et al.	1995	15–17	7 539	Multinational	Radiographic bone loss	0–35.7
Timmerman et al.	1998	15–25	225	Indonesia	CAL >2 mm	34

CAL, clinical attachment loss.

been performed on groups of children or adolescents with incipient periodontal destruction. The threshold of CAL measurements used in recent studies of adolescent populations has varied from 1 mm or less to 3 mm (Table 5.2).

In children with deciduous teeth the occurrence of a probable distance between the cementoenamel junction (CEJ) and the bottom of the gingiva may represent the progression of attachment loss caused by periodontal disease, but it may instead be a normal change associated with exfoliation of the deciduous tooth (Jamison, 1963). Keszthelyi and Szabó (1987) reported high rates (94%) of attachment loss when measuring the distance between CEJ and the most coronal attachment fibers on stained extracted deciduous teeth (Table 5.1), the mean loss of attachment being 0.26 mm, significantly larger on buccal sites compared with proximal and lingual sites. Apical migration of the junctional epithelium in the human deciduous dentition has also been demonstrated in histologic studies (Bimstein et al., 1985, 1988b). Furthermore, in one histologic study (Bimstein et al., 1988b) similar values to those reported by Keszthelyi and Szabó (1987) were reported. The small dislocation of the attachment apparatus reported in these studies may not necessarily represent attachment loss caused by periodontal diseases—it may also be related to the eruption and shedding processes (Bernick et al., 1951; Garguilo et al., 1961; Soskolne and Bimstein, 1977, 1989; Newman and Levers, 1979; Bimstein et al., 1988b).

Radiographic bone loss

Radiographs provide abundant information about the periodontal condition. Studies of periodontal disease in young populations have used radiographic methods to evaluate the presence or absence of the lamina dura over the alveolar bone crest (ABC), to measure the distance between the CEJ and the ABC, or both (Table 5.1). However, conventional radiographic assessments have shortcomings due to variations in projection geometry, exposure factors, and film processing (Jeffcoat, 1992; Benn, 1990). In addition, extensive changes in the bone structure may not be detectable by an unaided eye (Ortman et al., 1982), the consensus from the literature being that CAL precedes radiographic bone loss and radiographic analyses underestimate the loss of periodontal support (Goodson, et al., 1984; Albandar, 1989; Clerehugh and Lennon, 1984). On the other hand, evidence of partial loss of lamina dura over the ABC may not always indicate alveolar bone loss (Hausmann et al., 1991). Accordingly, only the complete loss of lamina dura in human deciduous teeth has been found to be associated with other signs of periodontal disease in primary teeth (Bimstein and Garcia-Godoy, 1994).

For the deciduous dentition, a threshold CEJ–ABC distance of more than 2 mm has been suggested for bone loss in the deciduous dentition (Table 5.1). However, CEJ–ABC distances in the deciduous dentition are not stable and their change does not necessarily imply ongoing periodontal disease. This distance seems to increase with age (probably due to facial growth and attrition), may normally be greater than 2 mm, and may decrease slightly in some teeth with the approximation of exfoliation (Bimstein and Soskolne, 1988; Sjödin and Matsson, 1992; Bimstein, 1995; Shapira et al., 1995; Needleman et al., 1997; Bimstein and Mattson, 1999). In addition, normal physiological conditions such as exfoliation of a neighboring deciduous tooth or eruption of an adjacent permanent tooth are associated with increased CEJ–ABC distances in the deciduous human dentition (Sjödin and Matsson, 1992). It may be concluded that alveolar bone loss in the deciduous human dentition in most cases is evidenced by the complete absence of lamina dura above the ABC and a CEJ–ABC distance greater than 2 mm. However, in particular cases, the clinician must take into consideration the possibility of normal CEJ–ABC distances exceeding 2 mm.

Radiographic assessment alone cannot discriminate between current disease and previous episodes of destructive periodontitis. Sjödin and Matsson (1994) showed that less than half of 26 patients expressing two or more sites with radiographic bone loss had other clinical signs of ongoing periodontal disease.

The borderline between health and disease in terms of the CEJ–ABC distance used in epidemiological studies in permanent teeth of adolescent populations has ranged from 1.5 mm to 3 mm (Davies et al., 1978; Latcham et al., 1983). In recent studies 2 mm has been used as a threshold for radiographic bone loss (Table 5.2). Källestål and Mattson (1989) found in a study of 18-year-old adolescents that the CEJ–ABC distance of sites without clinical attachment loss and gingival bleeding did not exceed 2 mm.

The validity of using radiological features, such as presence or absence of lamina dura or the widening of the periodontal ligament space, for early detection of destructive periodontal disease in adolescents has been debated (Jenkins et al., 1992). Waite et al. (1994) reported a correlation between radiographic features and maturation changes associated with the eruption of neighboring teeth. In the same study it was found that the above radiological signs also correlated with errors in radiographic technique. These factors may explain findings in longitudinal studies of adolescent cohorts where improvements in the alveolar bone have been registered in a significant proportion of the individuals (Albandar et al., 1991; Aass et al., 1994).

Loss of periodontal support in the deciduous dentition

Most studies of periodontal conditions in the deciduous dentition have focused on gingival inflammation. A number of studies on occurrence of attachment loss are summarized in Table 5.1. Older studies used clinical probing, while more recent studies used radiographic methods. There is a wide variation in prevalence, probably mainly explained by differences in criteria.

Factors associated with bone loss in the deciduous dentition

Caries, inadequate restorations, and subgingival calculus

The consensus from research in adult populations is that proximal caries, poor restorative dentistry, and subgingival calculus are associated with attachment and bone loss at adjacent sites. Though few studies have been performed, the same relationships have been established in children with deciduous teeth. In a group of 5-year-old New Zealand children, Bimstein et al. (1994) found that higher decayed, missing, and filled teeth (DMFT) rates were associated with higher prevalence of bone loss. Increased CEJ–ABC distances have also been associated with proximal decay, presence of stainless steel crowns, and poor amalgam fillings (Bimstein et

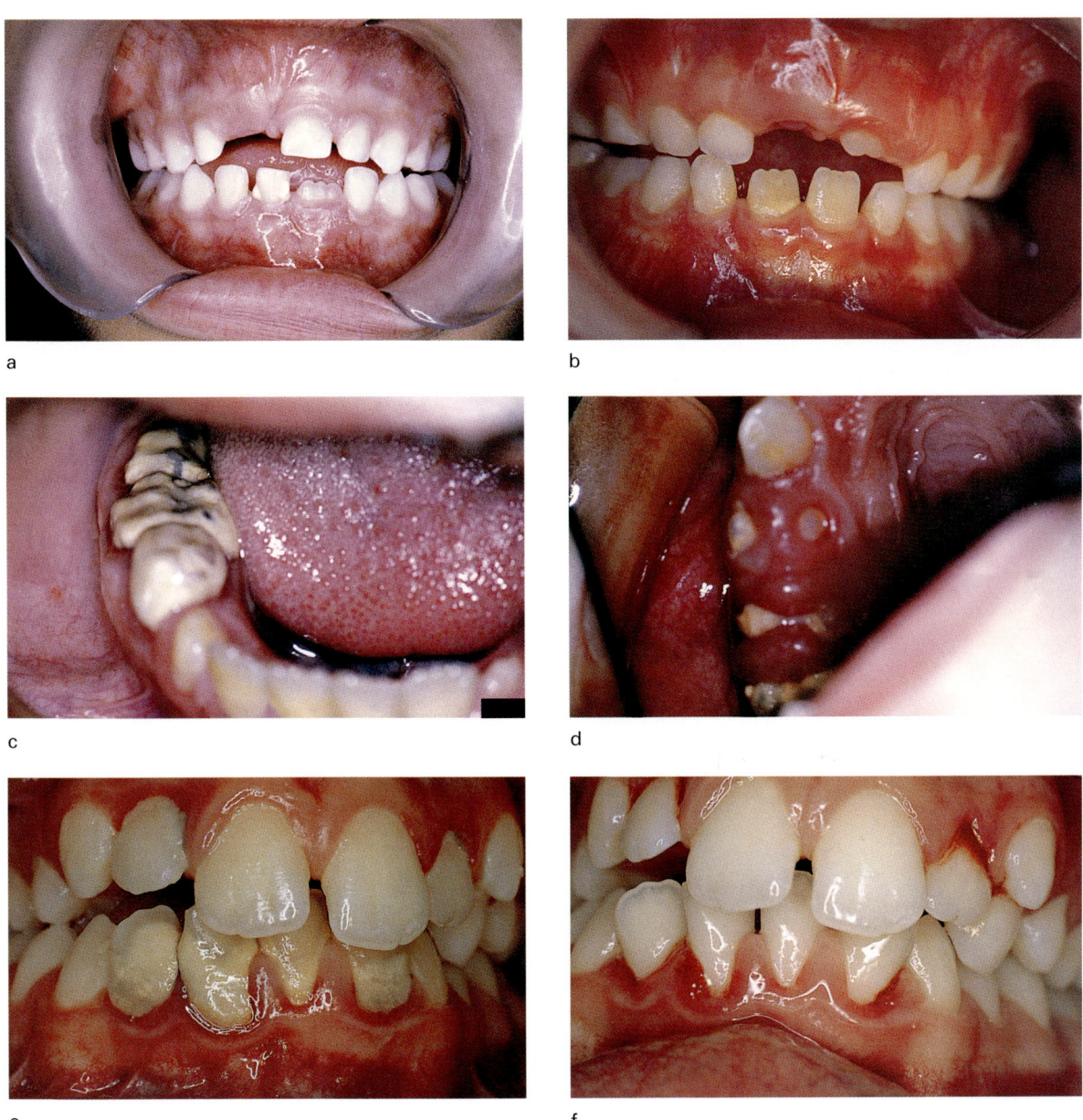

Figure 5.4

Calculus accumulation in children. Calculus accumulation in children related to insufficient function in: (a) a lower central deciduous incisor with increased normal mobility due to the shedding process and lack of antagonist; (b) a newly erupted permanent central incisor with no antagonist; (c) lower mandibular deciduous right molars, due to pain caused by deep carious lesions. (d) The antagonist teeth, in the same child in (c), with severe gingival inflammation. (e) Inadequate oral hygiene led to gingival inflammation with gingival bleeding in the mandibular anterior area of an adolescent. Due to fear from bleeding he avoided brushing the area and the extended negligence facilitated vast calculus formation. (f) The area in (e) immediately after scaling and brushing.

al., 1988a, 1992, 1993, 1994, 1996a, 1998; see Figure 1.2b). In addition, extensive proximal caries with contact loss was more often associated with bone defects compared with sites without contact loss, and in a significant proportion of the cases there was also indication that restoration of extensive proximal caries was followed by healing of bone defects (Bimstein, 1992). This finding implies that adequate restoration of carious lesions in children might be an important measure to prevent development of periodontal disease.

Occasionally, calculus unrelated to alveolar bone loss is found in areas with a reduced function, such as in recently erupted permanent teeth, missing antagonist, anterior teeth in open bite, and in cases in which pain prevents adequate mastication (Figure 5.4a–d; see also Figure 13.5b). Calculus may also be found in some children with extreme lack of oral hygiene (Figure 5.4e, f).

The periodontal destruction in patients with childhood periodontis and juvenile periodontitis has been considered to be out of proportion to the amount of local irritating factors, such as calculus (Baer, 1971). However, studies of groups of adolescent patients with juvenile periodontitis indicate that a notable proportion of the patients exhibit subgingival calculus (Bial and Mellonig, 1987; Sjödin et al., 1993; Albandar et al., 1998). Only a few case reports of childhood periodontitis specify the absence or presence of subgingival calculus. It seems that a small proportion of healthy children display subgingival calculus, the prevalence being higher in children with attachment loss: in a cross-sectional study of 2017 children aged 9 years, it was found that the prevalence of radiographically detected proximal subgingival calculus was 4% in children without bone loss, 13% in children with one bone loss site, and 42% in children with two or more bone loss sites (Sjödin and Matsson, 1994); however, the prevalence may vary with respect to different ethnic backgrounds (Matsson et al., 1995).

Not every case of extensive proximal decay, overfilling, or calculus is accompanied by bone defects. In contrast to the high frequencies of alveolar bone loss reported in some epidemiological studies, the number of children with severe periodontitis we meet in our daily dental work seems to be low. This uneven relation indicates that other etiologic or predisposing factors than those mentioned above may be the main cause in cases with severe periodontal disease in the deciduous dentition.

Ethnic origin

The association between alveolar bone loss and ethnic and/or socioeconomic factors has been investigated in a few studies. Sjödin and Matsson (1994) found that bone loss was four times more common in children of Asian origin aged 7–9 years compared with children of Scandinavian origin. In another study comparing Vietnamese immigrant children and Swedish children a significantly higher prevalence of alveolar bone loss and subgingival calculus was found among the Vietnamese (Matsson et al., 1995). Localized aggressive periodontitis in adolescents (formerly localized juvenile periodontitis) affects more African-Americans (1.5–2.1%) than whites (0.1–0.3%) (Löe and Brown, 1991; Cogen et al., 1992). On the other hand, when comparing 5-year-old European with non-European children in a New Zealand study using logistic regression analysis, Bimstein et al. (1994) found an association between presence of alveolar bone loss and DMFT rates, while no significant dependence to ethnic background was found. These findings do not necessarily contradict each other, since population characteristics may include differences modifying the ethnic influence on the periodontal tissues, such as diet, oral hygiene habits, caries prevalence and severity, and microbial composition of the dental plaque.

Microbiology

Overwhelming evidence indicates that microorganisms and bacterial substances of the bacterial plaque in the region of the gingival sulcus constitute the extrinsic causative agents of inflammatory gingivitis and periodontal disease. It seems reasonable to assume that the connections between alveolar bone loss and presence of decayed teeth, poor restorations, or subgingival calculus are due to plaque retention encouraged by these clinical conditions. Studies during the last decade have pointed out a few microorganisms as important in the pathogenesis of periodontal disease.

The frequent presence of *Actinobacillus actinomycetemcomitans* in juvenile cases as well as the potential virulence properties of this bacterium support the concept of specificity in periodontal disease. This bacterium has also been found in subgingival plaque samples from childhood periodontitis cases (Delaney et al., 1986; Crossner et al., 1990; Watanabe, 1990; López, 1992; Petit et al., 1993; Ram and Bimstein, 1994; Bimstein et al., 1997; Sixou et al., 1997; Kamma et al., 1998; Dibart et al., 1998a, b). Delaney et al. (1986) found this microorganism in 5 of 9 cases while Bimstein et al. (1997) reported the occurrence of *A. actinomycetemcomitans* in 4 of 5 diseased children and in 2 of 4 controls. In a study including 26 children with two or more sites with alveolar bone loss and 20 controls, *A. actinomycetemcomitans* was isolated in 14 of the cases while none of the controls harbored cultivable numbers of this microorganism. The presence of *A. actinomycetemcomitans* in childhood periodontitis cases is not consistent and some of the case presentations published report absence of cultivable proportions of this microbiota (D'Angelo et al., 1992; Linden et al., 1994; Yoshida-Minami et al., 1995; Bimstein et al., 1997). Although evidence suggests *A. actinomycetemcomitans* plays an important part in the disease process of juvenile periodontitis, its mere presence is not indicative of ongoing periodontal destruction. This bacterium is frequently found in healthy teenagers as well as in children with no clinical signs of periodontal disease (Zambon et al., 1983; Delaney, 1986; Abraham et al., 1990; Alaluusua et al., 1997; Bimstein et al., 1997; Timmerman et al., 1998). In adolescents it seems that occurrence of periodontal destruction may be related to the presence of high proportions of *A. actinomycetemcomitans* in the cultivable flora. Comparable data on prepubertal cases are sparse.

Other suspected periopathogens have been found in plaque samples from prepubertal cases and there are reports on the presence of black-pigmented *Bacteroides*, *Capnocytophaga*, *Prevotella intermedia*, *Fusobacterium*, *Porphyromonas gingivalis*, and others. Systematic longitudinal microbiological investigations on groups of children with periodontitis in the deciduous dentition are lacking.

The microbiology of periodontitis is discussed in Chapter 8.

Impaired host defense factors

The host defense against periodontal pathogens is similar to that for any local infection. Neutrophil polymorphonuclear leucocytes (PMNs) in the connective tissue and the epithelium provide the first line of defense against deleterious periodontal bacteria. Failure to control the pathogens leads to an engagement of local and systemic immunocompetent cells including antibody production. Deficiencies of the host defense system may result in development of destructive periodontal disease. This is demonstrated by increased susceptibility to periodontal disease in patients with diseases such as acquired immunodeficiency syndrome (AIDS), agranulocytosis, and neutropenia. The most significant finding of impaired host defense system in young individuals with periodontal disease is the association between juvenile periodontitis and depressed function of circulating PMNs and/or monocytes (for review see Van Dyke and Hoop, 1990). In fact, the chemotactic deficiency of the PMNs in JP patients forms a cornerstone of the hypothesis of impaired host defense in patients with severe periodontitis. Although infrequently investigated, chemotactic defects of the PMNs from otherwise healthy children with childhood periodontitis have been reported (Hara et al., 1986; Celenligil et al., 1987; Firatli et al., 1996). Watanabe et al. (1991) found that all of seven examined children with childhood periodontitis manifested reduced chemotactic function of their PMNs compared with adult controls but no difference was found when using age-matched controls. Additional reports describe prepubertal cases with normal PMN chemotaxis (Crossner et al., 1990; Lopez, 1992; Linden et al., 1994; Yoshida-Minami et al., 1995; Sixou et al., 1997).

Additional indications of host response dysfunction in individuals with childhood periodontitis stem from case reports including information on blood lymphocyte subpopulations. In patients with childhood periodontitis increased expression of CD11b/CD18 lymphocytes, reduced number of CD4 and CD8 cells, alterations in CD4/CD8 ratio, and elevation of the

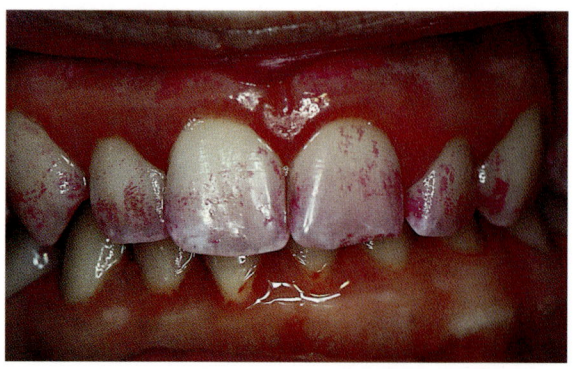

a

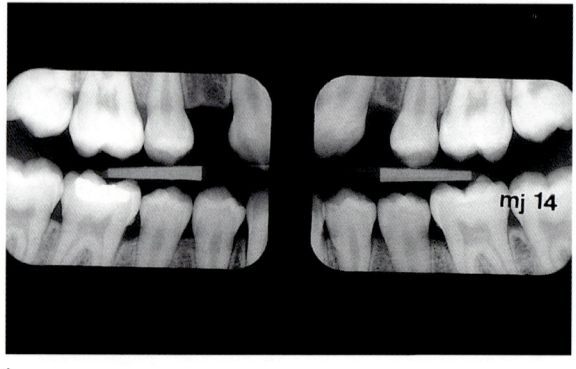

b

Figure 5.5

A 14-year-old boy with incidental attachment loss and subgingival calculus. (a) Clinical picture. (b) Bite-wing radiographs.

number of natural killer cells have been found (Celenligil et al., 1987; Watanabe et al., 1991; Katsuragi et al., 1994; Firatli et al., 1996). Information on immunological function or dysfunction in prepubertal cases is sparse, but future therapeutic strategies may depend upon recognition of the molecular pathogenic basis of the disease (see Chapter 7).

Cementopathia

Defects in cementum deposition have been suggested as an etiologic factor for periodontitis in systemically healthy young individuals (Gottlieb, 1928; Lindskog and Blomlöf, 1983). Page and Baab (1985) suggested that some children with childhood periodontitis could have had mild forms of hypophosphatasia with no other clinical sign of the disease than premature loss of deciduous teeth. Hypophosphatasia is a disorder caused by deficiency or low levels of serum alkaline phosphatase, and one of the clinical signs may be cementopathia. The authors also suggested an analogous etiology for some cases of juvenile or rapidly progressive periodontitis. However, Bimstein et al. (1998) did not reveal cementum aplasia in a histological examination of teeth from four childhood periodontitis cases. In a study of adolescents and young adults with aggressive periodontitis by

Machtei et al. (1994) the patients exhibited normal levels of alkaline phosphatase in blood and urinary levels of phosphoethanolamine were also within normal limits. Low levels of serum alkaline phosphatase and excretion of phospho-ethanolamine in urine are diagnostic findings. The same result was found in a study of 22 cases with bone loss in the deciduous dentition (Sjödin and Matsson, 1994).

Loss of periodontal support in the mixed and permanent dentition

Loss of periodontal support in the permanent dentition in adolescents

The occurrence of moderate or solitary attachment loss in adolescents has been termed incipient periodontitis, incidental attachment loss, incidental EOP, early periodontitis, or early adult periodontitis (Figure 5.5) (Davis et al., 1985; Delaney, 1986; Carlos et al., 1988; Clerehugh, 1991; Löe and Brown, 1991). It is the most prevalent form of periodontal disease in adolescents and young adults. It is generally not included in the EOP entity even though many patients eventually develop more severe destruction and thus show the characteristics of localized or generalized EOP. In a 6-year longitudinal study of the long-term outcome of EOP, a third of cases with localized juvenile periodontitis developed generalized juvenile periodontitis, 28% of the patients with incidental attachment loss developed localized or generalized juvenile periodontitis, while 30% of this group was reclassified as having no attachment loss (Albandar et al., 1997a). The authors suggested the use of the EOP forms "localized", "generalized", and "incidental" and a further subdivision according to progression patterns (slow or rapid).

Epidemiological studies on periodontal disease in adolescents more frequently focus on the permanent dentition. While most frequency studies of juvenile periodontitis have reported a prevalence well below 0.5%, incidental loss of attachment appears to be relatively frequent (Table 5.2). Most studies are cross-sectional although some adolescent cohorts have been followed longitudinally (Table 5.3). Results from the longitudinal studies indicate that adolescents exhibiting early bone or attachment loss are more prone to develop further loss (Clerehugh et al., 1990; Albandar et al., 1991). The risk of progression seems to be subject- rather than site-dependent (Albandar et al., 1991, 1997b). As in JP, the first molars are particularly likely to be involved (Clerehugh, 1991) (see Figures 1.3e, 5.1c, d, 5.2b, c, 5.3c).

Factors associated with loss of attachment in the permanent dentition of adolescents

Although dental plaque has a key role in initiation and progression of destructive periodontitis, the relationship at individual and site level is weak. The mere presence of plaque at a certain site will not necessarily be followed by loss of periodontal support, although there is ample evidence that local factors enhancing the accumulation of dental plaque predispose to the development and progression of adult periodontitis (Pennel and Keagle, 1977).

While oral hygiene training programs in adolescent populations may improve the oral hygiene and gingival status significantly, the impact on prevalence of attachment loss seems to be weak (Albandar et al., 1995b). A lack of relationship between oral hygiene and incidence of attachment loss does not necessarily mean that other determinants are more important than dental plaque. The etiology of periodontal disease is multifactorial and the degree of influence of different factors is not recognized. Findings in longitudinal studies of adolescent cohorts indicate that local factors facilitating plaque retention do influence the prevalence of attachment loss. Thus, in a 3-year longitudinal study of 227 children aged 13 years, Albandar et al. (1995a) found associations between the presence of untreated manifest caries lesions, non-defective and defective dental restorations, and progression of attachment loss. Teeth surfaces exhibiting these local factors were more prone to develop deterioration of their periodontal support. Also, the adjacent proximal surfaces of the neighboring teeth demonstrated increased loss of periodontal support.

In adolescent populations an association between the presence of subgingival calculus and attachment loss has been found. Adolescents with bone loss nearly twice as often exhibit proximal sites with subgingival calculus compared with adolescents without attachment loss (Källestål and Matsson, 1990; Clerehugh et

Table 5.3 Longitudinal studies on prevalence of attachment loss in adolescents.

Author(s)	Age when examined (years)	N	Country	Criteria	Prevalence (%)
Lissau et al., 1990		765	Denmark		
Clerehugh et al., 1990	14–16–19	167	Great Britain	CAL ≥ 1 mm	3–37–77
Albandar et al., 1991	14–15	422	Iraq	Radiographic bone loss <2 mm	13–24
Albandar et al., 1991	13–16	222	Brazil	Radiographic bone loss <2 mm	
Albandar et al., 1993			Iraq		
Aass et al., 1994	14–16–18–22	215	Norway	Radiographic bone loss <2 mm	

al., 1995; Albandar et al., 1998). However, in the latter studies the prevalence of subgingival calculus differed significantly between different populations and races. The method of registration may be a cause of the varying prevalence reported; radiographic techniques seem to underestimate the prevalence of calculus compared with probing. Two studies have reported a possible longitudinal impact of calculus on progression of loss of attachment. Clerehugh et al. (1990) found an association at site level between presence of subgingival calculus and future attachment loss in a British adolescent population. The same result was shown by Albandar et al. (1997b) who found a relationship between presence of subgingival calculus and progression of attachment loss in aggressive periodontitis patients. In localized and generalized forms of aggressive periodontitis this association was statistically significant, while there was a tendency (though not statistically significant) in individuals with incidental attachment loss. In this latter study analog associations between overt gingival inflammation and future attachment loss were found. The role of calculus in the initiation and progression of the periodontal lesions is unclear but it seems reasonable that this clinical finding may have a negative effect on healthy periodontal tissues (Mandel and Gaffar, 1986). Presence of subgingival calculus does not automatically imply that calculus is of etiologic importance for development of periodontal disease; other factors may be important in this regard.

Reports of microbiological findings in young individuals with periodontal disease have predominantly focused on cases with localized or generalized aggressive periodontitis. Strong evidence suggests that *Actinobacillus actinomycetemcomitans* plays a dominant role in the disease progression of the localized cases. A high percentage of individuals with localized juvenile periodontitis harbor this microorganism in their diseased pockets. In investigations including adolescents with incidental attachment loss the findings are not so unequivocal. While nearly 90% of cases with juvenile periodontitis harbor *A. actinomycetemcomitans* in the diseased pockets, recovery frequencies of 10–20% have been reported for individuals with incidental attachment loss (Van der Velden et al., 1989; Källestål et al., 1991; Albandar et al.,

1997b). The importance of eliminating this microorganism to secure healing in cases with localized aggressive periodontitis has been emphasized, but patients with incidental attachment loss seem to respond well to conventional therapy irrespective of the presence of *A. actinomycetemcomitans* (van Steenbergen et al., 1993). The importance of any specific microorganism in the pathogenesis of periodontal attachment loss has not been conclusively determined.

Screening for periodontal disease in young individuals

The objective of screening for periodontal disease in children and adolescents is to detect disease early enough to provide treatment that will alter its natural history. No clinical or biotechnical method of predicting who will suffer from periodontal disease is yet available, but primary prevention of periodontal disease in the young dentition could be achieved by detecting and treating gingivitis. Although gingivitis is a frequent finding in young children, only a small fraction of those affected will develop destructive periodontal disease in youth. Thus, the sensitivity of a screening method based on the gingival condition may be good but the specificity is very low. To implement preventive measures for a disease with a very low prevalence may not seem justified. The lack of distinct risk factors rules out the possibility of identifying high-risk groups and changes the focus to secondary prevention. Early findings of loss of periodontal support may be a possible way to identify high-risk patients. In adolescent populations a significant proportion of individuals—though certainly not all—with attachment loss will eventually develop further destruction, and disease progression among young subjects is a subject- rather than a site-dependent phenomenon (Albandar et al., 1991). Even if primary prevention may be preferable, there are indications that secondary prevention is more appropriate, and screening for early detection of signs of destructive periodontitis may be adequate to identify susceptible individuals (Albandar et al., 1997b).

Despite the absence of any longitudinal evaluation of the impact of early treatment on progression of attachment loss in children, the

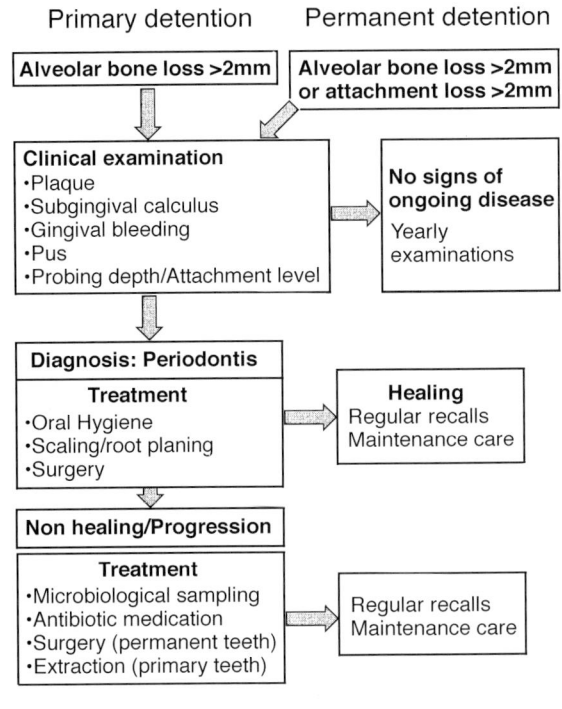

Primary detention   Permanent detention

Alveolar bone loss >2mm

Alveolar bone loss >2mm
or attachment loss >2mm

Clinical examination
•Plaque
•Subgingival calculus
•Gingival bleeding
•Pus
•Probing depth/Attachment level

No signs of
ongoing disease
Yearly
examinations

Diagnosis: Periodontis
Treatment
•Oral Hygiene
•Scaling/root planing
•Surgery

Healing
Regular recalls
Maintenance care

Non healing/Progression
Treatment
•Microbiological sampling
•Antibiotic medication
•Surgery (permanent teeth)
•Extraction (primary teeth)

Regular recalls
Maintenance care

Figure 5.6

Screening and treatment strategy for children and adolescents.

prevalence of incidental periodontitis in the permanent dentition seems to be lower in young populations receiving regular dental care. Prevalence studies from different districts in Denmark showed a higher prevalence of bone loss in districts without organized dental care for adolescents.

Figure 5.6 describes a strategy for screening and treatment of children and adolescents. The use of radiographic measurements is suggested in children since measurement of attachment loss may be difficult in the mixed dentition. The screening methods suggested for adolescents with permanent teeth include probing for proximal attachment loss and CEJ–ABC measurements on bite-wing radiographs. Eventually partial registration of probing pocket depths can be used. Registration of deep probing depths (6 mm or more) at proximal surfaces of molars and incisors will identify the great majority of

adolescents with proximal attachment loss (Källestål et al., 1991). Detection of bone or attachment loss leads to a comprehensive periodontal examination. If no other clinical sign of disease is found, the child is re-examined on a yearly basis. Any finding of other signs of periodontal disease leads to treatment. Standard procedures of treatment are suggested, although in cases with severe or progressive disease a microbiological examination as well as antibiotic medication is recommended. Severe cases of childhood periodontitis may require extraction of involved teeth.

New classification for periodontal disease in children and young adults

The classification of periodontal disease in children and young adults has evolved dramatically over time. This is due in part to improvements in molecular biology, immunologic methods, microbiologic techniques, and effective treatments. It is no longer acceptable to use arbitrary age-based criteria to diagnose destructive periodontal disease without taking into account clinical, radiographic, and laboratory findings as well as the historical and natural progression of the disease. Correct diagnosis is the key to successful treatment. It is important to recognize that each disease classification is not a static entity, but will continue to evolve as information is accumulated. Based on the current knowledge of periodontal disease, host response, pathophysiology, microbiology, and periodontal treatment, the following classification of periodontal diseases in children, adolescents, and young adults is offered:

I   Periodontal abscess
II Childhood periodontitis
    a. localized
    b. generalized
III Aggressive periodontitis
    a. localized
    b. generalized
IV Periodontitis associated with systemic disease and genetic abnormalities

a. Systemic diseases and conditions that enhance susceptibility for periodontitis
   i   diabetes mellitus
   ii   human immunodeficiency virus (HIV) and acquired immune deficiency syndrome (AIDS)
   iii tobacco use and drug abuse
   iv stress
   v   leukemias
   vi neutropenia and agranulocytosis
   vii Langerhans cell histiocytosis
   viii acrodynia
   ix genetic abnormalities
       a. trisomy 21 (Down syndrome)
       b. hypophosphatasia
       c. leukocyte adhesion deficiency
       d. Papillon–Lefèvre syndrome
       e. Chédiak–Higashi syndrome
       f. Ehlers–Danlos syndrome
b. Periodontitis that enhances the risk for certain systemic diseases and conditions
V Necrotizing ulcerative periodontitis

Periodontal abscess

A periodontal abscess is an acute suppurative inflammation of the deeper periodontal tissues caused by an infection of pyogenic bacteria (see Figure 1.3a–d). This results in a rapid destruction of the attachment apparatus and alveolar bone. Glickman (1979) suggested five mechanisms of abscess formation:

1. Extension of a pocket into the supporting periodontal tissues along the lateral aspect of the tooth root.
2. Lateral extension of the inner pocket surface into the connective tissue of the pocket wall.
3. In the sinuous pocket, an abscess may develop in the deeper portions due to the formation of a cul-de-sac.
4. Incomplete removal of calculus results in tissue shrinkage with subsequent occlusion of the pocket opening.
5. Following traumatic injury of a tooth or a perforation of the lateral wall of the root during endodontic treatment.

These lesions may also be caused by the traumatic introduction of bacteria or a foreign body into the periodontal tissues.

Periodontal abscesses are painful to palpation and frequently there is sensitivity of the associated tooth to occlusion, mastication or gentle percussion. The overlying gingiva and/or mucosa may be distended and edematous and the affected tissues will appear shiny with a red to reddish-blue hue. Frequently the affected tooth may extrude from its socket and exhibit increased mobility. Regional lymphadenopathy and slight elevation of body temperature have also been associated with the appearance of these lesions. Destruction of the periodontal attachment is rapid and deep pockets can form within a week.

Radiographically, a periodontal abscess will present as a distinct radiolucency along the lateral aspect of the affected tooth root (see Figure 1.3b, d). However, this finding is not diagnostic since the radiographic presentation may vary with the position and stage of the lesion, local bony morphology, and the extent of bone loss (Glickman, 1979). Microscopically, necrotic and lysed polymorphonuclear cells are evident and the predominant bacteria isolated in these lesions are Gram-negative anaerobic rods (Newman and Sims, 1979). Clinically, purulence can be expressed from the gingival margin with gentle pressure, demonstrating continuity between the lesion and the free gingival margin (see Figure 1.3a, c).

Treatment of periodontal abscess depends on the location of the lesion and its stage of development. The overall prognosis of the tooth including its periodontal attachment and its importance to the final treatment plan should be considered. The objective of treatment is drainage and debridement of the lesion, which will resolve the pain and other clinical symptoms. If the tooth is hopeless and local anesthesia can be achieved, extraction and debridement of the socket can quickly resolve the problem. Many abscesses can be treated by root planing through the gingival sulcus in a "closed" approach with optional irrigation of the lesion. However, incision and drainage or an open flap procedure should be used to treat lesions that are more extensive or not amenable to debridement through the sulcus. Periodontal abscesses are considered to have an excellent potential for repair of the attachment apparatus following treatment (Nabers et al., 1964).

Childhood periodontitis

Localized childhood periodontitis of children includes a form that is plaque-induced and modified by the presence of local factors; it also encompasses the description of LPP (Page et al., 1983b), with the caveat that there is no systemic condition superimposed on the disease process. Periodontal manifestations of systemic diseases are considered in Chapter 6. The generalized type follows the description of GPP, again without the presence of systemic modifiers.

Localized childhood periodontitis

In clinically healthy children and adolescents destruction of the attachment apparatus may proceed in a manner similar to that seen in "adult" periodontitis. This destruction may have a slow or moderate rate of progression but may exhibit periods of rapid breakdown. However, the amount of periodontal destruction is consistent with the amounts of local factors present and subgingival calculus deposits may be demonstrated. The bacterial plaque associated with the lesion is non-specific in terms of predominance of any particular periodontal pathogen, and this pathogenic plaque flora triggers an inflammatory cascade within the periodontium. If therapeutic intervention does not occur, this ultimately leads to the characteristic progressive loss of attachment and alveolar bone identified by pocket formation and/or gingival recession which may afflict both the deciduous and permanent dentitions.

Bacterial plaque is thought to be the primary etiologic factor of periodontal disease (Löe et al., 1965; Listgarten, 1986; Page, 1986). Therefore, it is possible to speculate that local factors that allow excessive plaque accumulation and impair proper oral hygiene have a secondary role in the pathogenesis of these diseases. Local irritants (Pennel and Keagle, 1977) such as unrestored carious lesions and defective or inferior restorative dentistry have been implicated in the progression of periodontal disease in children and adolescents (Jamison, 1963; Sweeney et al., 1987; Bimstein et al., 1988a 1996a; Albandar et al., 1995a).

Gross, untreated interproximal caries can cause loss of proximal contacts between teeth, facilitate food retention, allow excessive plaque accumulation, and act as an incurable reservoir of pathogenic bacteria. It has been demonstrated that unrestored caries are an etiologic factor in marginal alveolar bone loss in deciduous and permanent teeth of children (Bimstein et al., 1988a, 1993, 1994; Bimstein, 1992; Drummond and Bimstein, 1995). However, it was noted that alveolar bone loss did not occur in all cases of proximal caries, and that a greater percentage of children with loss of bone had destruction in more than one site (Bimstein et al., 1988a). Bimstein (1992) went on to quantify this phenomenon, finding bone loss in approximately 12% of quadrants with proximal caries and in 31% where some loss of interproximal contact had occurred. This suggests that some children may have an increased susceptibility to the development of periodontitis, but whether this is due to differences in the host or in pathologic flora has yet to be conclusively demonstrated (Bimstein et al., 1993, 1996b). Furthermore, evidence is required to demonstrate whether the presence of localized marginal periodontitis in the deciduous teeth facilitates the initiation of periodontitis in the newly erupted adjacent permanent teeth during the mixed dentition period. Bimstein (1992) also demonstrated spontaneous healing of some bony lesions subsequent to the restoration of carious defects, suggesting a possible connection between the presence and restoration of carious proximal surfaces and alveolar bone condition in children.

Poor or defective restorative dentistry may also play a role in localized attachment loss in both the deciduous and permanent dentition. These restorations are fabricated from foreign materials, none of which duplicates the physical properties of natural tooth structure, in an attempt to recreate proper tooth form. Stainless steel crowns with improper margins, contour, positioning, or retained cement have been associated with inflammatory changes in the periodontium (Webber, 1974; Myers, 1975; Ashraphi et al., 1981; Machen et al., 1981). Guelman et al. (1988) demonstrated that properly adapted stainless steel crowns on deciduous second molars did not adversely affect adjacent permanent first molars, while Bimstein et al. (1996a) found an increased prevalence of alveolar bone loss with inadequately placed crowns when compared with well-placed restorations. Albandar et al. (1995a) found a significant relationship

Table 5.4 Periodontitis in children, adolescents, and young adults.

	Childhood periodontitis		Aggressive periodontitis	
	Localized (LCP)	Generalized (GCP)	Localized (LAP)	Generalized (GAP)
Former disease entity	Incidental attachment loss Localized prepubertal periodontitis (w/o systemic involvement)	Generalized prepubertal periodontitis	Localized juvenile periodontitis	Generalized juvenile periodontitis Rapidly progressive periodontitis
Onset	Childhood–adolescence	Childhood	Adolescence	Adolescence
Teeth involved	Some primary and permanent teeth	All primary and permanent teeth	Permanent incisors and first molars	Several permanent teeth involved
Predisposing factors	Caries, faulty restorations	None	Neutrophil dysfunction Plaque and calculus are sparse Cementopathia (?)	Neutrophil dysfunction (?) Plaque and calculus are evident Cementopathia (?)
Familial history	Positive	Positive	Positive	Positive
Microbial association	Non-specific bacterial flora	Non-specific bacterial flora	*Actinobacillus actinomycetemcomitans* serotype b *Bacteroides* spp. (?)	Polymicrobial Predominantly Gram-negative anaerobes, including: *Porphyromonas gingivalis, A. actinomycetemcomitans, Prevotella intermedia, Bacteroides forsythus, Fusobacterium nucleatum, Campylobacter rectus, Eubacterium* spp., and several spirochete species
Humoral immune response	None	?	IgG2	?

between defective restorations and the loss of periodontal support in adolescents. Overhanging amalgam margins, especially when subgingival, can quickly lead to periodontal attachment loss (Hakkarainen and Ainamo, 1980; Rodriguez-Ferrer et al., 1980) and may have the potential to create an environment conducive for pathologic microflora (Brunsvold and Lane, 1990). Bimstein et al. (1996a) demonstrated that faulty amalgam restorations led to increased prevalence of alveolar bone loss in children when compared with adequately placed amalgams. Their data also demonstrated that loss of interproximal contact was a significant risk for localized bone destruction. Albandar and co-workers established that even clinically non-defective restorations can have a

detrimental effect on periodontal health in adolescents (Albandar et al., 1995a). This is a disturbing finding, restorative dentistry is widely used in children and adolescents, and suggests that clinicians must be circumspect when placing restorative materials.

According to Page et al. (1983b) LPP (actually localized childhood periodontitis-LCP) affects relatively few teeth in the deciduous dentition unless there is rampant gingival inflammation. However, tissue destruction proceeds at an accelerated rate despite the absence of facilitating factors. This form of prepubertal disease is considered amenable to antibiotic treatment and gingival curettage. It is important to stress that in this classification of periodontal diseases of children, adolescents, and young adults there can be no systemic modifiers superimposed upon the disease process. Bimstein et al. (1997) recognized that LCP may occur in seemingly healthy children, hence the rationale for inclusion of these patients in the new category of localized childhood periodontitis (LCP).

Generalized childhood periodontitis

Generalized childhood periodontitis (GCP) encompasses the disease entity formerly known as GPP (Page et al., 1983b). It is characterized by intense acute inflammation, a severe gingival response with spontaneous bleeding and recession, and rapid destruction of alveolar bone and exfoliation of deciduous teeth. This form affects both the deciduous and permanent dentition. Bimstein et al. (1997) provided evidence that this form of prepubertal disease can be found in systemically healthy patients. A brief comparison of LCP and GCP is given in Table 5.4.

Aggressive periodontitis

Aggressive periodontitis is a category of the American Academy of Periodontology's 1989 classification of EOP (AAP, 1989), consisting of the disease entities prepubertal periodontitis (localized and generalized), juvenile periodontitis (localized and generalized), and rapidly progressive periodontitis. Localized juvenile periodontitis, rapidly progressive periodontitis, and generalized juvenile periodontitis are now categorized as aggressive periodontitis. The basis for the division of the two entities is the relative early onset (adolescent years) and the clinical pattern of tissue destruction at presentation (localized to a few teeth, or generalized with several teeth involved).

Localized aggressive periodontitis

Localized aggressive periodontitis (LAP) replaces the previous terms localized juvenile periodontitis and juvenile periodontitis. This form of adolescent periodontitis presents with pocket formation, attachment loss and deep interproximal loss of the alveolar bone, limited to the first molars and incisor teeth in an otherwise clinically healthy patient. Radiographs reveal an arc-shaped pattern of destruction extending from the distal surface of the second premolar to the mesial surface of the second molar (Miller, 1948), often bilaterally distributed. Clinically there is little plaque accumulation and calculus formation (Baer and Benjamin, 1974), with little inflammatory change seen in the gingiva. Gottleib (1923) suggested defects in cementum to be a central cause of the disease. Ruben and Shapiro (1978) and Lindskog and Blomlof (1983) have since demonstrated abnormalities in cementum in healthy and diseased roots in LAP patients.

Analysis of plaque samples from patients afflicted with LAP revealed high populations of *Actinobacillus actinomycetemcomitans*, a Gram-negative anaerobic coccobacillus. It is suspected that this periopathogen, especially serotype b, is responsible for the destruction that is the hallmark of this disease (Listgarten et al., 1981; Mandell and Socransky, 1981; Haffajee et al., 1984; Zambon et al., 1983, 1996; van Winkelhoff et al., 1994; Asikainen et al., 1991). There are two good reasons for this belief. First, this bacterium possesses several virulence factors that can aid its colonization of susceptible hosts (Fives-Taylor et al., 1996): these include collagenases, bacteriocin, a fibroblast-inhibiting factor, and an endotoxin—all of which can adversely affect the host response. Serotype b also produces a potent leukotoxin (Berthold et al., 1992; Kolodrubetz, 1996; Lally et al., 1996), which is detrimental to leukocytes and monocytes. Second, patients with localized disease display higher antibody titers against this microorganism (Listgarten et al., 1981; Ebersole et al., 1982; Vincent et al., 1985; Lu et al., 1994; Tew et al., 1996). However, these data must be interpreted critically since *A. actinomycetemcomitans* can be isolated in other forms of periodontal disease (Crossner et al., 1990; Gunsolley et al., 1990a; Asikainen et al., 1995), or even in health, and may not always be isolated from patients with LAP (Okuda et al., 1984; Loesche et al., 1985; Moore et al., 1985). In addition, other bacterial species have been isolated in patients with this disease, including *Bacteroides* spp. (Kornman and Robertson, 1985). Also, elevated antibody titers to *A. actinomycetemcomitans* have not been a universal finding and there have been reports where this did not occur in LAP patients (Gunsolley et al., 1990b).

Sufferers of LAP also have been found with functional defects in their circulating polymorphonuclear cells. The influence of these abnormalities on disease susceptibility is currently unknown, but it is likely that this plays some role in the clinical manifestations of the disease. There is substantial evidence that patients with LAP have defective neutrophil chemotaxis and decreased phagocytic and bactericidal activity (Cianciola et al., 1977; Clark et al., 1977; Lavine et al., 1979; Van Dyke et al., 1980, 1982, 1985; Ellegaard et al., 1984; Page et al., 1984, 1985; Suzuki et al., 1985). It was later demonstrated that neutrophils from patients with LAP are deficient in cell surface receptors for chemoattractive ligands (Van Dyke et al., 1981, 1983, 1987). It was later found that these patients have decreased receptors for chemoattractant molecules. Other defects in neutrophil function include enhanced production of superoxide, abnormalities in signal transduction pathways, cellular metabolism, and impaired intracellular killing of *A. actinomycetemcomitans* (Kalmar et al., 1987; Noguchi et al., 1988; Agarwal et al., 1989; Agarwal and Suzuki, 1991; Tyagi et al., 1992; Daniel et al., 1993). Various molecular markers for LAP have also been studied: gp110, a cell surface glycoprotein that plays a role in leukocyte chemotaxis, has been shown to be decreased in LAP patients (Van Dyke et al., 1987). Wilson and Kalmar (1996) reported another potential marker, an alternative form of an IgG receptor, FcγRIIa, which may also play a role in the pathogenesis of LAP. Although there are many accounts of neutrophilic defects (De Nardin, 1996) in LAP, other research has failed to demonstrate any problems in these cells (Larjava et al., 1984; Kinane et al., 1989; Pederson, 1989; Repo et al., 1990). These differences probably reflect the character of the population studied (African-Americans, northern Europeans, etc.). Another current controversy is whether these defects are intrinsic—that is, genetically predetermined—or develop as a result of the disease process. Reviews by Schenkein and Van Dyke (1994), and Agarwal et al. (1996) on this subject summarize current information and point to the need for continued research.

Löe and Brown (1991) found that 0.53% of American children aged 14–17 years suffered from LAP, and other reports range from 0.1% to 15% in a variety of different age groups and populations (Saxen, 1980a, b; Kronauer et al., 1986; Harly and Floyd, 1988). Löe and Brown (1991) also demonstrated that African-American and Hispanic subjects had higher prevalence rates than whites. Schenkein et al. (1991) demonstrated that neutrophils from healthy African-Americans displayed lowered chemotaxis compared with whites, perhaps explaining the increased prevalence of LAP in this cohort. Löe and Brown (1991) also showed that males had a higher prevalence of the disease than females. This is contrary to the description of the disease by Baer (1971), who reported a 3:1 female to male ratio. However, the findings of Löe and Brown were supported by the work of Hart et al. (1991, 1992) which found the female to male ratio to be 1:1 when "proband ascertainment bias" was removed, and it also proved to be critical in disproving an X-linked dominant transmission pattern of the disease. A debate exists as to whether LAP is transmitted in an autosomal dominant or autosomal recessive mode and once again suggests a certain degree of heterogeneity in this disease entity.

Generalized aggressive periodontitis

The term "generalized aggressive periodontitis" (GAP) replaces the terms generalized juvenile periodontitis and rapidly progressive periodontitis. As evidenced by the two disease entities that it replaces, GAP is a heterogeneous condition, and as such it is difficult to determine its prevalence. Unlike LAP, there is marked plaque and calculus accumulation, and clinical signs of gingival inflammation are evident. There is also rapid destruction of periodontal tissues and exfoliation of teeth despite aggressive therapeutic intervention and antimicrobial treatment (Watanabe, 1991). The disease may evolve from defects in the periodontium, namely the cementum (Baab et al., 1985; Page and Baab, 1985), but this has yet to be confirmed.

The subgingival flora of GAP is much more complex than that seen in the localized form of the disease, and consists predominantly of non-motile, facultative, Gram-negative anaerobes (Moore et al., 1982; Slots, 1982; Zambon et al., 1983; Dzink et al., 1985; Kornman and Robertson, 1985). The bacteria most commonly isolated from these patients include some well-known periopathogens, including *Porphyromonas gingi-*

valis, *A. actinomycetemcomitans*, *Prevotella intermedia*, *Bacteroides forsythus*, *Fusobacterium nucleatum*, *Campylobacter rectus*, *Eubacterium* species, and several spirochetes. However, like LAP, the bacterial flora of GAP is not diagnostic for the disease since these pathogens can be isolated from other types of periodontal disease. Antibody levels to these bacteria are elevated in some patients with GAP, but this is not considered diagnostic since this immune response is not evident in all patients. Neutrophil dysfunction is also thought to play a role in the pathogenesis of GAP. Reports have shown that neutrophils from these patients may exhibit decreased chemotaxis (Van Dyke et al., 1982) while chemotactic markers such as gp100 appear at normal levels (Van Dyke et al., 1987, 1990).

Because of the similarities between LAP and GAP it may be that the generalized form is actually a continuation of the localized disease process. Cases have been reported in which the localized form progressed to GAP (Shapira et al., 1994; Gunsolley et al., 1995) but these seem to be anomalies. Gunsolley et al. (1995) noted differences in the clinical progressions of both LAP and GAP: the localized form was a stable lesion while the generalized type was prone to rapid loss of attachment and bone loss despite therapeutic measures. It is evident that continued investigation into these diseases is needed to characterize and fully understand these periodontal diseases.

et al., 1997). Disregarding the health of the patient, the loss of periodontal support seen in these individuals can be regarded as a manifestation of a systemic irregularity rather than a consequence of inflammatory periodontal disease. In cases of systemic problems manifesting with periodontal destruction, the progression of the disease is rapid and the extent of periodontal destruction is generalized and enormous. This clinical picture can be interpreted as (a) the periopathogenic flora is more aggressive in these individuals, and/or (b) the susceptibility of the patient to periodontal disease has been elevated.

Systemic disorders known to be associated with severe periodontitis and premature loss of deciduous and permanent teeth include AIDS, acrodynia, agranulocytosis, Chédiak–Higashi syndrome, Ehlers–Danlos syndrome, Langerhans cell histiocytosis (see Figure 1.7d), hypophosphatasia (see Figure 1.7b), type 1 diabetes (formerly insulin-dependent diabetes mellitus), leukemias, leukocyte adhesion deficiency, neutropenia, and Papillon–Lefèvre syndrome (see Figure 1.7e, f). A majority of these disorders are associated with an impaired host defense such as defective neutrophil function. However, alterations in the host tissues may be the cause of the rapid periodontal destruction. For example, in childhood hypophosphatasia, deficiencies in the cementum of the deciduous teeth are a consistent finding. Chapter 6 reviews the systemic and genetic disorders and their effects on the periodontium.

Periodontitis associated with systemic disease and genetic abnormalities

It is well recognized that some children, adolescents, and young adults with systemic disorders or genetic syndromes are afflicted with severe periodontal destruction. Almost all case reports of the previously defined disease entity, generalized prepubertal periodontitis, seem to describe medically compromised children. However, it has been suggested that even seemingly healthy children with severe periodontitis, whether localized or generalized, might suffer from some undetected systemic disorder or immunodeficiency (Watanabe, 1990; Watanabe et al., 1991; Bimstein

Necrotizing ulcerative periodontitis

Necrotizing ulcerative periodontitis (NUP) represents a severe and rapidly progressive disease characterized by extensive soft tissue necrosis and loss of interproximal bone without evidence of deep periodontal pocketing. This lesion is thought to develop after repeated bouts of acute necrotizing ulcerative gingivitis (ANUG) (Johnson and Engel, 1986). As in ANUG, the gingival tissues have areas of ulceration and necrosis and the pathognomonic sign of psuedomembrane formation. The lesion is painful and bleeds profusely upon provocation. In NUP, a neutrophilic inflammatory infiltrate extends from the gingiva and alveolar mucosa into the deeper periodontal tissues, resulting in rapid destruction of the attachment apparatus and deep osseous craters, typically discovered in the interdental regions. If this lesion is allowed to progress, exposure of the alveolar bone and sequestration may occur. Concurrent with the destruction of the attachment apparatus tooth mobility increases and eventual exfoliation may follow.

References

[AAP] American Academy of Periodontology (1996) Special issue: Periodontal diseases of children and adolescents. Guidelines. *J Periodontol* **67**: 57–62.

AAP (1989) Consensus report on periodontal diagnosis and diagnostic aids. *Proceedings of the World Workshop in Clinical Periodontics*. Chicago: American Academy of Periodontology; 1:23–1:31.

Aass AM, Tollefsen T, Gjermo P (1994) A cohort study of radiographic alveolar bone loss during adolescence. *J Clin Periodontol* **21**: 133–8.

Abraham J, Stiles HM, Kammerman LA, Forrester D (1990) Assessing periodontal pathogens in children with varying levels of oral hygiene. *ASDC J Dent Child* **57**: 189–93.

Agarwal S, Suzuki JB (1991) Altered neutrophil function in localized juvenile periodontitis: *intrinsic* cellular defect or effect of immune mediators? *J Periodont Res* **26**: 276–8.

Agarwal S, Reynolds MA, Dukkett LD, Suzuki JB (1989) Altered free cytosolic calcium changes and neutrophil chemotaxis in patients with juvenile periodontitis. *J Periodont Res* **24**: 149–54.

Agarwal S, Huang JP, Piesco NP et al. (1996) Altered neutrophil functions in Localized Juvenile Periodontitis: intrinsic or induced? *J Periodontol* **67**: 337–44.

Alaluusua S, Kivitie-Kallio S, Wolf J et al. (1997) Periodontal findings in Cohen syndrome with chronic neutropenia. *J Periodontol* **68**: 473–8.

Albandar JM (1989) Validity and reliability of alveolar bone level measurements made on dry skulls. *J Clin Periodontol* **16**: 575–9.

Albandar JM, Baghdady VS, Ghose LJ (1991) Periodontal disease progression in teenagers with no preventive dental care provisions. *J Clin Periodontol* **18**: 300–4.

Albandar JM, Buischi YAP, Axelsson P (1995a) Caries lesions and dental restorations as predisposing factors in the progression of periodontal diseases in adolescents. A 3-year longitudinal study. *J Periodontol* **66**: 249–54.

Albandar JM, Buischi YAP, Oliviera LB, Axelsson P (1995b) Lack of effect of oral hygiene training on periodontal disease progression over 3 years in adolescents. *J Periodontol* **66**: 255–60.

Albandar JM, Brown LJ, Genco RJ, Löe H (1997a) Clinical classification of periodontitis in adolescents and young adults. *J Periodontol* **68**: 545–55.

Albandar JM, Brown LJ, Löe H (1997b) Clinical features of early-onset periodontitis. *J Am Dent Assoc* **128**: 1393–9.

Albandar JM, Kingman A, Brown LJ, Löe H (1998) Gingival inflammation and subgingival calculus as determinants of disease progression in early-onset periodontitis. *J Clin Periodontol* **25**: 231–7.

Ashraphi MH, Durr DP, Duncan WK (1981) Inter-relationship between stainless steel crown, plaque accumulation and gingival health. *American Academy of Pedodontics Annual Meeting Reports*, Research Abstract R-26.

Asikainen S, Lai CH, Alauusua S, Slots J (1991) Distribution of *Actinobacillus actinomycetemcomitans* serotypes in periodontal health and disease. *Oral Microbiol Immunol* **6**: 115–18.

Asikainen S, Chen C, Slots J (1995) *Actinobacillus actinomycetemcomitans* genotypes in relation to serotypes and periodontal status. *Oral Microbiol Immunol* **10**: 65–8.

Baab DA, Page RC, Morton T (1985) Studies of a family manifesting premature exfoliation of deciduous teeth. *J Periodontol* **56**: 403–9.

Baer PN (1971) The case for periodontosis as a clinical entity. *J Periodontol* **42**: 516–20.

Baer PN, Benjamin S (1974) *Periodontal Diseases in Children and Adolescents*. Philadelphia: JP Lippincott.

Basu MK, Dutta AM (1963) Report of "Prevalence of periodontal disease in the adult population in Calcutta," by Ramfjord's technique. *J All-India Dent Assoc* **35**: 187–201.

Benn DK (1990) A review of the reliability of radiographic measurement in estimating alveolar bone changes. *J Clin Periodontol* **17**: 14–21.

Bernick S, Rutherford RL, Rabinowitch BZ (1951) The role of the epithelial attachment in tooth resorption of primary teeth. *Oral Surg Oral Med Oral Path* **4**: 1444–50.

Berthold P, Forti D, Kieba IR et al. (1992) Electron immunocytochemical localization of *Actinobacillus actinomycetemcomitans* leukotoxin. *Oral Microbiol Immunol* **7**: 24–7.

Bial JJ, Mellonig JT (1987) Radiographic evaluation of juvenile periodontitis (periodontosis). *J Periodontol* **58**: 321–6.

Bimstein E (1992) Frequency of alveolar bone loss adjacent to proximal caries in the primary molars and healing due to restoration of the teeth. *Pediatr Dent* **14**: 30–3.

Bimstein E (1995) Radiographic diagnosis of the normal alveolar bone height in the primary dentition. *J Clin Pediatr Dent* **19**: 269–71.

Bimstein E, Garcia-Godoy F (1994) The significance of age, proximal caries, gingival inflammation, probing depths and the loss of lamina dura in the diagnosis of alveolar bone loss in the primary molars. *ASDC J Dent Child* **61**: 125–8.

Bimstein E, Matsson L (1999) Growth and development considerations in the diagnosis of gingivitis and periodontitis in children. *Pediatr Dent* **21**: 186–91.

Bimstein E, Soskolne WA (1988) A radiographic study of interproximal alveolar bone crest between primary molars in children. *ASDC J Dent Child* **55**: 348–50.

Bimstein E, Lustmann J, Soskolne WA (1985) A clinical and histometric study of gingivitis associated with human deciduous dentition. *J Periodontol* **56**: 293–6.

Bimstein E, Delaney JE, Sweeney EA (1988a) Radiographic assessment of the alveolar bone loss in children and adolescents. *Pediatr Dent* **10**: 199–204.

Bimstein E, Soskolne WA, Lustmann J et al. (1988b) Gingivitis in the human deciduous dentition: a correlative clinical and block surface light microscopic (BSLM) study. *J Clin Periodontol* **15**: 575–80.

Bimstein E, Shanzer Y, Sgan-Cohen H (1989) Prevalence and severity of gingivitis in children aged 13–14 years in Jerusalem. *Commun Dent Oral Epidemiol* **17**: 331–2.

Bimstein E, Shapira L, Landau E, Sela MN (1993) The relationship between alveolar bone loss and proximal caries in children: prevalence and microbiology. *ASDC J Dent Child* **60**: 99–103.

Bimstein E, Treasure ET, Williams SM, Denver JG (1994) Alveolar bone loss in 5-year old New Zealand children: its prevalence and relationship to caries prevalence. Socioeconomic status and ethnic origin. *J Clin Periodontol* **21**: 447–50.

Bimstein E, Zaidenberg R, Soskolne AW (1996a) Alveolar bone loss and restorative dentistry in the primary molars. *J Clin Pediatr Dent* **21**: 51–4.

Bimstein E, Ram D, Naor R, Sela MN (1996b) The composition of subgingival microflora in two groups of children with and without primary dentition alveolar bone loss. *Pediatr Dent* **18**: 42–7.

Bimstein E, Sela MN, Shapira L (1997) Clinical and microbial considerations for the treatment of an extended kindred with seven cases of prepubertal periodontitis: a 2-year follow-up. *Pediatr Dent* **19**: 396–403.

Bimstein E, Wagner M, Nauman RK et al. (1998) Root surface characteristics of primary teeth from children with prepubertal periodontitis. *J Periodontol* **69**: 337–47.

Blankenstein R, Murray JJ, Lind OP (1978) Prevalence of chronic periodontitis in 13–15-year-old children. A radiographic study. *J Clin Periodontol* **10**: 37–45.

Boughman JA, Halloran SL, Roulston D et al. (1986) An autosomal-dominant form of juvenile periodontitis: its localization to chromosome 4 and linkage to dentino-genesis imperfecta and Gc. *J Craniofac Genet Dev Biol* **6**: 341–50.

Brown LJ, Albandar JM, Brunelle JA, Löe H (1996) Early-onset periodontitis: progression of attachment loss during 6 years. *J Periodontol* **67**: 968–75.

Brunsvold MA, Lane JJ (1990) The prevalence of overhanging dental restorations and their relationship to periodontal disease. *J Clin Periodontol* **17**: 67–72.

Buckley LA (1986) A radiographic study of alveolar bone loss in Irish schoolchildren. *J Ir Dent Assoc* **32**: 11–12.

Butler JH (1969) A familial pattern of juvenile periodontitis (periodontosis). *J Periodontol* **40**: 115–18.

Carlos JP, Wolfe JJ, Zambon JJ, Kingman A (1988) Periodontal disease in adolescents: some clinical and microbiologic correlates of attachment loss. *J Dent Res* **67**: 1510–14.

Carranza F, Garcia-Godoy F, Bimstein E (1998) Prevalence of marginal alveolar bone loss in children attending a university dental clinic in Mexico. *J Clin Pediatr Dent* **23**: 51–3.

Caton J (1989) Periodontal diagnosis and diagnostic aids. *Proceedings of the World Workshop in Clinical Periodontics*. Chicago: American Academy of Periodontology; 1:1–1:22.

Celenligil H, Kansu E, Eratalay K, Yavuzyilmaz E (1987) Prepubertal periodontitis. A case report with an analysis of lymphocyte populations. *J Clin Periodontol* **14**: 85–8.

Cianciola LJ, Genco RJ, Patters MR et al. (1977) Defective polymorphonuclear leukocyte function in human periodontal disease. *Nature* **265**: 445–7.

Clark R, Page RC, Wilde G (1977) Defective neutrophil chemotaxis in juvenile periodontitis. *Infect Immun* **18**: 694–700.

Clerehugh V (1991) Periodontal disease in children and adolescents. *Dent Update* **18**: 230–8.

Clerehugh V, Lennon MA (1984) The attachment level as a measure of early periodontitis. *Commun Dent Health* **1**: 33–40.

Clerehugh V, Lennon MA, Worthington HV (1990) 5-year results of a longitudinal study of early perio-dontitis in 14- to 19-year-old adolescents. *J Clin Periodontol* **17**: 702–8.

Clerehugh V, Worthington HV, Lennon MA, Chandler R (1995) Site progression of loss of attachment over 5 years in 14- to 19-year-old adolescents. *J Clin Periodontol* **22**: 15–21.

Cogen RB, Wright JT, Tate AL (1992) Destructive periodontal disease in healthy children. *J Periodontol* **63**: 761–5.

Crossner CG, Carlson J, Sjodin B et al. (1990) Periodontitis in the primary dentition associated with *Actinobacillus actinomycetemcomitans* infection and leukocyte dysfunction. A 3½ year follow up. *J Clin Periodontol* **17**: 264–7.

D'Angelo M, Margiotta V, Ammatuna P, Sammartino F (1992) Treatment of prepubertal periodontitis. A case report and discussion. *J Clin Periodontol* **19**: 214–19.

Daniel MA, McDonald G, Offenbacher S, Van Dyke TE (1993) Defective signal transduction in localized juvenile periodontitis. *J Periodontol* **64**: 617–21.

Davies AHJ, Downer MC, Lennon MA (1978) Periodontal bone loss in English secondary school children. A longitudinal radiological study. *J Clin Periodontol* **5**: 278–84.

Davis RM, Smith RG, Porter SR (1985) Destructive forms of periodontal disease in adolescents and young adults. *Br Dent J* **158**: 429–36.

Delaney JE (1986) Periodontitis in young children: current perspectives. *Dent Sch Quart* **2**: 7–11.

Delaney JE, Ratzan SK, Kornman KS (1986) Subgingival microbiota associated with puberty: studies of pre-, circum-, and postpubertal human females. *Pediatr Dent* **8**: 268–75.

De Nardin E (1996) The molecular basis for neutrophil dysfunction in early-onset periodontitis. *J Periodontol* **67**: 345–54.

Dibart S, Eftimiadi C, Socransky S et al. (1998a) Rapid evaluation of serum and gingival crevicular fluid immunoglobulin G subclass antibody levels in patients with early-onset periodontitis using checkerboard immunoblotting. *Oral Microbiol Immunol* **13**: 166–72.

Dibart S, Chapple IL, Skobe Z et al. (1998b) Microbiological findings in prepubertal periodontitis. A case report. *J Periodontol* **69**: 1172–5.

Drummond BK, Bimstein E (1995) Prevalence of marginal alveolar bone loss in children referred for treatment to the paediatric clinic at the School of Dentistry, University of Otago. *NZ Dent J* **91**: 138–40.

Durward CS, Wright FAC (1989) The dental health of Indo-Chinese and Australian-born adolescents. *Aust Dent J* **34**: 233–9.

Dzink JL, Tanner ACR, Haffajee AD, Scransky SS (1985) Gram negative species associated with active destruc-tive periodontal lesions. *J Clin Periodontol* **12**: 648–59.

Ebersole JL, Taubman MA, Smith IJ et al. (1982) Human immune responses to oral microorganisms. I. Association of localized juvenile periodontitis (LJP) with serum antibody responses to *Actinobacillus actinomycetemcomitans*. *Clin Exp Immunol* **47**: 43–52.

Ellegaard B, Borregaard N, Ellegaard J (1984) Neutrophil chemotaxis and phagocytosis in juvenile periodontitis. *J Periodont Res* **19**: 261–8.

Firatli E, Gurel N, Efeoglu A, Cebeci I (1996) Generalized prepubertal periodontitis. A report of 4 cases with the immunological findings. *J Clin Periodontol* **23**: 1104–11.

Fives-Taylor P, Meyer D, Mintz K (1996) Virulence factors of the periodontopathogen *Actinobacillus actinomycetemcomitans*. *J Periodontol* **67**: 291–7.

Garguilo AW, Wentz FM, Orban B (1961) Dimensions and relations of the dentogingival junction in humans. *J Periodontol* **32**: 261–7.

Glickman I (1979) *Clinical Periodontology*, 5th edn. Philadelphia: WB Saunders.

Goodson JM, Haffajee AD, Socransky S (1984) The relationship between attachment level loss and alveo-lar bone loss. *J Clin Periodontol* **24**: 348–53.

Gottlieb B (1923) Die diffuse Atrophie des Alveolarknochens. *Z Stomatol* **21**: 195–262.

Gottlieb B (1928) The formation of the periodontal pocket: diffuse atrophy of alveolar bone. *J Am Dent Assoc* **15**: 462–76.

Guelman M, Matsson L, Bimstein E (1988) Periodontal health at first permanent molars adjacent to primary molar stainless steel crowns. *J Clin Periodontol* **15**: 531–3.

Gunsolley JC, Ranney RR, Zambon JJ et al. (1990a) *Actinobacillus actinomycetemcomitans* in families affected with periodontitis. *J Periodontol* **61**: 643–8.

Gunsolley JC, Tew JG, Gooss CM et al. (1990b) Serum antibodies to periodontal bacteria. *J Periodontol* **61**: 612–19.

Gunsolley JC, Califano JV, Koertge TE et al. (1995) Longitudinal assessment of early onset periodontitis. *J Periodontol* **66**: 321–8.

Haffaje AD, Socransky SS, Ebersole JL, Smith DJ (1984) Clinical, microbiological and immunological features associated with treatment of active periodontosis lesions. *J Clin Periodontol* **11**: 600–18.

Hakkarainen K, Ainamo J (1980) Influence of overhanging posterior tooth restorations on alveolar bone height in adults. *J Clin Periodontol* **7**: 114–20.

Hara Y, Aono M, Maeda K et al. (1986) Immunohistological study with peroxidase-antiperoxidase staining in a case of generalized prepubertal periodontitis. *J Periodontol* **57**: 100–3.

Harly AF, Floyd PD (1988) Prevalence of juvenile periodontitis in schoolchildren in Lagos, Nigeria. *Commun Dent Oral Epidemiol* **16**: 299–301.

Hart TC, Marazita ML, Schenkein HA et al. (1991) No female preponderance in juvenile periodontitis after correction for ascertainment bias. *J Periodontol* **62**: 745–9.

Hart TC, Marazita ML, Schenkein HA, Diehl SR (1992) Reinterpretation of the evidence for X-linked dominant inheritance of juvenile periodontitis. *J Periodontol* **63**: 169–73.

Hart TC, Shapira L, Van Dyke TE (1994) Neutrophil defects as risk factors for periodontal diseases. *J Periodontol* **65**: 521–9.

Hausmann E, Allen K, Clerehugh V (1991) What alveolar crest level on a bite-wing radiograph represents bone loss? *J Periodontol* **62**: 570–2.

Jamison HC (1963) Prevalence of periodontal disease of the deciduous teeth. *J Am Dent Assoc* **66**: 207–15.

Jeffcoat MK (1992) Radiographic methods for detection of progressive alveolar bone loss. *J Periodontol* **63**: 367–72.

Jenkins SM, Dummer PM, Addy M (1992) Radiographic evaluation of early periodontal bone loss in adolescents. An overview. *J Clin Periodontol* **19**: 363–6.

Johnson BD, Engel D (1986) Acute necrotizing ulcerative gingivitis. A review of diagnosis, etiology and treatment. *J Periodontol* **57**: 141–51.

Källestål C, Matsson L (1989) Criteria for assessment of interproximal bone loss on bite-wing radiographs in adolescents. *J Clin Periodontol* **16**: 300–4.

Källestål C, Matsson L (1990) Periodontal conditions in a group of Swedish adolescents. (II) Analysis of data. *J Clin Periodontol* **17**: 609–12.

Källestål C, Matsson L, Persson S (1991) Proximal attachment loss in Swedish adolescents. *J Clin Periodontol* **18**: 760–5.

Kalmar JR, Arnold RR, Van Dyke TE (1987) Direct interaction of *Actinobacillus actinomycetemcomitans* with normal and defective (LJP) neutrophils. *J Periodont Res* **22**: 179–81.

Kamma JJ, Lygidakis NA, Nakou M (1998) Subgingival microflora and treatment in prepubertal periodontitis associated with chronic idiopathic neutropenia. *J Clin Periodontol* **25**: 759–65.

Katsuragi K, Takashiba S, Kurihara H, Murayama Y (1994) Molecular basis of leukocyte adhesion molecules in early-onset periodontitis patients with decreased CD11/CD18 expression on leukocytes. *J Periodontol* **65**: 949–57.

Keszthelyi G, Szabó I (1987) Attachment loss in primary molars. *J Clin Periodontol* **14**: 448–51.

Kinane DF, Cullen CF, Johnson FA, Evans CW (1989) Neutrophil chemotactic behaviour in patients with early-onset forms of periodontitis. I. Leading front analysis of Boyden chambers. *J Clin Periodontol* **16**: 242–6.

Kolodrubetz D (1996) Molecular genetics and the analysis of leukotoxin in *A. actinomycetemcomitans*. *J Periodontol* **67**: 309–16.

Kornman KS, Robertson PB (1985) Clinical and microbiological evaluation of therapy for juvenile periodontitis. *J Periodontol* **56**: 443–6.

Kronauer E, Borsa G, Lang NP (1986) Prevalence of incipient juvenile periodontitis at age 16 years in Switzerland. *J Clin Periodontol* **13**: 103–8.

Lally ET, Kieba IR, Golub EE et al. (1996) Structure/function aspects of *Actinobacillus actinomycetemcomitans* leukotoxin. *J Periodontol* **67**: 298–308.

Larjava H, Saxen L, Kosunen T, Gahmberg CG (1984) Chemotaxis and surface glycoproteins of neutrophil granulocytes from patients with juvenile periodontitis. *Arch Oral Biol* **29**: 935–9.

Latcham NL, Powell RN, Jago JD et al. (1983) A radiographic study of chronic periodontitis in 15-year-old Queensland children. *J Clin Periodontol* **10**: 37–45.

Lavine WS, Maderazo EG, Stolman J et al. (1979) Impaired neutrophil chemotaxis in patients with juvenile and rapidly progressing periodontitis. *J Periodont Res* **14**: 10–19.

Lennon MA, Davies RM (1974) Prevalence and distribution of alveolar bone loss in a population of 15-year-old schoolchildren. *J Clin Periodontol* **1**: 175–82.

Linden G, Fleming P, Coulter W, Lynn G (1994) Localized prepubertal periodontitis in a 5-year-old child: investigations and clinical observations over a 3-year period. *Int J Paed Dent* **4**: 47–53.

Lindskog S, Blomlof C (1983) Cementum hypoplasia in teeth affected by juvenile periodontitis. *J Clin Periodontol* **10**: 443–51.

Listgarten MA (1986) Pathogenesis of periodontitis. *J Clin Periodontol* **13**: 418–25.

Listgarten MA, Lai CH, Evian CI (1981) Comparative antibody titres to *Actinobacillus actinomycetemcomitans* in juvenile periodontitis, chronic periodontitis and periodontally healthy subjects. *J Clin Periodontol* **8**: 155–64.

Löe H (1993) Periodontal diseases: a brief historical perspective. *Periodontol 2000* **2**: 7–12.

Löe H, Brown LJ (1991) Early onset periodontitis in the United States of America. *J Periodontol* **62**: 608–16.

Löe H, Theilade E, Jensen SB (1965) Experimental gingivitis in man. *J Periodontol* **36**: 177–87.

Loesche WJ, Syed SA, Schmidt E, Morrison EC (1985) Bacterial profiles of subgingival plaques in periodontitis. *J Periodontol* **56**: 447–56.

López NJ (1992) Clinical, laboratory, and immunological studies of a family with a high prevalence of generalized prepubertal and juvenile periodontitis. *J Periodontol* **63**: 457–68.

Lu H, Wang M, Gunsolley JC et al. (1994) Serum immunoglobulin G subclass concentrations in periodontal healthy and diseased individuals. *Infect Immun* **62**: 1677–82.

Machen E, Rapp R, Baumhammers A, Zullo T (1981) The effect of stainless steel crowns on gingival tissue. *American Academy of Pedodontics Annual Meeting Reports*, Research Abstract R-27.

Machtei EE, Ben-Yehouda A, Zubery Y, Sela BA (1994) Lack of evidence for hypophosphatasia as a factor in the pathogenesis of early-onset periodontitis. *J West Soc Periodontol Periodontal Abstr* **42**: 113–17.

Mandel ID, Gaffar A (1986) Calculus revisited. A review. *J Clin Periodontol* **13**: 249–57.

Mandell RL, Socransky SS (1981) A selective medium for isolation of *Actinobacillus actinomycetemcomitans* and the incidence of the organism in periodontosis. *Infect Immun* **45**: 778–80.

Marazita ML, Burmeister JA, Gunsolley JC et al. (1994) Evidence for autosomal dominant inheritance and race-specific heterogeneity in early onset periodontitis. *J Periodontol* **65**: 623–30.

Matsson L, Hjersing K, Sjodin B (1995) Periodontal conditions in Vietnamese immigrant children in Sweden. *Swed Dent J* **19**: 73–81.

McCall J (1938) Gingival and periodontal disease in children. *J Periodontol* **9**: 7–15.

Miller SC (1948) Precocious advanced alveolar atrophy. *J Periodontol* **19**: 146–58.

Miyazaki H, Hanada N, Andoh MI et al. (1989) Periodontal disease prevalence in different age groups in Japan as assessed according to the CPITN. *Commun Dent Oral Epidemiol* **17**: 71–4.

Moore WEC, Holderman LV, Smibert RM et al. (1982) Bacteriology of severe periodontitis in young adult humans. *Infect Immun* **38**: 182–92.

Moore WEC, Holdeman LV, Cato EP et al. (1985) Comparative bacteriology of juvenile periodontitis. *Infect Immun* **48**: 507–19.

Myers DR (1975) A clinical study of the response of the gingival tissue surrounding stainless steel crowns. *ASCD J Dent Child* **42**: 33–6.

Nabers JM, Meadeor HL, Nabers CL, O'Leary TJ (1964) Chronology, an important factor in the repair of osseous defects. *Periodontics* **2**: 304–7.

Needleman HL, Ku TC, Nelson L et al. (1997) Alveolar bone height of primary and first permanent molars in healthy seven- to nine-year-old children. *ASDC J Dent Child* **64**: 188–96.

Newman HM (1992) The classification of periodontal diseases. In: Newman HM, Ress TD, Kinane DF (eds) *Diseases of the Periodontum*. A pre-IADR Symposium at The Royal College of Physicians and Surgeons in Glasgow. pp. 1–26.

Newman HM, Levers BGH (1979) Tooth eruption and function in an early Anglo-Saxon population. *J R Soc Med* **72**: 341–50.

Newman M, Sims T (1979) The predominant cultivable microbiota of the periodontal abscess. *J Periodontol* **50**: 350–54.

Ngan PWH, Tsai CC, Sweeney E (1984) Advanced periodontitis in the primary dentition: case report. *Pediatr Dent* **7**: 255–8.

Noguchi K, Morita I, Ishikawa I, Murota SI (1988) Impaired polymorphonuclear leukocyte 15–lipoxygenase activity in juvenile and rapidly progressive periodontitis. *Prost Leukot Essent Fatty Acids* **33**: 137–41.

Novak MJ, Novak KF (1996) Early-onset periodontitis. *Curr Opin Periodontol* **3**: 45–58.

Okuda K, Naito Y, Ohta K et al. (1984) Bacteriological study of periodontal lesions in two sisters with juvenile periodontitis and their mother. *Infect Immun* **45**: 118–21.

Orban B, Weinmann JP (1942) Diffuse atrophy of the alveolar bone (periodontosis). *J Periodontol* **13**: 31–45.

Ortman LF, McHenry K, Hausmann E (1982) Relationship between alveolar bone measured by ^{125}I absorptiometry with analysis of standardized radiographs: 2 Bjorn technique. *J Periodontol* **53**: 311–14.

Page RC (1986) Current understanding of the aetiology and progression of periodontal disease. *Int Dent J* **36**: 153–61.

Page RC, Baab DA (1985) A new look at the etiology and pathogenesis of early-onset periodontitis. Cementopathia revisited. *J Periodontol* **57**: 748–51.

Page RC, Schroeder H (1982) *Periodontitis in Man and Other Animals. A Comparative Review.* Basel: Karger.

Page RC, Altman L, Ebersole J et al. (1983a) Rapidly progressive periodontitis—a distinct clinical condition. *J Periodontol* **54**: 197–209.

Page RC, Bowen T, Altman L (1983b) Prepubertal periodontitis. 1. Definition of a clinical disease entity. *J Periodontol* **54**: 257–71.

Page RC, Sims TJ, Geissler F et al. (1984) Abnormal leukocyte motility in patients with early-onset periodontitis. *J Periodont Res* **19**: 591–4.

Page RC, Vandesteen GE, Ebersole JL et al. (1985) Clinical and laboratory studies of a family with a high prevalence of juvenile periodontitis. *J Periodontol* **56**: 602–10.

Papapanou P (1996) Periodontal disease: epidemiology. *Ann Periodontol* **1**: 1–36.

Pederson MM (1989) Chemotactic response of neutrophil polymorphonuclear leukocytes in juvenile periodontitis measured by the leading front method. *Scand J Dent Res* **96**: 421–7.

Pennel BM, Keagle JG (1977) Predisposing factors in the etiology of chronic periodontal disease. *J Periodontol* **48**: 517–32.

Petit MD, Van Steenbergen TJ, De Graaff J, Van der Velden U (1993) Transmission of *Actinobacillus actinomycetemcomitans* in families of adult periodontitis patients. *J Periodont Res* **28**: 335–45.

Pilot T, Barmes DE, Leclercq MH et al. (1987) Periodontal conditions in adolescents, 15–19 years of age: an overview of CPITN data in the WHO Global Oral Data Bank. *Commun Dent Oral Epidemiol* **15**: 386–8.

Ram D, Bimstein E (1994) Subgingival bacteria in a case of prepubertal periodontitis, before and one year after extractions of the affected primary teeth. *J Clin Pediatr Dent* **19**: 45–7.

Ramfjord SP (1961) The periodontal status of boys 11 to 17 years old in Bombay, India. *J Periodontol* **32**: 237–48.

Ranney RR (1991) Diagnosis of periodontal diseases. *Adv Dent Res* **5**: 21–36.

Ranney RR (1993) Classification of periodontal diseases. *Periodontol 2000* **2**: 13–25.

Repo H, Saxen L, Jaatela M et al. (1990) Phagocyte function in juvenile periodontitis. *Infect Immun* **58**: 185–92.

Rodriguez-Ferrer HJ, Strahan JD, Newman HN (1980) Effect on gingival health of removing overhanging margins of interproximal subgingival amalgam restorations. *J Clin Periodontol* **7**: 457–62.

Ruben PM, Shapiro A (1978) Analysis of root surface changes in periodontal disease—a review. *J Periodontol* **48**: 89–91.

Russell AL (1971) The prevalence of periodontal disease in different populations during the circumpubertal period. *J Periodontol* **42**: 508–12.

Sakamoto FO, Hackman A, Horton JE (1984) Familial involvement by aggressive (prepubertal and rapid) forms of periodontal disease [abstr. 312]. *J Dent Res* **63**: 205.

Saxen L (1980a) Juvenile periodontitis. *J Clin Periodontol* **7**: 1–19.

Saxen L (1980b) Prevalence of juvenile periodontitis in Finland. *J Clin Periodontol* **7**: 177–86.

Schenkein HA, Van Dyke TE (1994) Early-onset periodontitis: systemic aspects of etiology and pathogenesis. *Periodontol 2000* **6**: 7–25.

Schenkein HA, Best AM, Gunsolley JC (1991) The influence of race and periodontal clinical status on neutrophil chemotactic responses. *J Periodont Res* **26**: 272–5.

Shapira L, Shmidt A, Van Dyke TE et al. (1994) Sequential manifestation of different forms of early-onset periodontitis. A case report. *J Periodontol* **65**: 631–5.

Shapira L, Tarazi E, Rosen L, Bimstein E (1995) The relationship between alveolar bone height and age in the primary dentition. A retrospective longitudinal radiographic study. *J Clin Periodontol* **22**: 408–12.

Sixou JL, Robert JC, Bonnaure-Mallet M (1997) Loss of deciduous teeth and germs of permanent incisors in a 4-year-old child. An atypic prepubertal periodontitis? A clinical, microbiological, immunological and ultrastructural study. *J Clin Periodontol* **24**: 836–43.

Sjödin B, Matsson L (1992) Marginal bone level in the normal primary dentition. *J Clin Periodontol* **19**: 672–8.

Sjödin B, Matsson L (1994) Marginal bone loss in the primary dentition. A survey of 7–9-year-old children in Sweden. *J Clin Periodontol* **21**: 313–19.

Sjödin B, Crossner CG, Unell L, Östlund P (1989) A retrospective radiographic study of alveolar bone loss in the primary dentition in patients with juvenile periodontitis. *J Clin Periodontol* **16**: 124–7.

Sjödin B, Matsson L, Unell L, Egelberg J (1993) Marginal bone loss in the primary dentition of patients with juvenile periodontitis. *J Clin Periodontol* **20**: 32–6.

Slots J (1982) Importance of black-pigmented *Bacteroides* in human periodontal disease. In: Genco RJ, Mergenhagen SE (eds) *Host-Parasite Interactions in Periodontal Diseases*. Washington: American Society for Microbiology, pp. 27–45.

Soskolne AW, Bimstein E (1977) Histomorphological study of the shedding process of human deciduous teeth at various chronological ages. *Arch Oral Biol* **22**: 331–5.

Soskolne AW, Bimstein E (1989) Apical migration of the junctional epithelium in the human primary dentition. *J Pedodont* **13**: 239–42.

Spektor MD, Vandesteen GE, Page RC (1985) Clinical studies of one family manifesting rapidly progressive, juvenile and prepubertal periodontitis. *J Periodontol* **56**: 93–101.

Stamm JW (1986) Epidemiology of gingivitis. *J Clin Periodontol* **13**: 360–6.

Suzuki JB (1988) Diagnosis and classification of the periodontal diseases. *Dent Clin North Am* **32**: 195–216.

Suzuki JB, Risom L, Falker WA et al. (1985) Effect of periodontal therapy on spontaneous lymphocyte response and neutrophil chemotaxis in localised and generalised juvenile periodontitis. *J Clin Periodontol* **12**: 124–34.

Sweeney EA, Alcoforado GAP, Nyman S, Slots J (1987) Prevalence and microbiology of localized prepubertal periodontitis. *Oral Microbiol Immunol* **2**: 65–70.

Tew JG, Zhang JB, Quinn S et al. (1996) Antibody of the IgG2 subclass, *Actinobacillus actinomycetemcomitans*, and early-onset periodontitis. *J Periodontol* **67**: 317–22.

Thoma KH, Goldman HM (1940) Wandering and elongation of the teeth and pocket formation in paradontosis. *J Am Dent Assoc* **27**: 335–41.

Timmerman MF, Van der Weijden GA, Armand S et al. (1998) Untreated periodontal disease in Indonesian adolescents. Clinical and microbiological baseline data. *J Clin Periodontol* **25**: 215–24.

Tyagi SR, Uhlinger DJ, Lambeth JD et al. (1992) Altered diacylglycerol levels and metabolism in localized juvenile periodontitis neutrophils. *Infect Immun* **60**: 2481–7.

Van der Velden U, Abbas F, Van Steenbergen TJM et al. (1989) Prevalence of periodontal breakdown in adolescents and presence of *Actinobacillus actinomycetemcomitans* in subjects with attachment loss. *J Periodontol* **60**: 604–10.

Van Dyke TE, Hoop GA (1990) Neutrophil function and oral disease. *Crit Rev Oral Bio Med* **1**: 117–33.

Van Dyke TE, Schenkein HA (1996) Research objectives for the study of early-onset periodontitis. A summary of the working groups for the early-onset periodontitis workshop. *J Periodontol* **67**: 279–81.

Van Dyke TE, Horoszewicz HU, Cianciola LJ, Genco RJ (1980) Neutrophil chemotaxis dysfunction in human periodontitis. *Infect Immun* **26**: 124–32.

Van Dyke TE, Levine MJ, Tabak LA, Genco RJ (1981) Reduced chemotactic peptide binding in juvenile periodontitis: a model for neutrophil function. *Biochem Biophys Res Commun* **100**: 1278–84.

Van Dyke TE, Horoszewica HU, Genco RJ (1982) The polymorphonuclear leukocyte (PMNL) locomotor defect in juvenile periodontitis: a study of random migration, chemokinesis and chemotaxis. *J Periodontol* **53**: 682–7.

Van Dyke TE, Levine MJ, Genco RJ (1983) Periodontal disease and neutrophil abnormalities. In: Genco RJ, Mergenhagen SE (eds) *Host–Parasite Interactions in Periodontal Diseases*. Washington: American Society for Microbiology; pp. 235–45.

Van Dyke TE, Schweinebraten M, Cianciola LJ et al. (1985) Neutrophil chemotaxis in families with localized juvenile periodontitis. *J Periodont Res* **20**: 503–14.

Van Dyke TE, Wilson-Burrows C, Offenbacher S, Henson P (1987) Association of an abnormality of neutrophil chemotaxis in human periodontal disease with a cell surface protein. *Infect Immun* **55**: 2262–7.

Van Dyke TE, Warbington M, Gardnner M et al. (1990) Neutrophil surface protein markers as indicators of defective chemotaxis in LJP. *J Periodontol* **61**: 180–4.

Van Steenbergen TJ, van der Velden U, Abbas F, de Graaff J (1993) Microbiological and clinical monitoring of non-localized juvenile periodontitis in young adults: a report of 11 cases. *J Periodontol* **64**: 40–7.

Van Winkelhoff AJ, de Groot P, Abbas F, de Graaff J (1994) Quantitative aspects of the subgingival distribution of *Actinobacillus actinomycetemcomitans* in a patient with localized juvenile periodontitis. *J Clin Periodontol* **21**: 199–202.

Vincent JW, Suzuki JB, Fakler WA Jr, Cornett WC (1985) Reaction of human sera from juvenile periodontitis, rapidly progressive and adult periodontitis patients with selected periodontopathogens. *J Periodontol* **56**: 464–9.

Waite IM, Furniss JS, Wong WM (1994) Relationship between clinical periodontal condition and the radiographic appearance at 1st molar sites in adolescents. *J Clin Periodontol* **21**: 155–60.

Waldrop TC, Anderson DC, Hallmon WC et al. (1987) Periodontal manifestations of the heritable MAC-1, LFA-1 deficiency syndrome—clinical, histopathologic, and molecular characteristics. *J Periodontol* **58**: 400–16.

Wannenmacher E (1938) Umschau auf dem Gebiete der Paradentose. *Dtsch Zahnarztl Mund Kieferheilk* **3**: 81–96.

Watanabe K (1990) Prepubertal periodontitis: a review of diagnostic criteria, pathogenesis, and differential diagnosis. *J Periodont Res* **25**: 31–48.

Watanabe K (1991) Generalized juvenile periodontitis in a thirteen-year-old child. *ASDC J Dent Child* **58**: 390–5.

Watanabe K, Lambert LA, Niederman LG et al. (1991) Analysis of neutrophil chemotaxis and CD11b expression in pre-pubertal periodontitis. *J Dent Res* **70**: 102–6.

Webber DL (1974) Gingival health following placement of stainless steel crowns. *J Child Dent* **41**: 186–9.

Wei SHY, Yang S, Barmes DE (1986) Needs and implementation of preventive dentistry in China. *Commun Dent Oral Epidemiol* **14**: 19–23.

Wilson ME, Kalmar JR (1996) FcγRIIa (CD 32): a potential marker defining susceptibility to localized juvenile periodontitis. *J Periodontol* **67**: 323–31.

Wolfe MD, Carlos JP (1987) Periodontal disease in adolescents: epidemiologic findings in Navajo Indians. *Commun Dent Oral Epidemiol* **15**: 33–40.

Yoshida-Minami I, Kishimoto K, Suzuki A et al. (1995) Clinical, microbiological and host defense parameters associated with a case of localized prepubertal periodontitis. *J Clin Periodontol* **22**: 56–62.

Zambon JJ, Christersson LA, Slots J (1983) *Actinobacillus actinomycetemcomitans* in human periodontal disease: prevalence in patient groups and distribution of biotypes within families. *J Periodontol* **54**: 707–11.

Zambon JJ, Haraszthy VI, Hariharan G, Lally ET, Demuth DR (1996) The microbiology of early-onset periodontitis: association of highly toxic *Actinobacillus actinomycetemcomitans* strains with localized juvenile periodontitis. *J Periodontol* **67**: 282–90.

6

The relationship between periodontitis and systemic diseases and conditions in children, adolescents, and young adults

Roy C. Page, Tom J. Sims, Andrew J. Delima, Enrique Bimstein, Howard L. Needleman, and Thomas E. Van Dyke

There are valid reasons for including a chapter on the relationship between periodontal disease and systemic diseases and conditions in a book focusing on periodontal health and disease in children, adolescents, and young adults. It is during childhood and young adulthood that the foundations are laid for either lifelong periodontal and general health, or development of periodontal and systemic diseases later in life. While it has long been known that certain systemic diseases such as diabetes mellitus significantly enhance the risk of development of periodontitis, it has also been shown that having periodontitis, especially at a young age, significantly enhances the risk of several systemic diseases and conditions including low birth-weight infants, atherosclerosis, heart attack, stroke, complications of diabetes mellitus, and osteoporosis and pneumonia in the elderly.

While bacteria are essential for the development of periodontitis, bacteria alone are insufficient; a susceptible host is also necessary (Page, 1998). It is now clear that environmental, acquired, and genetic factors that enhance risk are the major determinants of the probability of onset of adult periodontitis and its progress and severity. Notably, roughly half of the risk of developing periodontitis later in life is genetically determined (Michalowicz, 1994) and therefore is present in childhood. Tobacco smoking, a habit that is most frequently acquired during childhood or young adulthood, outweighs by far all other acquired and environmental factors that enhance risk for adult periodontitis (Page, 1998).

Systemic diseases and conditions that enhance the risk of periodontitis

Many systemic diseases and conditions, often genetically transmitted, enhance the risk of periodontitis (Table 6.1). The association between these diseases and periodontitis has been reviewed (Sofaer, 1990; Löe, 1993; Oliver and Tervonen, 1993).

A notable characteristic of all of these entities (except Ehlers–Danlos syndrome and hypophosphatasia) is abnormal phagocytic cell function, especially neutrophil function. It is well documented that the phagocytic cells, especially neutrophils, operating in conjunction with

Table 6.1 Genetically transmitted traits predisposing for periodontitis.

Cyclic neutropenia	Chédiak–Higashi syndrome
Chronic idiopathic neutropenia	Diabetes mellitus
Papillon–Lefèvre syndrome	Trisomy 21
Leukocyte adherence deficiency	Ehlers–Danlos syndrome
	Hypophosphatasia

specific antibody and complement, are the primary host defense against the microbial challenge presented by pathogenic bacteria in dental plaque and subgingival microbial biofilms (Page, 1998). It seems likely that abnormalities in phagocytic cell function may be the common thread linking these diseases to an enhanced risk of periodontitis. Although there are several possible mechanisms linking periodontitis and diabetes mellitus, many diabetic patients also manifest abnormalities in neutrophil function which make them more susceptible to periodontal and other infections.

Diabetes mellitus

Diabetes mellitus and its complications are major disease problems, affecting 30–40 million persons in the USA. The American Academy of Periodontology has taken the following position regarding an association between diabetes mellitus and periodontal disease (AAP, 1996):

> The incidence of periodontitis increases among diabetic subjects after puberty and as the patient population ages. Periodontal disease may be more frequent and severe in diabetic individuals with more advanced systemic complications. Increased suscepti-bility does not correlate with levels of plaque and calculus. There is a relationship between periodontal disease and diabetes mellitus especially in patients with poorly controlled disease or hyperglycemia.

An association between diabetes and periodontitis has been long suspected and has now been reasonably well documented for both type 1 insulin-dependent diabetes mellitus (IDDM) and type 2 non-insulin-dependent diabetes mellitus (NIDDM). An imbalance in blood glucose levels which occurs in some children and adolescents with type 1 diabetes appears to predispose to gingival inflammation (Karfalainen and Knuuttila, 1996). In a study of 263 type 1 diabetes patients, 59 non-diabetic siblings, and 149 non-diabetic controls, Cianciola et al. (1982) observed an increased risk for development of periodontitis with age; the sever-ity of disease increased with increasing duration of diabetes. Diabetic subjects under poor metabolic control lost more attachment and bone than well-controlled patients. The same

conclusions were reached by Firatli (1997) in a study of 44 type 1 diabetes children and adoles-cents and 20 healthy control subjects over 5 years. Similarly, Thorstensson (1995) observed that a greater proportion of individuals with type 1 diabetes manifested advanced periodontal disease, and advanced disease appeared at an earlier age than in non-diabetic individuals. In addition, diabetic patients with advanced periodontitis had a higher prevalence of renal disease and cardiovascular complications includ-ing angina, myocardial infarct and stroke than diabetic patients with minor periodontal disease (Thorstensson et al., 1996).

Similar results are reported for individuals with type 2 diabetes. In a study of Pima Indians (N = 3219), Shlossman et al. (1990) found that irrespective of age, subjects with type 2 diabetes were 2.8 times more likely than non-diabetic subjects to have periodontal disease as defined by clinical attachment loss, and 3.4 times more likely to exhibit disease as defined by radio-graphic bone loss. In the same population, for individuals 15 years of age and older, prevalence of periodontal disease was 60% for diabetics compared with 36% in non-diabetics (Nelson et al., 1990). The rate of development of periodon-titis was 2.6 times that seen in non-diabetic subjects. More recently, Collin et al. (1998) reported 40% of a group of 25 type 2 diabetic patients 58–76 years of age had advanced periodontitis compared with 12.5% of 40 non-diabetic controls. As pointed out by Soskolne (1998), much of our knowledge about periodon-titis in type 2 diabetes comes from studies of the Pima Indians who have an extraordinarily high prevalence of type 2 diabetes and a high preva-lence of severe periodontitis even among non-diabetic individuals. Those data, therefore, may not be generalizable to other populations.

In children with type 1 diabetes lacking adequate metabolic control, periodontal compli-cations usually start with the onset of gingivitis in the circumpubertal period. Without diligent intervention to reduce the presence of microbial plaque on the teeth, caries and severe periodon-titis may follow. In addition to destructive inflam-matory responses to microbial etiologic agents that are linked with all forms of periodontitis, systemic manifestations of the diabetes such as microangiopathy, impaired immune response, abnormal collagen metabolism, and enhanced matrix metalloproteinases activity may also contribute to the pathogenesis of diabetes-associated periodontal disease. Furthermore, observed differences in the flow rate and composition of the saliva in children with type 1 diabetes relative to healthy controls may explain in part why they are at greater risk of developing caries and periodontal infections. Saliva from children with type 1 diabetes is higher in peroxidase, glucose, magnesium, and calcium, while the pH, flow rate, and buffer capacity are lower, compared with healthy controls. Because these conditions may increase plaque accumulation, instruction in oral hygiene and frequent visits to the dentist to deal with calculus and plaque should be part of the overall treatment plan for these children (Iughetti et al., 1999).

The pathogenesis of diabetes mellitus and periodontitis involves both environmental and genetic factors. The common pathogenic mechanism in all forms of diabetes mellitus is an absolute or relative lack of insulin resulting in hyperglycemia or an inability of cells in various tissues to utilize insulin. In the case of periodontitis, all forms of the disease involve the destruction of tissues supporting the teeth through the activation of host-derived mediators of inflammation by toxic components of Gram-negative bacteria found in subgingival biofilms (Page and Kornman, 1997). Genetic predisposition of the host is an apparent prerequisite of pathogenesis in both periodontitis and diabetes mellitus. For example, in the case of periodontitis, individuals with a specific polymorphism in genes coding for interleukin-1 have greatly enhanced risk of development of adult periodontitis (Kornman et al., 1997). However, in the absence of microbial challenge coupled with other environmental factors such as smoking, the genetically susceptible individual may remain healthy. In the case of type 1 diabetes, genetic susceptibility is linked with the HLA system (specifically the HLA *DR* and *DQ* alleles), but pathogenesis in individuals genetically predisposed to type 1 diabetes will not start in the absence of environmental factors such as viral infections, early exposure to certain dietary constituents (cow's milk), and other acquired factors that initiate destructive autoimmune responses against the insulin-producing β cells of the pancreas.

Genetic factors are even more important in type 2 diabetes, but they are not linked with the HLA system. There appears to be a strong racial component in the patterns of genetic susceptibility to type 2 diabetes (Löe, 1993; Martin-Iverson et al., 1999). In this form of diabetes genetic susceptibility is related to certain secretory disorders and/or insulin resistance, while obesity, due in part to diet, is strongly linked with intensification of these problems (Felig et al., 1995). The role of diabetes as a risk factor for periodontitis therefore may involve both environmental and genetic components.

Although there is sufficient evidence to conclude that diabetes is a risk factor for severe periodontitis (Löe, 1993), the role that severe periodontitis may play in exacerbating diabetes or making metabolic control of the disease more difficult is poorly understood and not well documented. However, a recently proposed hypothetical model seems plausible based on what is known about the involvement of mediators of inflammation in the pathogenesis of both diseases (Grossi and Genco, 1998). The advanced glycation end-products (AGE) that occur in people with diabetes are the result of the non-enzymatic reaction of glucose with proteins such as collagen and hemoglobin. Production of AGE is accelerated by hyperglycemia. The macrophage is the primary cell type involved in cytokine synthesis in both periodontitis and diabetes mellitus. The Gram-negative bacteria and substances derived from them such as lipopolysaccharide (LPS) may chronically upregulate cytokine synthesis and this may amplify production of the destructive cytokines. In the case of diabetes, cytokine synthesis and release is stimulated when the receptor for glycation end-products (RAGE) on the macrophage surface binds AGE. The proponents of this model suggest that this dual pathway of Gram-negative bacterial infection and cytokine upregulation could explain the increase in tissue destruction seen in patients with diabetes-associated periodontitis, and it could also explain how chronic periodontal infection could amplify the severity of diabetes and hamper metabolic control. As pointed out by Lalla et al. (1998), the role of AGE–RAGE interactions in diabetic periodontitis could be elucidated using murine models in which RAGE expression has been genetically altered.

There is general agreement that diabetes is a true risk factor for severe periodontitis and that periodontitis is a serious complication of diabetes (Löe, 1993). The American Dental Association recently put forth a consensus report, which outlined and interpreted the current research literature. The panel of experts stated:

> The biomedical literature supports the conclusion that diabetes is associated with a reduced ability to cope with infections and impaired wound healing. These alterations are associated with both genetic and metabolic factors. The periodontal disease literature in this area is limited. PMN dysfunction in IDDM appears to be linked to the severity of periodontal disease. The medical literature indicates that resolution of infection improves diabetic control. Limited data show that initial therapy of periodontal disease may have at least a transient beneficial effect on the metabolic control of diabetes.
>
> (ADA, 1998)

Although conventional periodontal therapy is considered to be effective in diabetic patients, not all experts believe a convincing case has been made that periodontal therapy has clinically significant effects on metabolic control of diabetes (Gustke, 1999).

Human immunodeficiency virus infection and AIDS

The acquired immune deficiency syndrome (AIDS) is a defined pathologic entity caused by infection with a retrovirus—human immunodeficiency virus (HIV). Infection with HIV has been found in increasing prevalence in children and adolescents since 1983 (Oleske et al., 1983; Shannon and Ammann, 1985); although much information is available for adult populations (Murray, 1994), there are relatively few reports on younger cohorts. However, this group seems to be rapidly growing because more HIV-infected women are of childbearing age (Pizzo, 1990).

The virus preferentially attacks the immune system, specifically lymphocytes and macrophages, and renders them non-functional. This causes a progressive and eventually irreversible immunosuppression that allows a variety of potentially fatal opportunistic infections, malignancies, and rare autoimmune diseases to occur. Early symptoms of HIV infection in infants may be weight loss and failure to thrive, chronic diarrhea, lymphadenopathy, hepatosplenomegaly, oral

candidiasis, interstitial pneumonitis, and recurrent infections. Neurological disturbances have also been reported in children with HIV (Black, 1985; Epstein et al., 1985; Ho et al., 1985). Marion et al. (1986) described developmental abnormalities in the facial features of HIV-infected infants which may include a prominent forehead, flat bridge of the nose, long palpebral fissures, a prominent triangular philtrum, microencephaly, and a prominent upper lip.

Oral lesions in HIV-infected patients are of diagnostic importance, since they are common and may often be the first clinical symptoms of the disease. Findings include salivary gland enlargement, sialoadenitis, herpes labialis, buccal petechiae (Valdez et al., 1994) and increased caries rate (Valdez et al., 1994; Madigan et al., 1996; Vieira et al., 1998). The most common oral manifestation of HIV in infected children is oral candidiasis (OC) (Ketchem et al., 1990; Tovo et al., 1992; Katz et al., 1993; Moniaci et al., 1993; Ramos-Gomez et al., 1996). There are four major types of OC: pseudomembranous, hyperplastic, erythematous, and angular cheilitis, with the pseudomembranous type most commonly seen. Oral candidiasis in children with AIDS tends to be chronic or frequently recurring and is refractory to antifungal therapy (Ketchem et al., 1990; Leggott, 1992). The prominent species of *Candida* in OC of HIV/AIDS patients is *Candida albicans*, followed by several other *Candida* species, including *C. glabrata*, *C. tropicalis*, *C. parapsilosis*, *C. dubliniensis* and *C. krusei*. *Candida* has also been isolated from the subgingival flora of AIDS patients (Zambon et al., 1990).

According to the EEC Clearinghouse on Oral Problems Related to HIV Infection (EEC, 1990, 1993), three major forms of periodontal diseases are strongly correlated with HIV infection: linear gingival erythema (LGE), necrotic ulcerative gingivitis (NUG), and necrotic ulcerative periodontitis (NUP). Although these destructive entities are commonly seen in adults, it is debatable whether they affect children and adolescents. Gingivitis in HIV-positive children has been described (Moniaci et al., 1993; Vieira et al., 1998), yet other reports found no increased incidence (Schoen et al., 1995; Valdez et al., 1994). It is also believed that severe periodontal lesions do not occur in HIV-positive children

(Ketchem et al., 1990; Moniaci et al., 1993; Fonseca, 1996; Schoen et al., 1995). However, San Martin et al. (1992) demonstrated HIV gingivitis and HIV periodontitis in HIV-infected children, and Soubry et al. (1995) chronicled 84 cases of necrotizing periodontal disease in 84 patients. Differences in these studies may be due to the cohorts studied or the parameters used to measure the disease, but continued research clearly is needed to prove a link between HIV/AIDS infection and destructive periodontal disease in children and adolescents.

Tobacco use and drug abuse

There is a well-documented link between smoking and periodontal disease. Arno et al. (1959) found an increase in alveolar bone loss with increasing amounts of smoking. Several recent studies found cigarette smoking to be one of the most important risk factors for the development of periodontal disease (Locker and Leake, 1992; Bergstrom and Preber, 1994; Grossi et al., 1994). Smoking also has a detrimental effect on healing following both non-surgical and surgical therapies (Cortellini et al., 1996; Kaldahl et al., 1996).

The relationship between smokeless tobacco and oral cancer has been well documented (Wray and McGuirt, 1993), but its role in destructive periodontal disease is much more controversial. Individual cases of gingivitis, gingival recession, and periodontitis have been reported in habitual smokeless tobacco users (Christen et al., 1979; Hoge and Kirkham, 1983; Offenbacher and Weathers, 1985; Cullen et al., 1986; Robertson et al., 1990). One study reported a significant increase in localized areas of periodontal destruction (Robertson et al., 1990) usually on mandibular buccal areas adjacent to the site of habitual placement of tobacco in the buccal vestibule. Therefore, chronic assaults of smokeless tobacco may play a role in this localized attachment loss. This is important because of the resurgence in popularity of smokeless tobacco, particularly among adolescent males (Connolly et al., 1986; Creath et al., 1991).

Recreational drug usage is an increasing problem affecting people of all ages and socio-economic backgrounds. Two particularly popular agents of abuse are cocaine and cannabis. Oral usage of cocaine may cause gingival erosions, epithelial damage, and periodontitis in some cases (Dello Russo and Temple, 1982; Gargiulo et al., 1985; Yukna, 1991; Parry et al., 1996). Likewise, excessive marijuana intake results in gingival enlargement and possibly alveolar bone loss (Darling and Arendorf, 1992). The mechanisms of tissue destruction have not been investigated.

Stress

Periodontal diseases are thought to represent bacterial infections of pathogenic species that colonize the gingival crevice. However, it is evident that systemic and local factors may modify the host's response to the presence of these periopathogens. Psychosocial factors may represent another group of modifiers that can alter the host's capacity to contend effectively with these noxious bacteria. Stress can be defined as a condition of altered or threatened homeostasis (Chrousos and Gold, 1992) and it may represent a significant disruptive force in the homeostatic regulation between the oral flora and the host immune system (Genco, 1992; Seymour et al., 1993; Ainamo and Ainamo, 1996; Breivik et al., 1996).

There has been increasing interest in the link between psychosocial attributes and periodontitis. Green et al. (1986) demonstrated an association between negative, stressful life events and periodontal disease severity. Unfortunately, the study was not controlled and other modifying factors such as smoking status, age, and oral hygiene levels were not taken into account by the authors. da Silva et al. (1995) in a controlled study found that subjects with severe periodontitis had an elevated incidence of depression and psychosocial stress. Linden et al. (1996) related increasing attachment level loss to occupational stress factors, while Freeman and Goss (1993) demonstrated a similar relation between stress and pocket probing depth. Axtelius et al. (1998) tested the role of a stress system disorder (Chrousos and Gold, 1992) in the pathogenesis of therapy-resistant periodontitis, and showed that individuals who were not responsive to periodontal treatment displayed elevated levels of psychosocial tension and a passive-dependent personality. This suggests that stress factors may also play a role in periodontal disease that is not responsive to therapy.

Genco and co-workers, in a cross-sectional study, followed 1426 patients aged 25–74 years in Erie County, New York (Genco et al., 1998, 1999). They attempted to evaluate a relationship between levels of stress, emotional distress, and coping behaviors, and the severity of periodontal disease. The large cohort was adjusted for known periodontal risk factors, including age, sex, systemic health, smoking, and level of oral hygiene. They found that financial strain and emotional depression are additional risk factors for more severe periodontal disease. They also suggested that patients with adequate coping behaviors in comparison with those with highly emotion-focused behavior (an inadequate form of coping behavior) could potentially neutralize this stress-related risk.

The mechanism by which psychosocial stress can detrimentally influence oral health has yet to be fully elucidated, but Ballieux (1991) noted that psychosocial factors can influence immune functions by two distinct pathways: the nervous "wiring system", and the "soluble connection" of the neuroendocrine system. How stress affects these two pathways is still largely unknown.

Genco et al. (1998) believes that two different models may explain how stress can influence the response to infectious agents. The first is a biologic model, in which stress affects the hypothalamic–pituitary–adrenal axis to cause hormonal changes. The second is a behavioral model, in which stress leads to detrimental behavioral changes such as smoking and cessation of oral hygiene practices.

Leukemias

The leukemias comprise a group of malignant neoplasias characterized by an uncontrolled proliferation of leukocytic stem cells. Normal bone marrow is progressively replaced by proliferating neoplastic leukemic cells. In most cases, high levels of abnormal immature white cells are found in the circulating blood and may infiltrate the liver, spleen, lymph nodes, and other tissues throughout the body (Robbins et al., 1989).

The leukemias are classified according to the cell type of origin and as acute or chronic. Both lymphocytic and myelocytic cell types can become leukemic and both can be acute or chronic. Monocytic leukemia is extremely rare. Acute leukemias typically have a rapid clinical course and, without effective treatment, result in death within a few months; they mostly occur in individuals under the age of 20 years or over the age of 60 years. Chronic leukemias are characterized by relatively well-differentiated leukocytes and a prolonged clinical course, and typically occur in individuals over 40 years of age.

Oral manifestations in chronic leukemia are rare; the following descriptions refer almost exclusively to acute leukemia. Oral manifestations are more commonly found in non-lymphocytic leukemias. Although acute leukemia is the most commonly occurring form in childhood, it is least likely to produce oral lesions. Symptoms include local lymphadenopathy, mucous membrane petechiae and ecchymoses, gingival bleeding and hypertrophy, pallor, and nonspecific ulceration—see Figure 1.7a (Lynch and Ship, 1967; Curtis, 1971; Michaud et al., 1977).

Leukemic cells are capable of infiltrating the gingiva and (less frequently) the deeper periodontal tissues. The gingival infiltration of the corium can lead to leukemic gingival hyperplasia, resulting in gingival pockets, which can become inflamed and deepen when colonized by bacteria. The gingiva may appear cyanotic, with blunting of the gingival margins and hyperplasia beginning in the interproximal papillae. Gingival bleeding is a common finding; it is secondary to thrombocytopenia resulting from the replacement of the normal bone marrow by leukemic cells. Lynch and Ship (1967) reported oral bleeding as a presenting sign in 17.7% of patients with acute leukemia and in 4.4% of those with chronic leukemia. The bleeding tendency found in leukemic patients may also be manifested as petechiae distributed throughout the alveolar mucosa. Granulocytopenia, which develops secondarily to leukemia, results in a decreased resistance to pathogenic microorganisms and leads to ulceration and infection of the oral tissues.

Carranza et al. (1965) and Brown et al. (1969) investigated the periodontal changes in a murine model, using mice that spontaneously develop leukemia. They reported the presence of an infiltrate in the periodontal ligament (PDL), resulting in destruction of the alveolar bone, disappearance of the periodontal fibers, and exfoliation of the teeth. The disease follows a similar course in humans where generalized loss of trabeculation in the bone, loss of the lamina dura, widening of the PDL space, displacement of developing tooth buds, and possible exfoliation of the teeth may occur (Worth, 1966; Curtis, 1971; Roistacher, 1973).

Neutropenia and agranulocytosis

Normal, healthy individuals have circulating neutrophil counts between 5000 cells/mm³ and 10 000 cells/mm³ (5–10 × 10⁹/l). A person is considered neutropenic if the number of circulating neutrophils decreases to below 2000 cells/mm³ (2 × 10⁹/l). Agranulocytosis occurs if this count drops below 500 cells/mm³ (0.5 × 10⁹/l) (Zancharski et al., 1971). Neutropenia and agranulocytosis can be symptoms of systemic disease or pathologic conditions in their own right. The causes of these entities are diverse: drug-induced, radiation-induced, disease- or infection-induced, or autoimmune responses directed against the neutrophil. Most systemic neutropenias appear to be idiopathic, but may have a genetic component. Individuals with neutropenia or agranulocytosis manifest a greatly enhanced risk for destructive generalized periodontitis (Baehni et al., 1983; Lamster et al., 1987; Carrassi et al., 1989; Stabholz et al., 1990; Van Dyke and Hoop, 1990; Hart et al., 1994).

Recurrent infections and severe periodontitis have been observed in patients with chronic idiopathic neutropenia and cyclic neutropenia (Vaughn et al., 1990). Cyclic neutropenia is a disease of unknown etiology characterized by a regular 7–day period of depression in the number of the neutrophils, occurring every 21 days. Patients have recurrent fever, malaise, mucosal ulcers, and episodes of life-threatening infections. Oral manifestations include oral mucosal ulceration, severe gingivitis, and periodontitis (Cohen and Morris, 1961; Chadwick et al., 1989). The periodontal destruction can affect both the primary and permanent dentition (Prichard et al., 1984) and can lead to premature exfoliation of teeth. Periodontal destruction is usually more severe if the cyclic neutropenia starts in infancy and childhood.

Agranulocytosis is characterized by high fever, prostration, and necrotic lesions of the mouth, rectum, and vagina. Some cases are idiopathic and are considered a rarity; more commonly the disease is a secondary manifestation of drugs or radiation. Oral symptoms consist of hyperplastic, severely inflamed gingiva. Radiographs demonstrated extensive bone loss around the first molars and incisors. The oral manifestations vary between gingivitis and severe periodontitis and there is a potential for loss of primary teeth (Bauer, 1946; Zubery et al., 1991).

Langerhans cell histiocytosis

The histiocytoses are a puzzling group of diseases which present as a result of the accumulation and/or proliferation of one of the cell types of histiocytes (Pritchard and Broadbent, 1994). They are currently divided into four classes: class I (Langerhans cell histiocytosis) and class II (hemophagocytic lymphohistiocytosis) are the most common (Pritchard and Broadbent, 1994). In the past these disorders were known as Hand–Schuller–Christian syndrome, Letterer–Siwe disease, and eosinophilic granuloma. However, in 1953 Lichtenstein proposed that these three disorders were actually a continuum of one disease process for which he coined the term "histiocytosis X" (Lichtenstein, 1953). This term was abandoned when Nezelof et al. (1973) identified a Langerhans-like cell as diagnostic of this pathologic process, and in 1987 the term "Langerhans cell histiocytosis" was adopted by the Histiocyte Society. Langerhans cell histiocytosis is of importance to the dental profession because oral soft tissue and bony lesions are common and may be the earliest manifestation of the disease (Sigala et al., 1972; Hartman, 1980). Cranin and Rockman (1981) described three cases in which the oral manifestations were the first symptoms to appear. These included loosened teeth, "periodontosis-like" symptoms, and premature eruption of the primary teeth with gingival bleeding. Filocoma et al. (1993) reported that 29% of a patient cohort of 45 children with histiocytosis exhibited oral symptoms at diagno-

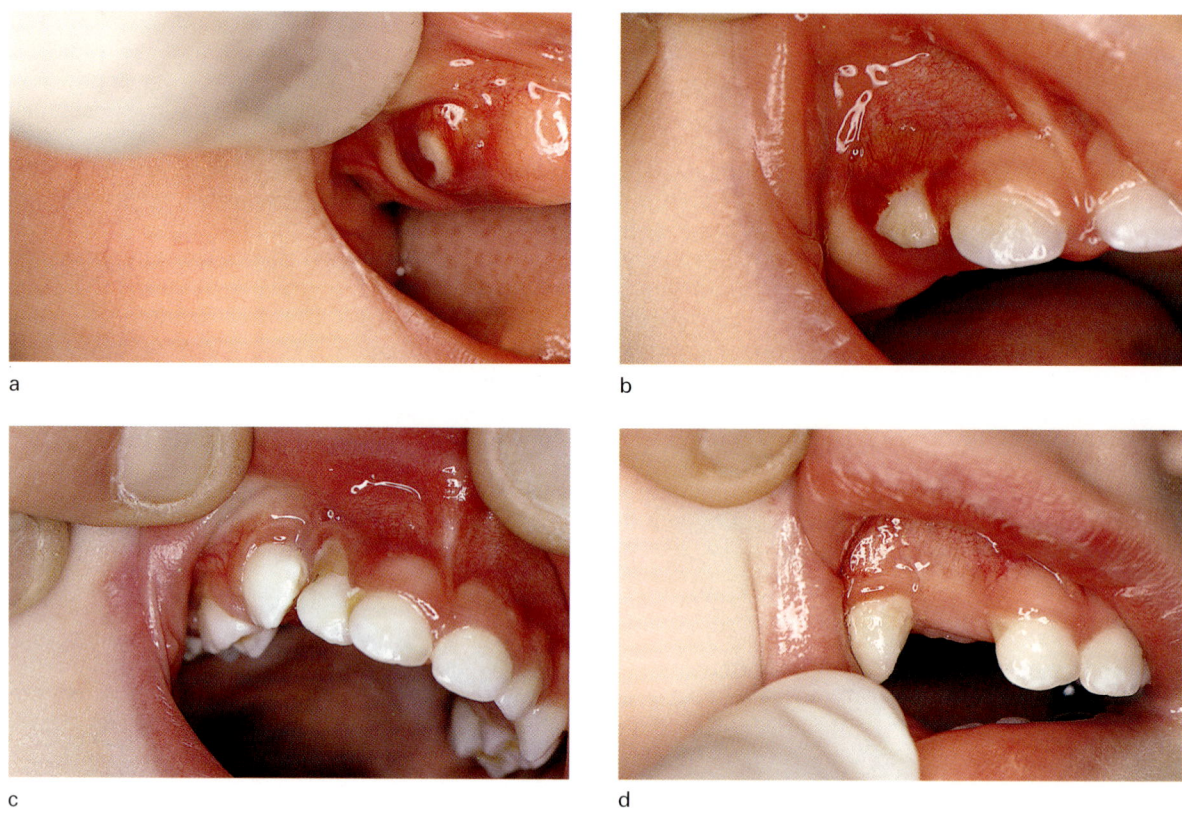

Figure 6.1

(a) Gingival ulceration and inflammation in an 8-month-old boy with Langerhans cell histiocytosis, exposing the unerupted maxillary left primary lateral incisor. (b) Five months later, with continued gingival inflammation and eruption of the maxillary left primary lateral incisor. (c) One year after (a), with exposure of the root of the maxillary left primary lateral incisor. (d) Two years after (a), with normal gingival tissue after extraction of the maxillary left primary lateral incisor.

sis and nearly 45% had some oral manifestations during the natural course of the disease. In addition, the children with oral symptoms required longer treatment periods and more systemic therapy when compared with children without oral complications.

Oral soft tissue invasion by the Langerhans cells can present as gingival inflammation, ulceration, or hypertrophy (Figure 6.1) and is often associated with a bad taste or halitosis. This cell invasion is associated with various degrees of alveolar bone destruction. In severe cases, the bone loss is so extensive that the involved teeth present with exposed roots and increased mobility, and primary teeth will eventually exfoliate

prematurely if left untreated. The radiographic appearance of affected molars has classically been described as "floating teeth" (see Figure 1.7d). Frequent oral sites of involvement include the palatal shelves of the maxillary molars and the buccal or lingual surfaces of the mandibular molars (Needleman HL, personal communication).

Treatment and prognosis depend on the staging of the disease, which includes the age at onset, presence or absence of organ dysfunction, and the extent of organ involvement (Lahey, 1962, 1975, 1981). If the systemic involvement is minimal, local therapy (surgery and radiation) is often sufficient since the disease will usually spontaneously regress. In more severe cases, chemotherapy with vinblastine has been proved to reduce both mortality and morbidity in children (Greenberger et al., 1981; Lipton, 1983). Dental management consists of optimizing oral hygiene, particularly of involved areas, and removal of teeth with extensive bony involvement. These local regimens along with chemotherapy will result in the return of healthy oral soft tissues and the cessation of alveolar bone destruction.

Acrodynia

Acrodynia (pink disease) was first described by Selter (1903) and is a hypersensitivity reaction to mercury (Warkany and Hubbard, 1948; Akabane, 1992) usually seen in infancy and early childhood. Clinical manifestations vary and can progress from listlessness to severe sweating, irritability, anorexia, insomnia, profuse perspiration, photophobia, hypertension, tachycardia, a red to pink coloration of the skin (especially hands, feet, nose, and cheeks), desquamation, hypotonia, and itching. Oral symptoms include increased salivation, sore mouth, gingival hyperplasia, alveolar bone destruction, and mobility of the deciduous teeth (Obura, 1965). Premature tooth loss occurs only in extreme cases. Children with acrodynia have an increased susceptibility.

Genetic abnormalities that enhance the risk for periodontitis

Trisomy 21 (Down syndrome)

The genetic disorder first described in 1866 by John Langdon Down is caused by an autosomally inherited trisomy of chromosome 21 (LeJeunne et al., 1959), band q22 (Jones, 1988). Trisomy 21 is the most frequently occurring genetic disorder with a frequency of approximately 1 in 700 live births. It is characterized by an atypical orofacial appearance including flattened facial profile with epicanthic folds, expanded bridge of the nose, opened mouth, and a protruding, fissured tongue (Cohen et al., 1961). Growth of the middle face is stunted while the mandible is oversized with a protrusive dentition. Affected children also demonstrate a myriad of other difficulties including growth retardation, mental deficiency, muscle hypotonia, joint hyperflexibility, and congenital heart disease. Patients with Down syndrome are also prone to infections, suggesting a defective immune system. These symptoms previously limited the life expectancy of stricken individuals, but advances in medicine have been able to prolong and increase the quality of these patients' lives.

It has long been recognized that affected individuals frequently manifest an aggressive form of periodontal disease affecting both the primary and permanent dentition (Cohen et al., 1961; Johnson and Young, 1963; Saxen et al., 1977; Snajder et al., 1968; Svatum and Gjermo, 1978) which may lead to the early exfoliation of the teeth. The periodontal destruction is characterized by the formation of deep periodontal pockets associated with heavy plaque accumulation and intense gingival inflammation. Saxen et al. (1977) measured alveolar bone loss on orthopantograms and found that 69% of trisomy 21 patients were affected by destructive periodontal disease. Interestingly, alveolar bone loss was observed only in patients over 18 years of age. Periodontal destruction is often generalized although lesions are most severe around the lower anterior teeth (Johnson and Young, 1963; Baer and Benjamin, 1974; Agholme et al., 1999). Other investigators (Saxen and Aula, 1982) found the most bone loss around the lower first molars. Although bacterial plaque, calculus, and other potential local irritants are present and oral hygiene is frequently poor owing to the physical and mental limitations of these patients, the severity of periodontal destruction far exceeds that explainable by these local factors alone (Ulseth et al., 1991).

It has been repeatedly shown that individuals with trisomy 21 are more susceptible to periodontal disease relative to normal, age-matched control groups and other mentally impaired patients. Dow (1951) reported that over 90% of afflicted children, aged 8–12 years, demonstrated some form of periodontal disease. Subsequent studies also reported the prevalence of periodontal disease to be 90–100% in trisomy 21 patients (Kisling and Krebs, 1963; Cohen and Goldman, 1960; Johnson and Young, 1963).

Reuland-Bosma et al. (1986) used an experimental gingivitis model to show that gingival inflammation was induced more rapidly and with a greater severity in patients than in normal control subjects. Orner (1976) compared the periodontal status of affected children with their normal siblings and reported that periodontal diseases ranging from gingivitis to severe periodontitis were present in trisomy 21 children. He also reported that the periodontal index of children with Down syndrome was nearly 4.5 times greater than that of their siblings. Numerous other studies have demonstrated a higher prevalence of periodontal disease in trisomy 21 patients than in other patients with learning difficulties (Johnson and Young, 1963; Snajder et al., 1968; Cutress, 1971; Brown, 1973; Reuland-Bosma and van Dijk, 1986; Cichon et al., 1998). Swallow (1964) demonstrated a higher prevalence of periodontal disease in institutionalized Down syndrome patients compared with those residing at home.

Factors proposed to explain the high prevalence and increased severity of periodontal destruction observed in trisomy 21 patients include reduced local resistance to infection and defects in the host response. Common abnormalities in the host response are decreased numbers of T lymphocytes and functional defects in neutrophils and monocytes resulting in both impaired chemotaxis and phagocytosis (Kahn et al., 1975; Barkin et al., 1980a, b; Sohol et al., 1992). Reuland-Bosma et al. (1986) used an experimental gingivitis model to demonstrate that leukocytic infiltration of the periodontium in affected individuals increased slightly during the first week of the study and then stabilized. Conversely, control subjects showed a slower increase in leukocyte infiltration but significantly higher numbers of leukocytes were found after 2 weeks and 3 weeks. Izumi et al. (1989) showed that individuals with the most severe forms of periodontal disease had a lower chemotactic index than patients with mild bone destruction, suggesting that defective host response can influence the periodontal destruction seen in trisomy 21 patients.

Another area of intense research is concerned with the microflora of patients with trisomy 21 and how this may predispose to the increased prevalence of periodontal disease. Meskin et al. (1968) found a significantly elevated number of black-pigmented anaerobic rods in the supragingival plaque of trisomy 21 patients. More specifically, Bacteroides melaninogenicus (today known as Prevotella or Porphyromonas sp.) was found in 71% of patients and in only 10% of control subjects. Other investigations (Barr-Agholme et al., 1992; Santos et al., 1996; Morinushi et al., 1997; Cichon et al., 1998) have reported an increased prevalence of Actinobacillus actinomycetemcomitans, Porphyromonas gingivalis, Bacteroides forsythus, Fusobacterium spp. Prevotella intermedia, Peptostreptococcus micros, Campylobacter spp., and spirochetes in plaque from periodontally diseased sites in trisomy 21 patients. Conversely, Cutress (1971) found no discernible difference between plaque samples of mentally retarded patients (including trisomy 21 patients) and normal subjects.

Hypophosphatasia

Hypophosphatasia is a rare familial disease, characterized by incomplete bone mineralization. This condition was first described by Rathbun (1948) and is characterized by low levels of serum, liver, kidney, and bone alkaline phosphatase and elevated levels of phosphoethanolamine in serum and urine (Watanabe et al., 1993). Skeletal abnormalities (rickets, osteomalacia, poor cranial bone formation, and craniostenosis) and premature loss of the primary teeth are also common findings. The disorder shows no racial or sexual predilection. It can be diagnosed by taking samples of the gingival crevicular fluid (Chapple et al., 1992) or by molecular genetic analysis (Watanabe et al., 1999), but there is no effective treatment for this condition (Chapple, 1993).

Three clinical forms of the disease were originally described (Fraser, 1957), based on age of onset and degree of severity. However, these categories are not conclusive and some cases do not fit neatly into any one case type. Type 1 (infantile form), considered to be the most severe form of the disease, usually manifests within the first 6 months of life and is characterized by bony ossification abnormalities, hypercalcemia, and failure to thrive. This form of hypophosphatasia is usually fatal in the neonatal period (Greenberg et al., 1990). Type 1 is found in approximately 1 out of 100 000 births (Fraser, 1957) with a mortality rate of over 50%.

Type 2 (childhood or juvenile form) manifests from 6–24 months up to adulthood, and is less severe than the infantile form. Premature loss of the primary teeth in the absence of bone pathology is the hallmark of this form of hypophosphatasia and is often the first clinical symptom (Bruckner et al., 1962; Beumer et al., 1973; Cheung, 1987; Lundgren et al., 1991). These teeth are exfoliated in the absence of plaque and periodontal disease (Baer et al., 1964; Kjellman et al., 1973), with the mandibular central and lateral incisors most frequently shed, followed by the maxillary incisors, while the posterior teeth are least likely to be lost (see Figure 1.7b). These patients also demonstrate craniosynostosis and rachitic symptoms, but premature exfoliation of teeth may be the only overt sign (Pimstone et al., 1966). Sobel et al. (1953) coined the term "odontohypophosphatasia" to describe the premature primary tooth loss in the absence of other systemic manifestations, implying that it was a separate clinical entity, but this has proved to be incorrect. The permanent teeth may also be affected in type 2 hypophosphatasia (Silverman, 1962).

Radiographically, the teeth appear to have a characteristic "shell" appearance due to the widening of the pulp chamber and root canal systems. Other common findings include loss of alveolar bone (Jedrychowski and Duperon, 1979), poorly formed and haphazardly organized PDL (Listgarten and Houpt, 1969), and hypoplasia (Beumer et al., 1973) or aplasia of cementum (Casson, 1969).

Type 3 or adult hypophosphatasia is an uncommon form of the disease. It manifests in early adult life and is characterized by bone pain and pathologic fractures. However, there may be no overt clinical symptoms—only laboratory findings of decreased serum levels of alkaline phosphatase, elevated serum phosphate levels (Chodirker et al., 1990), and increased levels of phosphoethanolamine in the urine. There may be exfoliation of the permanent teeth but the primary dentition is more commonly affected.

Bixler et al. (1974) described a possible fourth category of the disease, in which the levels of alkaline phosphatase are not as markedly reduced as with the other types. There is early exfoliation of the incisors but the bone is unaffected (Bixler, 1976; Berkovitz et al., 1982). In 1984, Terheggen and Wischermann modified Fraser's original classification and described four different groups: "perinatal or lethal", "infantile", "childhood", and "adult". Once again the prognosis depended on the severity of the bone lesions and the age of onset of the disease.

The pathologic alterations in the periodontium are thought to be due to insufficient levels of alkaline phosphatase. This enzyme is a key step in the production of a competent organic matrix in both bone and cementum. The decreased production and activity of this enzyme is likely to result in the accumulation of inorganic phosphate, which inhibits mineralization (Whyte, 1989). This leads to defective osteogenesis and cementogenesis and the formation of an incompetent attachment apparatus, making the teeth more prone to exfoliation and the root surfaces more susceptible to bacterial colonization (Baab et al., 1986).

The diverse phenotype presented in hypophosphatasia suggests that this disease is a heterogeneous entity (Chapple, 1993). Early studies (Fraser, 1957; Sobel et al., 1958) suggested an autosomal recessive mode of inheritance, which has been confirmed in the more severe perinatal and infantile forms of the disease. However, the transmission of the childhood and adult forms is still not fully elucidated and some reports indicate an autosomal dominant mode of inheritance (Eastman and Bixler, 1982, 1983; Silverman, 1962).

Leukocyte adhesion deficiency syndrome

Leukocyte adhesion deficiency (LAD) syndrome is used to denote a heterogeneous group of rare disorders characterized by abnormal leukocyte function and decreased cellular adhesion. Clinically, these patients present with recurrent, necrotic, and non-purulent bacterial infections, generally involving the skin and subcutaneous tissues, middle ear, and the oropharynx. Infants afflicted with this syndrome have delayed separation of the umbilical cord (Crowley et al., 1980) and delayed wound healing. Infections appear to be due to the inability to mobilize neutrophils and monocytes to migrate from the blood vessels to the sites of injury and bacterial challenge (Todd and Freyer, 1988), and there are deficiencies of cell-to-cell interactions, phagocytosis, and antibody-mediated cytotoxicity. A large proportion of LAD patients die of overwhelming sepsis despite antibiotic therapy (Harlan, 1993; Paller et al., 1994; Waldrop et al., 1987; Fischer et al. 1983).

Two forms of LAD have been described. Type 1 (LAD-1) is an autosomal disorder characterized by defects in critical leukocyte antigens Mac-1 (the CRbi complement receptor), lymphocyte function-associated antigen 1 (LFA-1), and the p150/95 glycoprotein; LFA-1 (CD11a/CD18) is involved in cytotoxic T cell responses and T helper cell function, as well as antibody-dependent cellular toxicity and phorbol ester-stimulated lymphocyte aggregation. Antibodies against LFA-1 block the mixed leukocyte reaction and both adhesion and phagocytosis of polymorphonuclear cells, monocytes, and macrophages. The Mac-1 (CD11b/CD18) antigen is found on monocytes, macrophages, PMNs, and granular lymphocytes. It is associated with the C3bi receptor, which aids in phagocytosis and degradation of C3–opsonized microorganisms. It also mediates adherence, spreading, aggregation, chemotaxis and antibody complement-dependent cellular cytotoxicity of PMNs. The glycoprotein gp150/95 (CD11c/CD18) is found on monocytes, macrophages, PMNs, and lymphocytes, and is involved in granulocyte adherence and aggregation. It is also a ligand for stimulated endothelial cells.

These cell surface antigens are members of the integrin family of receptors which are involved in many cell-to-cell adhesion processes, particularly in the immune system (Springer, 1990; Hemler, 1990). These glycoproteins are normally found on granulocyte, monocyte and/or lymphocyte cell surfaces and are believed to be essential for the tight adhesion of neutrophils to activated endothelial cells and for neutrophil transepithelial migration into extravascular inflammatory sites (Mackay and Imhof, 1993; McEver, 1992). All three of these receptors are composed of two non-covalently bound subunits—an α and a β subunit (Anderson et al., 1985; Anderson and Springer, 1987). In LAD-1 there is an abnormal expression of the β_2 subunit (CD18), which is common to LFA-1, Mac-1, and gp150/95. This deficiency is profound and level of integrin expression correlates with disease severity in

individuals with LAD-1. Anderson and Springer (1987) defined two phenotypes based on integrin expression: a severe form, resulting from a homozygous expression in which no integrins are detected, and a moderate type, from heterozygous expression, where integrin levels are between 3% and 30%. Several reported aberrant precursors of the β subunit (Kishimoto et al., 1987) and mutations in the CD18 gene (Arnaout et al., 1990; Corbi et al., 1992; Matsuura et al., 1992; Sligh et al., 1992) have been suggested as the molecular basis of the cellular defect.

One of the most dramatic findings in LAD is severe periodontal disease. Periodontal findings include rapid bone loss leading to the exfoliation of teeth, gingival clefting and recession associated with fiery-red gingiva, profuse bleeding, and other signs of generalized destruction (Waldrop et al., 1987). Oral hygiene and antimicrobial therapy do little to arrest the disease process (Waldrop et al., 1987; Roberts and Atkinson, 1990; Majorana et al., 1999). Periodontal destruction begins during or immediately after the eruption of the primary teeth. Extremely acute inflammation and proliferation of the gingival tissues with rapid destruction of the bone are seen. Profound defects in peripheral blood neutrophils and monocytes and an absence of neutrophils in the gingival tissues have been noted. The extent of the disease process is related to whether one or two defective alleles are present (Waldrop et al., 1987): homozygotes have generalized periodontitis of both the primary and permanent dentitions, while heterozygotes have normal prepubertal status although "post-LJP lesions" may be seen in adults. Clinical and radiographic appearances can resemble generalized juvenile periodontitis (Hormand and Frandsen, 1979), but are more closely similar to generalized prepubertal periodontitis (Page et al., 1983). Other reported oral findings include stomatitis, ulcerations of the mucous membranes, and facial cellulitis (Anderson and Springer, 1987; Majorana et al., 1999).

Leukocyte adhesion deficiency type 2 (LAD-2) is a selectin ligand deficiency, with a failure to express sialo-Lewis-x which is the ligand for the E and P selectins (Etzioni, 1994, 1996). As a result, neutrophil rolling does not increase in response to inflammatory stimulus since the affected cells can no longer bind to endothelial selectins. Individuals with this deficiency suffer from recurrent bacterial infections, neutrophilia, and severe early onset periodontitis (Price et al., 1994).

Papillon–Lefèvre syndrome

The syndrome originally described by Papillon and Lefèvre (1924) is a rare, autosomal recessive genetic disease (Haneke, 1971; Giansanti et al., 1973) characterized by severe periodontitis and hyperkeratosis of the skin. The skin abnormalities are usually limited to the palms and soles of the feet (palmoplantar hyperkeratosis), but may be found on areas of the skin that withstand minor trauma. Lesions associated with this disease begin to manifest at approximately age 2–4 years and there is rapid destruction of the periodontium resulting in the premature exfoliation of the deciduous teeth, usually in the order of their eruption (Gorlin et al., 1964; Carvel, 1969; Brownstein and Skolnik, 1972; Baer and Benjamin, 1974; Bimstein et al., 1990). The gingiva appears to be erythematous and swollen with deep periodontal pockets, which bleed easily upon provocation and may be suppurative. There is increasing mobility of the primary teeth and radiographs demonstrate advanced alveolar bone loss by age 4–5 years. After exfoliation of the teeth, the gingiva resumes a typically healthy clinical appearance until the eruption of the permanent dentition. A similar clinical course is seen in the permanent dentition (see Figure 1.7e, f), perhaps with increased severity, until all the permanent teeth are lost, at which point the gingiva once again reverts to normal (Carvel, 1969). Glenwright and Rock (1990) chronicled a patient who lost both primary and permanent teeth despite antimicrobial therapy and supportive periodontal therapy. Conversely, Nazzaro et al. (1988) found that they could retain the permanent dentition by early intervention with acitretin.

The immunopathology of Papillon–Lefèvre syndrome (PLS) is still under debate. It has been hypothesized that phagocytic defects are responsible for the disease (Haneke et al., 1975); however, there have been reports of normal (Lyberg, 1982) and diminished neutrophil activity (Djawari, 1978; Van Dyke et al., 1984; Schroeder et al., 1988). Van Dyke et al. (1984) studied a family of two siblings afflicted with PLS. The affected children showed severe periodontal disease and diminished neutrophil chemotaxis. These children also harbored elevated levels of *Actinobacillus actinomycetemcomitans* and increased immunoglobulin G antibody levels to this periodontal pathogen. Chemotaxis was normal in the mother but depressed in the father, suggesting a familial mode of inheritance. Another non-affected sibling also had normal chemotaxis, and neither the parents nor this sibling showed antibodies to or colonization by *A. actinomycetemcomitans*. Bimstein et al. (1990) further indicated the presence of elevated levels of *A. actinomycetemcomitans* in a child with PLS. Sutton (1989) suggested defective collagen formation as the impetus for tooth exfoliation. Increased plaque control and a regular recall schedule seem to prevent the loss of teeth (Preus and Gjermo, 1987), while extraction of the primary teeth allowed for the maintenance of the permanent dentition as well (Preus and Gjermo, 1987; Tinanoff et al., 1986).

Chédiak–Higashi syndrome

Chédiak–Higashi syndrome (CHS) is a rare autosomal disease caused by a lysosomal defect, leading to anomalies of blood cells and neutrophil dysfunction (Clark and Kimball, 1971). This disease presents with variable oculocutaneous albinism, strabismus, photophobia, nystagmus, and recurrent cutaneous and respiratory infections (Blume and Wolff, 1972). The increased vulnerability to bacterial infections demonstrated in CHS patients often proves to be fatal (death before age 5 years is common), despite the fact that both humoral and cellular immunity are completely intact. The onset of the disease for the majority of patients occurs before the age of 10 years, with a mean of 5.9 years (Blume and Wolff, 1972). Neutropenia, gingivitis, and severe periodontal disease have also been described as characteristic of this disease (Tempel et al., 1973). Early onset with severe periodontal destruction is a frequent finding, leading to rapid loss of periodontal attachment, severe mobility, and premature exfoliation of teeth (Hamilton and Giansanti, 1974).

On a cellular level, leukocytes have large lysosomal granules caused by fusion of azurophil and specific granules. Additionally, normal functions of neutrophils and other leukocytes are compromised (Root et al., 1972). The importance of the cellular defects in the pathogenesis of CHS has been demonstrated in several animal models (Davis and Douglas, 1972; Gallin et al., 1975; Lavine et al., 1976).

Ehlers–Danlos syndrome

Ehlers–Danlos syndrome (EDS) is a heterogeneous group of at least ten distinct disease types (McKusick, 1972). This syndrome is an inherited disorder of connective tissue characterized by hyperextensibility of the joints, increased fragility and stretchability of the skin, bleeding tendencies, skeletal deformities, ocular fragility, and possible rupture of the intestines or arteries (Ehlers, 1901; Danlos, 1908). Early onset periodontitis has been recognized in EDS type VIII, which is also characterized by skin hyperextensibility, ecchymotic pretibial lesions, "cigarette paper" scars, and minimal to moderate joint hypermobility. It is believed that an autosomal dominant mode of transmission is found in this genetic syndrome (Linch and Acton, 1979; Stewart et al., 1977).

Except for the early onset periodontitis, EDS VIII closely resembles EDS type IV, which also presents with hyperextensive skin, pretibial lesions, cigarette paper scars, easy bruisability, joint hypermobility, pes planus, and arterial or intestinal ruptures. Byers et al. (1983) have suggested that periodontal disease may also be a component of type IV EDS. Genetic defects in type III collagen are considered pathognomonic for type IV EDS, but this finding has not been consistently established in all type VIII patients— some demonstrate this defect (Lapiere and Nusgens, 1981) while others do not (Hartsfield and Kousseff, 1990). This defect of type 3 collagen is thought to compromise the integrity of the periodontium since 9% of gingival collagen and approximately 20% of the periodontal ligament are of this type (Narayanan and Page, 1983).

In light of the phenotypic similarities between EDS IV and VIII, it might be reasonable to regard EDS VIII as a form of EDS IV. On the other hand, patients with early onset periodontitis and apparent EDS IV may actually have EDS type VIII. This dilemma calls for better biochemical diagnosis of the two phenotypes.

Periodontitis as a risk factor for systemic disease

The concept that oral and dental infections may be related to various systemic diseases and conditions originated under the name "focal infection" just after the turn of the twentieth century. Following introduction of X-rays as a diagnostic tool, dentists for the first time were able to detect tooth-associated granulomas, abscesses, and other lesions in the alveolar bone that were not clinically apparent. Physicians began ordering the extraction of any teeth with such lesions as well as of teeth with root canal fillings—and in many cases all of the teeth, diseased or not—even in young individuals, in an effort to resolve obscure, undiagnosed or misdiagnosed, systemic problems. The practice gradually ceased by the 1920s because of lack of evidence.

The major development in periodontology in the 1990s was the acquisition of evidence for the idea that periodontitis, especially severe forms, enhances risk for a number of systemic diseases and conditions: these include atherosclerosis, myocardial infarction, stroke, complications from diabetes mellitus, preterm low-birthweight infants, osteoporosis, and pneumonia (especially in elderly individuals).

Periodontitis and risk of cardiovascular disease

For many years, infection and inflammatory diseases have been thought to be important factors in atherosclerosis, coronary heart disease, myocardial infarction, and stroke (Valtonen, 1991; Valtonen et al., 1993). Evidence has now accumulated to support this idea, as well as demonstrating a link between periodontitis and these diseases, especially in men aged 40–50 years (Seymour and Steele, 1998). Several cross–sectional, case-control, retrospective and prospective longitudinal studies have been conducted.

Persons with cardiovascular disease have poor oral and dental health

There is strong evidence that after adjusting for age and other relevant factors, individuals with cardiovascular disease have worse oral health than otherwise normal persons. Mattila et al. (1989) reported the results of two case–control studies of a total of 100 patients with acute myocardial infarction and 102 controls selected at random. After adjusting for age, social class, smoking, serum lipid concentrations, and diabetes, dental health assessed by two independent dental disease indices was significantly worse in patients than in controls using both indices. Another study of 100 individuals who had been referred for diagnostic coronary angiography provided evidence for a link between atheromatosis and severity of dental infections determined using pantomography. Mean pantomograph score was 3.0 for males in the highest tertile of coronary atheromatosis, compared with 0.0 among the remaining male participants (P = 0.003). The relationship remained after adjusting for age, blood lipid level, body mass index, hypertension, smoking, and social class (Mattila et al., 1993). A similar outcome was reported from a case–control study by Grau et al. (1997). A total of 166 consecutive patients with acute cerebrovascular ischemia and 166 age-matched controls were studied. Patients had more severe periodontitis (P = 0.05) and periapical lesions (P = 0.03) than controls, and poor dental status was independently associated with cardiovascular ischemia with an odds ratio (OR) of 2.6.

Preliminary data are also available from a case–control study of over 3600 individuals in four communities (Offenbacher et al., 1999a). Subjects studied included 100 individuals with coronary heart disease (cases), 227 individuals with subclinical atherosclerosis, and 329 controls. Periodontal disease (defined as more than 60% of sites with attachment loss of 3 mm or greater) was significantly greater in the cardiovascular disease cases (20%) and subclinical cases (17.8%) than in controls (7.3%); P = 0.03

and 0.02, respectively. Cardiovascular disease subjects tended to be diabetic, male, less well educated, and current or previous smokers, compared with controls.

Loss of natural teeth may enhance the risk of cardiovascular disease

Periodontal and periapical infections are the major causes of tooth extraction. Tooth loss is associated with enhanced risk of cardiovascular disease. In a randomly sampled group of 1287 men and 1330 women aged 25–64 years, more unfavorable risk factors for cardiovascular disease were observed in the edentulous group than in those with natural dentition (Johansson et al., 1994). Morrison et al. (1999) demonstrated a relative risk of 1.90 (95% CI 1.17 to 3.10) between edentulism and death from cardiovascular disease and stroke. In another study, the number of missing teeth in 1384 men aged 45–64 years was a weak but statistically significant independent factor for ischemic heart disease (P = 0.037) (Paunio et al., 1993). Lopatin et al. (1999) have provided preliminary evidence for a significant association between the presence of periodontal pathogens in the subgingival flora and salivary IgA antibodies to their antigens, and congestive heart failure in a group of US veterans.

Oral and dental infections may enhance the risk of stroke

Syrjanen et al. (1989) studied 40 patients with acute cerebral infarction and 40 age- and sex-matched controls. Oral health was measured using an index taking into account carious teeth, periodontal disease, and the number of periapical lesions. Poor oral health was associated with cerebral infarction in men. Recent infections including dental infection had occurred in 40% of the patients but in only 5% of the controls. Additional support for a link between dental disease and cerebral vascular disease was provided by a study of US veterans 60 years and older (Loesche et al., 1998). In that study, dependent-living individuals who reported that they did not have their teeth cleaned at least once a year were 4.76 times more likely to have had a cerebral vascular accident. Notably, the results of

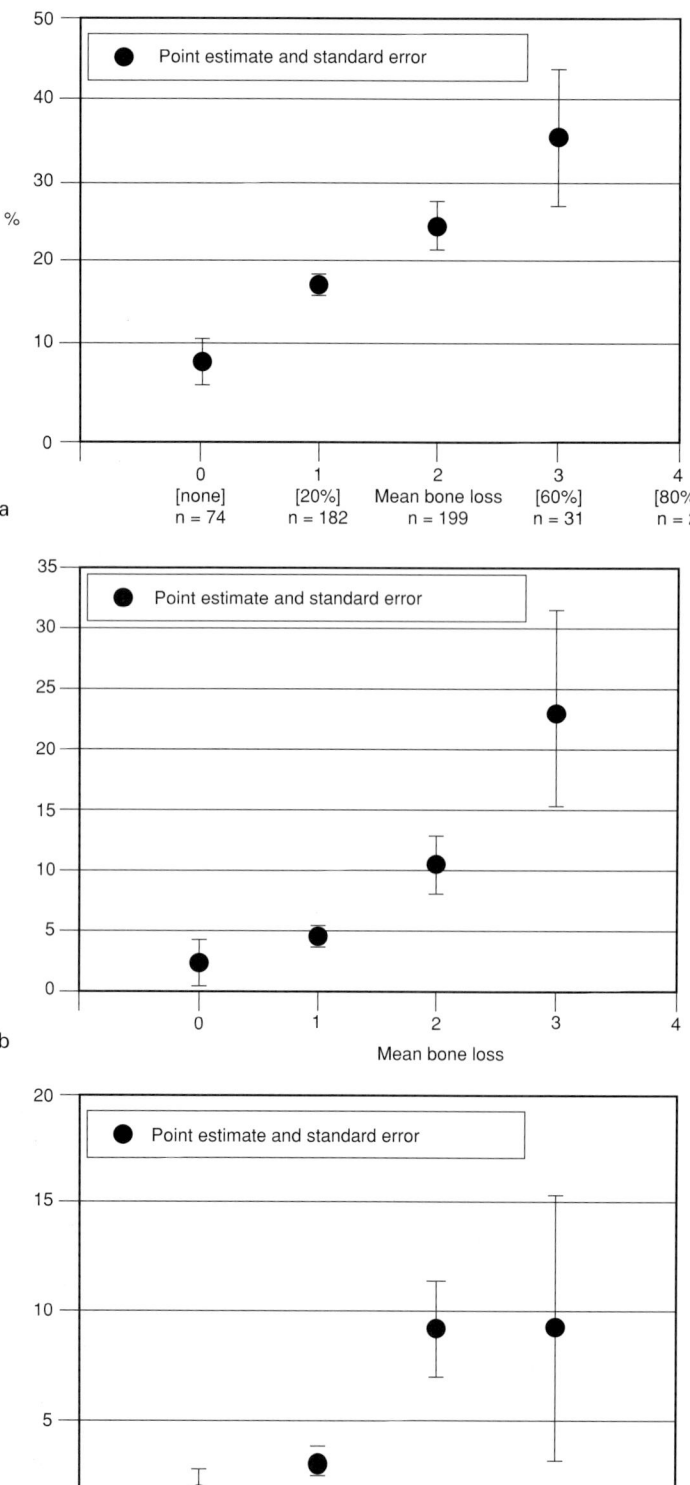

a

b

c

Figure 6.2

Age-adjusted level of alveolar bone loss (a measure of periodontitis), from Beck et al. (1996), with permission. (a) Cumulative percentage incidence of coronary heart disease. (b) Fatal heart disease. (c) Stroke.

this study may not be generalizable since the investigators used a convenience sample of older veterans and the dental data were collected after the cardiovascular event had occurred. Both male and female ischemic stroke patients had fewer teeth and more bone loss around the remaining teeth than controls (Young et al, 1999).

Persons with periodontitis have enhanced risk of cardiovascular disease and of death from cardiovascular disease

Several longitudinal studies, some of which were prospective, have been conducted. A prospective study monitoring approximately 10 000 American adults over a period of 17 years was reported by DeStefano et al. (1993). Those with periodontitis had a 25% increased risk of coronary heart disease. This was associated with poor oral hygiene, but not with caries or missing teeth. Those under 50 years of age at baseline had a 50% increased risk, and risk of dying was increased by almost 300%. Those with the most severe periodontitis were older, non-white men, who were less well educated, unmarried, and smokers. Notably, these are risk factors for both periodontitis and heart disease. Another longitudinal study of 9760 individuals over a period of 14 years revealed a positive correlation between dental infections and risk of cardiovascular heart disease. Severity of dental infection correlated with the extent of coronary atheromatosis. Patients with dental infection also had high levels of blood fibrinogen, leukocytes, and von Willebrand factor (Mattila et al., 1993).

Another prospective study was conducted by Beck et al. (1996). Of 1147 men studied, 207 developed coronary heart disease, 59 died from the disease, and 40 had strokes. Odds ratios for an association of periodontitis with cardiovascular disease were 1.5 for total coronary heart disease, 1.9 for fatal coronary heart disease and 2.8 for stroke. In this study, evidence for a biological gradient was observed for the cumulative incidence of coronary heart disease, fatal coronary heart disease, and stroke (Figure 6.2). Demonstrating a biologic gradient provides strong support for the validity of the observed associations.

Joshipura et al. (1998) performed a prospective cohort study of 44 110 male professionals aged 40–75 years with no history of coronary heart disease, cancer, or diabetes at baseline. Over a 6-year period, 757 cases of the disease occurred. An increased relative risk of 1.67 (95% CI 1.03 to 2.71) was seen in those with antecedent periodontitis with ten or fewer teeth after adjusting for other factors. When the number of teeth was not considered, no relationship was found.

A retrospective study beginning in 1970 was conducted on male and female participants aged 35–84 years without self-reported coronary heart disease (10 368) or cerebrovascular disease (11 251) (Morrison et al., 1999). By 1993, analyzable data were available for 416 deaths from cardiovascular disease and 182 from cerebrovascular disease. After adjusting for age, sex, diabetes, serum cholesterol, smoking, hypersensitivity status, and province, the relative risk for fatal coronary heart disease was 2.15 (95% CI 1.25 to 3.72) for severe gingivitis.

Preliminary results are available from another longitudinal study performed on 697 older adults. Subjects were judged to have periodontitis if they had two or more sites with 3 mm or more attachment loss over a 2-year interval. Individuals with periodontitis died at a rate 3.3 (95% CI 1.2 to 9.7) times higher than individuals with fewer attachment loss events (Elter et al, 1999).

Beck et al. (1999) reported preliminary cross-sectional data from a longitudinal study looking for association of periodontitis with intimal wall thickness (IMT) of carotid arteries, a preclinical measure of atherosclerosis. The results were based on 3937 persons aged 52–76 years. Periodontitis was defined as 3 mm or more attachment loss on 60% or more of sites plus plaque scores of 1 or more at each of these sites. After adjusting for risk factors common to both diseases including age, male sex, educational level, diabetes status, and years of cigarette smoking, individuals with periodontitis had 1.76 times the odds of having elevated carotid IMT as those not having periodontitis. They also had higher levels of prostaglandin E_2 and interleukin-1 in the gingival crevicular fluid (GCF) and higher levels of systemic markers of inflammation such as C-reactive protein.

Periodontitis and fetal health

Low-birthweight (LBW) babies are a significant health problem worldwide. In 1991 in the USA,

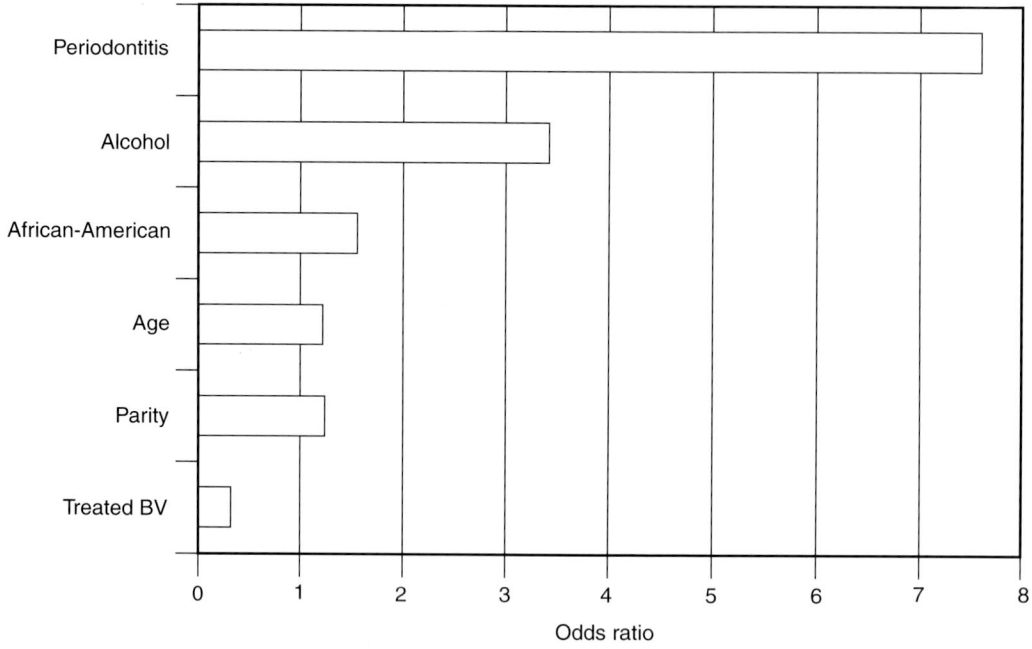

Figure 6.3

Multivariate logistic regression model demonstrating that periodontitis is a significant risk factor for all mothers of preterm, low-birthweight (PLBW) infants. The odds ratio is shown for each risk factor along with the 95% confidence interval. From Offenbacher et al. (1998), with permission.

13.6% of all Afro-American births and 5.8% of all white births were LBW (National Center for Health Statistics, 1993). A significant portion of these were very low-birthweight babies, who have lifelong health problems. Low-birthweight babies impose an enormous burden on the health-care system. In 1988 it was estimated that 35% of all expenditure on health care for babies in the USA involved LBW infants (Lewit et al., 1995).

Bacterial infection in the mother has long been suspected as an important risk factor for LBW babies. Vaginosis, a condition characterized by replacement of the predominantly Gram-positive vaginal flora by an overgrowth of a complex of mostly Gram-negative bacteria, is a risk factor for LBW infants. In a study of 271 pregnant women with vaginosis, relative risk for preterm low birth-weight (PLBW) was 3.3 (95% CI 1.2 to 9.1, P = 0.02) and for premature rupture of membranes 3.8 (95% CI 1.6 to 9.0, P = 0.002) (McGregor et al., 1994). Frequently, subspecies of *Fusobacterium nucleatum* and *Capnocytophaga* spp., typically not found in the vagina but rather in the oral cavity, can be isolated (Hill, 1998). For example, Dixon et al. (1994) described a case of a 23-year-old woman with preterm labor at 24 weeks gestation from whom subchorionic placental cultures yielded *F. nucleatum* and *Capnocytophaga* spp.

Evidence is accumulating that periodontitis in the mother is associated with LBW babies. A case–control study of 124 pregnant or postpartum women (Offenbacher, 1996) demonstrated that periodontal disease is a clinically significant risk factor for PLBW infants. The adjusted odds ratio for all mothers was 7.9 and for primiparous mothers 7.5. It has been suggested that periodontitis in the mother may account for about 18% of all premature LBW babies (Offenbacher et al., 1998).

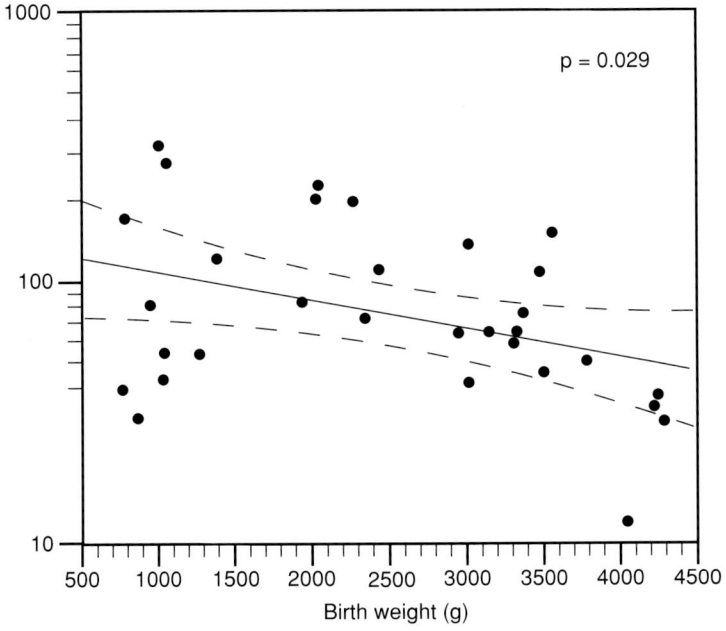

Figure 6.4

For primiparous mothers, the log value of PGE_2 in the gingival crevicular fluid is inversely related to current birthweight ($P < 0.029$). The smaller and more premature babies were born to mothers with the higher GCF PGE_2 levels. From Offenbacher et al. (1998), with permission.

The odds ratios for periodontitis and the other known risk factors for PLBW for all mothers in the study are illustrated in Figure 6.3. The odds ratio for periodontitis is more than double that for alcohol consumption.

There is evidence that both infection by periodontopathic bacteria and pathogenic effects of inflammatory mediators, specifically prostaglandin E_2 (PGE_2) produced in response to infection, may comprise the links between periodontitis and LBW babies (Offenbacher et al., 1998). In a case–control study of 48 subjects, GCF levels of PGE_2 were significantly higher in PLBW mothers (131.4 ± 21.8 µg/ml) than in controls (62.6 ± 10.3 µg/ml) ($P = 0.02$). In addition, within primiparous PLBW mothers, there was a significant inverse association between birth age (as well as gestational age) and GCF PGE_2 levels, with $P = 0.023$. *Bacteroides forsythus, Actinobacillus actinomycetemcomitans, Porphyromonas gingivalis* and *Treponema denticola* were detected at higher levels in the subgingival flora of PLBW mothers compared with mothers of normal birthweight babies (Offenbacher et al., 1998). There is a close relationship between PGE_2 levels in the

GCF and in amniotic fluid in pregnant women. Damare et al. (1997) collected samples of GCF and amniotic fluid during the early mid-trimester of 18 women undergoing routine amniocentesis and measured PGE_2 levels. Pairwise regression analysis revealed that PGE_2 levels in GCF were positively associated with intra-amniotic levels at $P = 0.018$. Furthermore, for primiparous mothers, the log GCF PGE_2 levels were inversely related to current birthweight (Figure 6.4). In other words, the smaller and more premature infants were born to mothers with the higher GCF PGE_2 levels.

Additional evidence for a role for periodontal bacteria in preterm low birthweight comes from preliminary studies in which samples of immunoglobulin M purified from cord blood of preterm and full-term babies were examined for specific antibodies reactive with periodontal pathogens. Of the ten samples from full-term babies, one was weakly positive for antibodies reactive with *Campylobacter rectus*. Among the ten preterm babies, two samples had antibodies reactive with multiple periodontal pathogens including *Porphyromonas gingivalis, Prevotella intermedia, B. forsythus, F. nucleatum,*

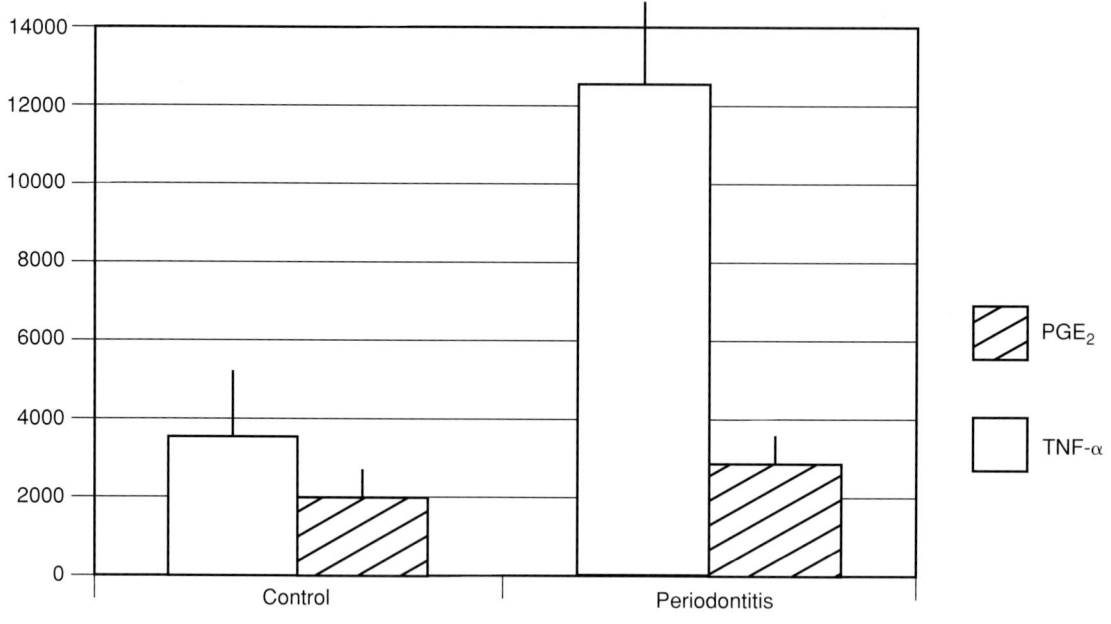

Figure 6.5

Effects of experimental periodontitis on intra-amniotic inflammatory mediator levels in pregnant hamsters. In the periodontitis group, there was a significant elevation in levels of both TNF-α and PGE$_2$ in intra-amniotic fluid relative to groups who did not develop periodontitis ($P < 0.03$ and $P < 0.05$ respectively). From Offenbacher et al. (1998), with permission.

Campylobacter rectus, *Eikenella corrodens*, *Capnocytophaga ochracea* and *Capnocytophaga gingivalis*. Thus, for some preterm babies, exposure to components from periodontopathogenic bacteria may have occurred in utero (Offenbacher et al., 1999b).

There is also experimental evidence supporting a role for infection with *Porphyromonas gingivalis* and the resulting production of inflammatory mediators in fetal toxicity. Using hamsters that had been injected with heat-killed *P. gingivalis* prior to mating, Collins et al. (1994) implanted subcutaneous chambers. On the eighth day of gestation, *P. gingivalis* was injected into the chambers. On days 1 and 5, chamber contents were assayed for PGE$_2$ and tumor necrosis factor alpha (TNF-α). By day 5, PGE$_2$ concentrations had risen from 4.7 pg/ml to 362 pg/ml, and TNF-α levels from 26.4 pg/ml to 724 pg/ml. Relative to controls, fetal weight

was decreased by 24%, embryo lethality increased by 26.5%, and embryo resorption increased to 10.6%. Increasing concentrations of both PGE$_2$ and TNF-α were associated with fetal growth retardation and embryo lethality ($P < 0.001$). The effect of experimental periodontitis in hamsters on increasing intra-amniotic levels of TNF-α and PGE$_2$ are shown in Figure 6.5. Thus in this animal model, infection with *P. gingivalis* adversely affected the pregnancy with severity related to the rise in inflammatory mediators.

The case for a causative relationship between periodontitis in the mother and premature membrane rupture and LBW babies is now sufficiently well documented that action needs to be taken. Practitioners need to provide information to all women patients of childbearing age and to ensure continuing periodontal health for prospective mothers. Women who have periodontitis and who are already pregnant require periodontal therapy, at least thorough scaling and root planing using coverage by an appropriate antibiotic. Dentists, periodontists, and dental staff have the opportunity to dramatically reduce the estimated 18% incidence of premature LBW infants thought to be associated with periodontitis.

All-cause mortality

Periodontitis may enhance the risk of mortality from all causes. A longitudinal study by Garcia et al. (1998) provided the first evidence for such a link. Over a 6-year period, 166 of the 804 dentate subjects studied died. After adjusting for age, smoking, alcohol use, education, body mass index, cholesterol, white blood cell count, blood pressure, family history of heart disease, and number of teeth present, for each 20% increment in mean whole-mouth alveolar bone loss, the subject's relative risk (RR) for death increased by 51% (RR 1.51, 95% CI 1.11 to 2.04). Increased risk attributable to periodontal status was comparable with that attributable to cigarette smoking (RR 1.52, 95% CI 1.06 to 2.19). The population quintile with the highest percentage of alveolar bone loss had a 1.85-fold increase in risk of death (95% CI 1.25 to 2.74).

Preliminary results have been reported from another longitudinal study of mortality in older adult subjects who were judged to have periodontitis if they had two or more sites with 3 mm or more attachment loss. The rate of deaths from all causes was 1.9 (95% CI 1.1 to 2.8) times higher in the group with periodontitis than in the periodontally normal group. The rate remained 1.7 (95% CI 1.0 to 2.9) times higher after controlling for race, sex, diabetes, education, and smoking (Elter et al., 1999). Preliminary data from a study of subjects drawn from the same population after controlling for race, sex, age, tobacco use, education, gingival recession, and physical impairment, show that subjects with a root caries event died from all causes at a rate 1.7 (95% CI 1.2 to 2.4) times higher than subjects not having such an event.

Whether or not a true association exists between periodontitis and all-cause mortality remains unclear. Furthermore, interpretation of all-cause mortality data can be fraught with problems. If a true association does exist, it seems probable that much of the periodontally related enhanced risk for all-cause mortality may result from deaths from cardiovascular disease, since heart disease and stroke are the leading causes of death in many countries.

Mechanisms linking periodontitis and systemic disease

Characteristics of periodontitis

Periodontitis is caused by bacterial biofilms that form on the surfaces of the teeth, enter the gingival sulcus, and extend apically along the surfaces of the roots of the teeth (Page, 1998). These biofilms consist of large numbers of bacterial species embedded in matrix material which they create (Darveau et al., 1997). A small group of predominantly anaerobic, Gram-negative bacteria including *Porphyromonas gingivalis*, *Bacteroides forsythus* and *Actinobacillus actinomycetemcomitans* present in the biofilms initiate and perpetuate an immunoinflammatory response that results in tissue destruction (Haffajee and Socransky, 1994). Clinical and radiographic features of advanced periodontitis are shown in Figure 6.6a, b. The gingival tissues are swollen and highly acutely inflamed; in some cases of longstanding disease, they may be fibrotic. Because of advanced bone loss and very deep periodontal pockets the teeth are mobile and splay apart. Radiographically, it is apparent that, in this case, 50–100% of the alveolar bone around various teeth has been resorbed. Anatomic results of the bone resorption are shown in Figure 6.6c, with exposure of approximately half of the total root length and opening of the furcation areas between the roots.

Histologic features of a periodontal pocket containing calculus with highly ulcerated pocket epithelium can be seen in Figure 6.6d. Strands of pocket epithelium extend deeply into the

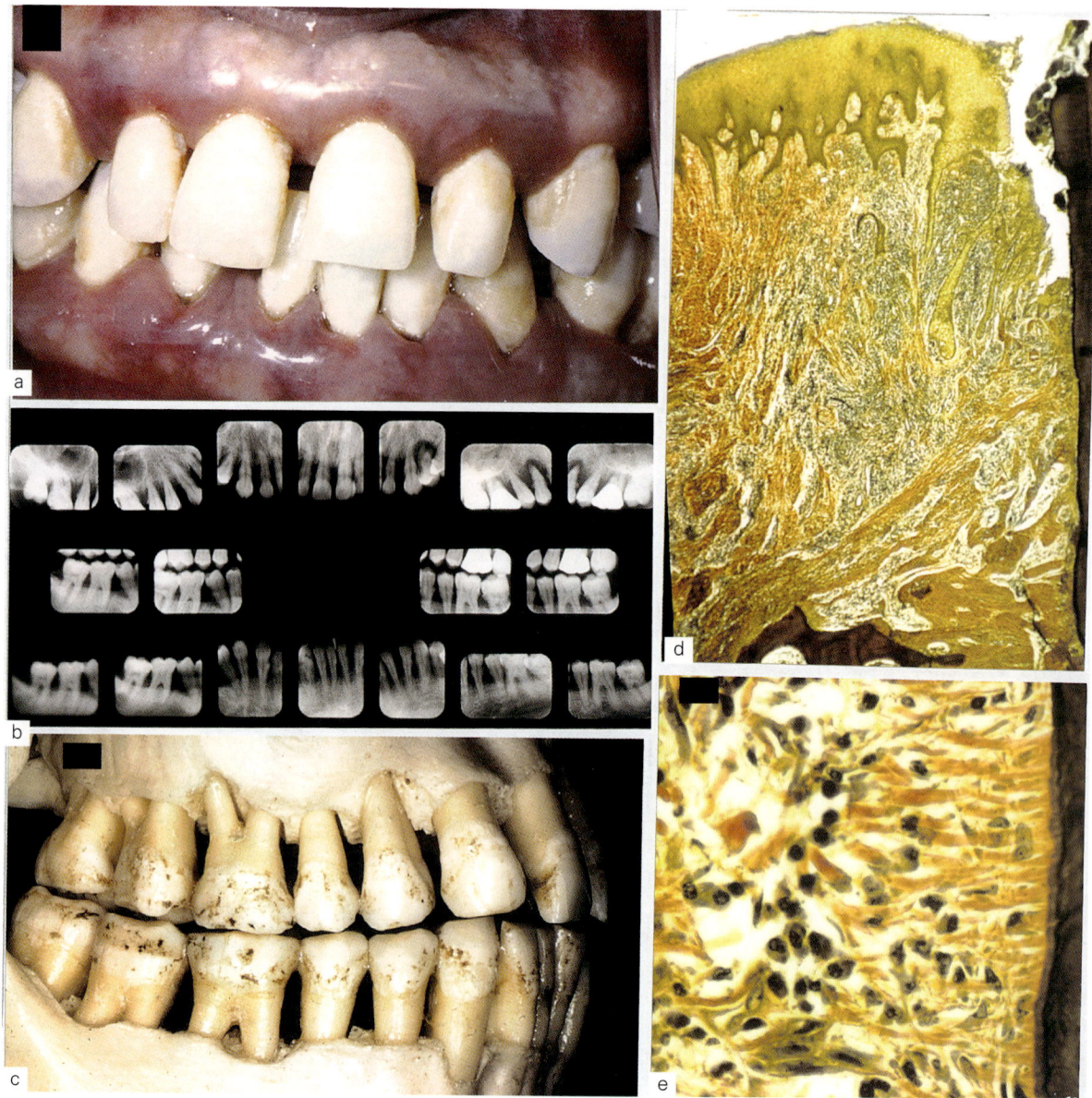

Figure 6.6

(a) Advanced periodontitis. The gingival tissues are highly inflamed. Note microbial plaque on the interproximal surfaces of the teeth and calculus at the gingival margin of the lower incisors. (b) Radiographs of the same patient showing extensive alveolar bone resorption. (c) Alveolar bone and dentition of a skull with advanced alveolar bone loss. (d) Histologic features of a human periodontal pocket. (e) Collagen fibers of the periodontal ligament have been disrupted and partially destroyed.

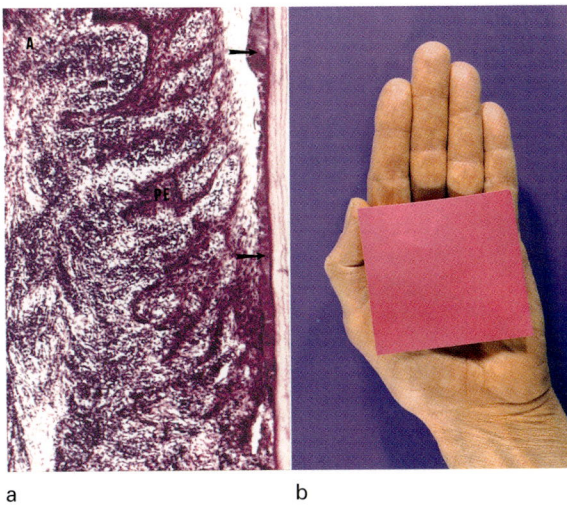

a   b

Figure 6.7

(a) Apical portion of a periodontal pocket around the incisors of sheep. The subgingival biofilm (arrows) extends to near the apical terminus of the pocket and it is in contact with strands of thin pocket epithelium (PE). Note the dense inflammatory infiltrate and paucity of collagen fibers. Although not seen here, the pocket epithelium is frequently ulcerated. From Page (1998), with permission. (b) Estimated area of ulcerated pocket epithelium in contact with subgingival biofilms in a patient with 5–6 mm pockets around all of the teeth. The total area would be about 72 cm², the size of the paper square. When the pockets are deeper the area could be much bigger. From Page (1998), with permission.

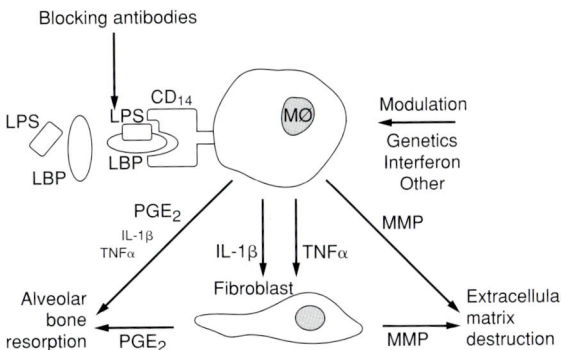

Figure 6.8

Activation of monocyte/macrophages by binding of the lipopolysaccharide–lipid binding protein (LPS–LBP) complex to the CD14 receptor, resulting in production of PGE_2, IL-1β, TNF-α, and matrix metalloproteinases (MMP). Although not shown, additional mediators including IL-6 and INF-γ are also produced. Resident fibroblasts become activated by binding IL-1β and TNF-α resulting in their production of additional PGE_2 and MMP. The latter mediate destruction of the connective tissues, and PGE_2 causes osteoclastic bone destruction. The process of monocyte/macrophage activation may be modulated by genetic factors and mediators such as TGF-β and IFN-γ. From Page (1998), with permission.

inflammatory infiltrate and the gingival collagen fibers have been disrupted and destroyed. The periodontal ligament collagen fibers inserted into the root cementum are disrupted by infiltrating inflammatory cells (Figure 6.6e). Additional details near the bottom of a periodontal pocket are shown in Figure 6.7a. The subgingival biofilm on the root surface extends to the pocket bottom, and is in intimate contact with the pocket epithelium which is very thin and highly permeable. Bacteria from the subgingival biofilms and components such as lipopolysaccharides (LPS) and metabolites derived from them have ready access to the periodontal connective tissues and the circulation through which they can become widely disseminated. The surface area in contact with the biofilms can be large (Figure 6.7b).

Bacterial substances such as LPS activate macrophages and other cells in the inflammatory infiltrate to produce and secrete large amounts of prostaglandins, especially PGE_2, and cytokines including IL-6, IL-1, TNF-α, interferon gamma (INF-γ), and matrix metalloproteinases (MMP) (Figure 6.8). Some of these may reach concentrations as high as 1–3 μM in the inflamed tissues (Offenbacher, 1996). Prostaglandin E$_2$ and (to a much lesser extent) IL-1β, TNF-α and IL-6 mediate resorption of the alveolar bone (Schwartz et al., 1997); and MMPs produced by the activated macrophages and fibroblasts destroy the connective tissues of the gingiva and periodontal ligament (Reynolds and Meikle, 1997).

There is evidence that periodontal bacteria, along with substances such as LPS derived from them and high levels of prostaglandins and cytokines produced by the gingival tissues in response to bacterial substances, may link periodontitis to enhanced risk of various systemic diseases and conditions.

Bacterial infection

Subgingival biofilms constitute an enormous and continuing bacterial load. They are a continually renewing reservoir of LPS, other toxic bacterial substances, and living Gram-negative bacteria, with ready access to the periodontal tissues and circulation. A sample harvested from one pocket by a single pass with a curette may yield up to 10^7–10^8 bacteria. All three of the major periodontal pathogens are Gram-negative and they continuously shed vesicles rich in LPS. The biofilms are difficult to destroy, and once destroyed they tend to reform rapidly.

As gingival and periodontal pockets form, the pocket epithelium is the only barrier between the biofilms and connective tissues. The strands of thin, frequently ulcerated epithelium are easily broached, allowing bacterial access to the connective tissue and blood vessels (see Figure 6.7a). In patients with moderate to severe periodontitis, the total area of pocket epithelium in direct contact with subgingival biofilms is surprisingly large: it may be about the size of the palm of the human hand (see Figure 6.7b), or much larger in cases of advanced disease.

There is evidence that significant doses of viable Gram-negative bacteria, LPS and other soluble bacterial components enter the circulation frequently. Treatment procedures such as scaling and root planning result in bacteremia as manifested by induction of humoral immune responses (Chen et al., 1991; Sjöstrom et al., 1994). Such simple manipulations as tooth brushing and flossing (Sconyers et al., 1973; Carroll and Sebor, 1980; Silver et al., 1980)—even chewing—result in bacteremia. Approximately 55% of patients with severe periodontitis manifested positive blood cultures after chewing paraffin (Murray and Moonsnick, 1941).

Porphyromonas gingivalis and other periodontal bacteria appear to play a role in the formation, maturation, and eventual rupture of atherosclerotic plaques; *P. gingivalis* can actively invade vascular endothelial cells (Desphande et al., 1998), and pathogenic bacteria can be found in atherosclerotic lesions. Using species-specific DNA probes and polymerase chain reaction techniques, Haraszthy et al. (1998) found bacterial DNA in 40% of carotid and 38% of coronary artery atheroma surgical specimens. Both *A. actinomycetemcomitans* and *P. gingivalis* were detected. In similar specimens, Chiu (1998) detected several species of periodontopathic bacteria using specific monoclonal antibodies. Notably *P. gingivalis* and other species were found in the shoulder region of the fibrous cap, an area that is most susceptible to rupture. Since *P. gingivalis* produces large amounts of proteolytic enzymes, especially cysteine proteases, it seems probable that enzyme activity may weaken the tissues, making rupture more likely.

Some bacteria from dental plaque have the capacity to induce platelet aggregation (Herzberg and Meyer, 1996, 1998). The phenomenon is mediated by a platelet aggregation-associated protein (PAAP) located on the cell surfaces of these bacteria. Both *Streptococcus sanguis* and *P. gingivalis* express PAAP. Following the intravenous infusion of PAAP-positive *S. sanguis* in rabbits, changes were observed in the electrocardiogram, heart rate, blood pressure, and cardiac contractility consistent with the occurrence of myocardial infarction. These events did not occur when PAAP-negative bacteria were infused. These bacteria could contribute to cardiovascular changes during periodontitis.

Systemic challenge with Gram-negative bacteria or LPS induces major vascular responses including an inflammatory cell infiltrate in the vessel walls, vascular smooth muscle proliferation, vascular fatty degeneration, and intravascular coagulation (Mattila et al., 1989; Marcus and Hajjar, 1993). Lipopolysaccharide upregulates expression of endothelial cell adhesion molecules, and secretion of IL-1, TNF-α and thromboxane, which results in platelet aggregation and adhesion, formation of lipid-laden foam cells, and deposits of cholesterol and cholesterol esters. Diseased aortas manifest large numbers of monocytes (Pearce et al., 1992). Adhesion molecule expression results in adherence of monocytes and their incorporation into plaques where they became loaded with cholesterol. Low-density lipoprotein activates monocytes to secrete IL-1β and TNF-α, and high-density lipoprotein suppresses secretion (Salbach et al., 1992; Foster and Jackson, 1993; Jambou et al., 1993). Several investigators have concluded that infections of unknown origin may contribute to atherogenesis and cardiovascular disease; periodontal infections may be responsible (Beck et al., 2000; Mattila et al., 1993; Lopes-Virella and Virella, 1985).

Inflammation and acute phase reactants

The pathogenesis of periodontitis and that of systemic diseases such as atherosclerosis, coronary heart disease, and stroke appear to hold many features in common. Pro-inflammatory cytokines, TNF-α, IL-1β and IFN-γ, as well as PGE_2, reach high concentrations in the range 1–3 µMol in the tissues in periodontitis (Offenbacher et al., 1996). The periodontium can, therefore, serve as a renewing reservoir for overspill of these mediators into the circulation where they may induce and perpetuate systemic effects. There is a strong correlation between PGE_2 in GCF and PGE_2 levels in amniotic fluid (Damare et al, 1997). Interleukin-1 and PGE_2 levels are elevated in GCF samples from individuals who have more cardiovascular disease as assessed by intimal wall thickness (Beck et al, 2000). Interleukin-1β favors coagulation and thrombosis and retards fibrinolysis (Clinton et al., 1991). Interleukin-1, TNF-α, and thromboxane can cause platelet aggregation and adhesion, formation of lipid-loaded foam cells, and deposition of cholesterol. These same mediators emanating from the diseased periodontium may also account for preterm labor and LBW infants.

The acute phase response by the liver is a systemic feature of inflammation (Slade et al, 2000; McCarty, 1999). Interleukin-6 produced by activated monocytes and armed Th2 lymphocytes acts on hepatocytes to induce production of acute phase reactants, including C-reactive protein and haptoglobin, which increase blood viscosity and promote thrombus formation. Interleukin-6 also acts on bone cells to generate and activate osteoclasts, resulting in bone resorption. Elevated white blood cell counts are another feature of infectious inflammatory diseases such as periodontitis. Measurement of C-reactive protein (CRP) levels is a convenient way to assess inflammation.

Acute phase reactants are elevated in the blood of patients with periodontitis. Ebersole et al. (1997) measured CRP and haptoglobin in sera from adult periodontitis patients and controls. Levels of both proteins were significantly increased in the patient group: serum values for CRP were 9.12 ± 1.61 mg/l versus 2.17 ± 0.41 mg/l ($P < 0.001$) and for haptoglobin were 3.68 ± 0.37 g/l versus 1.12 ± 0.78 g/l ($P < 0.001$). Levels of both were highest in individuals with more frequent episodes of periodontal disease activity.

Slade et al. (2000) measured levels of CRP in the sera of a random sample of the US population and in a group of 1817 edentulous persons. Individuals with periodontitis (more than 10% of sites with periodontal pockets 4 mm or more) had an approximately 33% elevation in mean CRP levels and a doubling in the prevalence of elevated levels compared with periodontally normal persons. These findings persisted after adjusting for other factors known to cause elevated CRP levels ($P < 0.01$). For unexplained reasons, levels were also elevated in edentulous persons. These results are especially important as they represent data on the entire US population. The acute phase reactants may provide a link between periodontitis and various systemic diseases and conditions.

There is evidence that an elevated level of CRP is a risk factor for cardiovascular disease. A prospective study was conducted over a period exceeding 8 years on 543 apparently healthy men who developed myocardial infarction, stroke, or venous thrombosis, and an equal number of controls (Ridker et al., 1997). Levels of CRP at baseline were higher in men who had myocardial infarction (1.51 mg/l versus 1.13 mg/l; $P < 0.001$) or ischemic stroke (1.38 mg/l versus 1.13 mg/l; $P = 0.02$), but not venous thrombosis. Men in the highest quartile had three times the risk of myocardial infarction (RR 2.9; $P < 0.001$) and two times the risk for ischemic stroke (RR 1.9; $P = 0.02$). Aspirin reduced the risk of myocardial infarction by 55.7%. Risks were independent of other lipid-related and non-lipid-related risk factors. In an additional prospective, nested, case–control study, levels of serum CRP were measured in the blood of 144 apparently healthy men who subsequently developed peripheral arterial disease (Ridker et al., 1998). After controlling for body mass index, hypercholesterolemia, hypertension, diabetes, and family history of premature atherosclerosis, mean CRP levels at baseline were significantly higher in those who subsequently developed peripheral artery disease (1.34 mg/l versus 0.99 mg/l; $P = 0.04$). A dose effect was demonstrated. These data support the idea that chronic inflammation is an important determinant in the pathogenesis of atherothrombosis.

Elevated levels of fibrinogen and white blood cell counts may provide another link between periodontitis and myocardial infarction. Three prospective cohort studies were conducted by Phillips et al. (1992). In a total of 28 181 middle-aged men who were monitored for 6–12 years, l768 had a non-fatal myocardial infarction or died from coronary heart disease. In all three cohorts after adjusting for age, total serum cholesterol, diastolic blood pressure, and number of cigarettes smoked per day, there was a positive and significant correlation between leukocyte count at baseline and risk for subsequent major coronary heart disease events. In another study of 50 patients 25–50 years of age with periodontal disease and 50 age-matched controls with relatively healthy periodontal tissues, significantly higher levels of fibrinogen and elevated white blood cell counts were observed in the patients relative to controls (Kweider et al., 1993). Dental indices correlated significantly with these two factors, which are risk factors for cardiovascular disease.

Kannel et al. (1992) performed a prospective cohort study with a 12-year follow-up of 1393 men and 1401 women 30–59 years of age at baseline, who were free of cardiovascular disease at the beginning of the study. There were 180 cardiovascular disease events in the men and 80 in the women. In non-smoking men with white blood cell counts within the normal range, for each $1.0 \times 10^9/l$ difference in cell count, the cardiovascular disease risk increased by 32%. The value in women was 17%, but only in smokers. White blood cell counts were strongly associated with number of cigarettes smoked per day. It was concluded that the white blood cell count is a marker for increased risk for cardiovascular disease and the risk is partially explained by cigarette smoking.

Hyperinflammatory monocytes

Beck et al. (1996) and Offenbacher et al. (1999a) presented a hypothetical model based on the existence in some individuals of a hyperinflammatory monocyte phenotype to account in part for the association between periodontitis and systemic diseases and conditions, especially cardiovascular diseases and diabetes mellitus (Figure 6.9). They suggest that the innate or acquired presence of this monocyte phenotype places individuals at risk of both periodontitis and cardiovascular disease. Considerable evidence exists in support of this hypothesis.

Individuals vary greatly in the capacity of their monocytes to produce and secrete proinflammatory mediators such as IL-1β, TNF-α, IL-6, and prostaglandins, following activation with LPS. Amounts of inflammatory mediators produced may be 3–10 times greater than normal and they are stable over time. The responsiveness of blood monocytes to activation by LPS as measured by PGE_2 production is highly correlated with levels observed in gingival crevicular fluid (Offenbacher and Salvi, 1999) and presumably, therefore, in the tissues. The hyperinflammatory monocyte phenotype has been identified in patients including those with early onset and refractory periodontitis and those with type 1 diabetes mellitus (Shapira et al., 1994, Hernichel-Gorbach et al., 1994). The hyperinflammatory monocyte phenotype could provide a link between periodontitis and diabetes mellitus as well as cardiovascular diseases through the overproduction of inflammatory mediators which participate in atheroma formation, PGE_2 which mediates resorption of alveolar bone in periodontitis, and by perpetuation of the inflammatory response in diabetes.

Conclusions

There can no longer be any doubt that oral health and systemic health are strongly linked. This fact, when it becomes widely understood by practitioners, will significantly change the practice of dentistry and periodontics. Not only do certain systemic diseases such as abnormalities in phagocytic cell function enhance the risk of periodontitis, but also—possibly even more importantly—periodontitis especially at a young age enhances the risk of several serious and potentially fatal systemic diseases and conditions. These include atherosclerosis, coronary

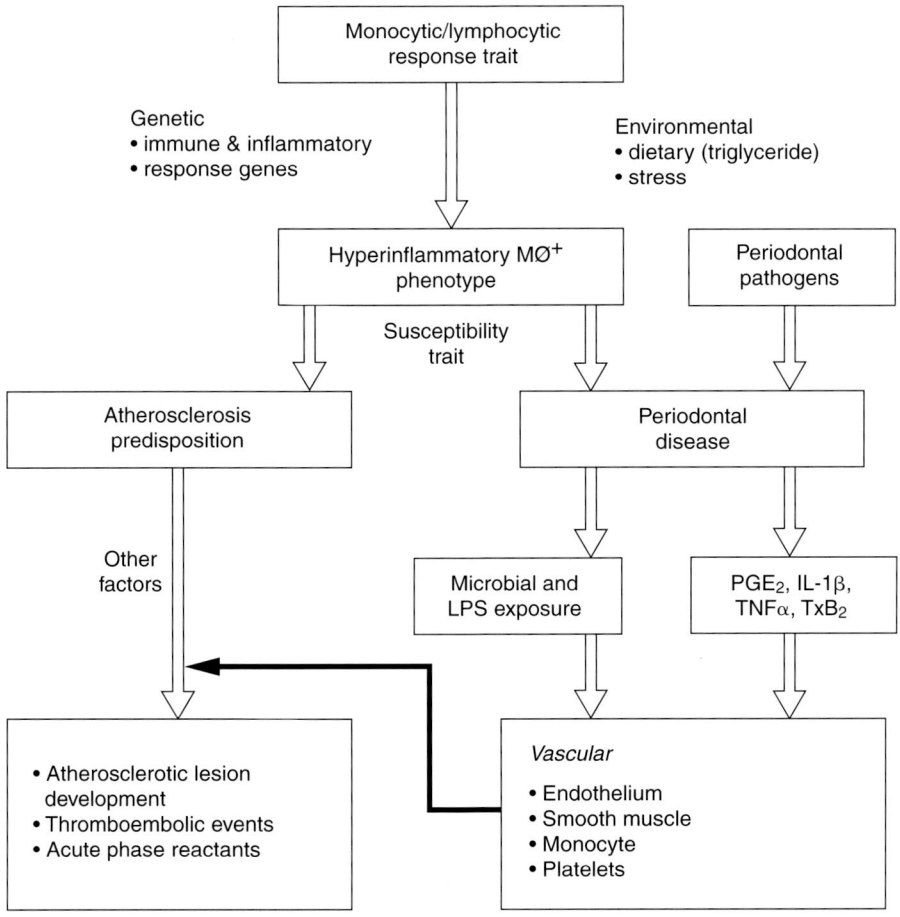

Figure 6.9

Hyperinflammatory monocyte model. The authors suggest that a hyperinflammatory monocytic phenotype can result from a genetic trait or may be induced by environmental factors such as triacylglycerols or stress. Following activation by bacterial substances or cytokines, such cells produce several-fold greater amounts of proinflammatory mediators that predispose to development of atherosclerotic lesions. In the case of periodontitis the excess proinflammatory mediators in the presence of LPS and other bacterial factors damage vascular endothelial and smooth muscle cells, enhance thromboembolic events, and activate the acute phase response to enhance development of atherosclerotic lesions. From Beck et al. (1996), with permission.

heart disease, myocardial infarction, stroke, osteoporosis, and pneumonia. In addition, periodontitis in women greatly enhances the risk of preterm, LBW infants. These relationships between oral and systemic diseases mandate that practitioners caring for children, adolescents, and young adults redouble their efforts to prevent the onset of periodontitis, and take aggressive measures to resolve the disease in those who already have gingivitis or periodontitis.

Focusing efforts aimed at prevention of periodontal disease on children is likely to provide major lifelong oral and systemic health benefits. Advances are being made rapidly in identifying genetic traits that enhance susceptibility for periodontitis. A test is now commercially available that identifies individuals who carry a specific polymorphism in the interleukin-1 gene family whcih enhances susceptibility for adult periodontitis about 19–fold (Kornman et al., 1997). It has been suggested that individuals who are positive for this test plus those who smoke can account for about 85% of all cases of adult periodontitis. It is likely, although not yet proved, that appropriate monitoring, vigorous efforts at prevention, and early intervention in children can negate the genetically enhanced susceptibility in individuals who are gene-test positive. Such an approach, combined with efforts to prevent acquisition of the tobacco smoking habit in young people, may be expected to prevent periodontitis in a large proportion of the population. In light of the documented strong influence of periodontitis on enhancing susceptibility for several potentially death-dealing diseases, preventing periodontitis in children will have lifelong health consequences extending far beyond oral health.

References

[AAP] American Academy of Periodontology (1996) Diabetes and periodontal diseases. Position paper. *J Periodontol* **67**: 166–76.

ADA (1998) Consensus Report. Periodontal diseases: pathogenesis and microbial factors. *J Am Dent Assoc* **129** (suppl.): 58S–62S.

Agholme MB, Dahllof G, Modeer T (1999) Changes of periodontal status in patients with Down syndrome during a 7-year period. *Eur J Oral Sci* **107**: 82–8.

Ainamo J, Ainamo A (1996) Risk assessment of recurrence of disease during supportive periodontal care. Epidemiological considerations. *J Clin Periodontol* **23**: 232–9.

Akabane T (1992) Mercury. In: Berman RE (ed.) *Nelson's Textbook of Pediatrics*, 14th edn. Philadelphia: WB Saunders.

Anderson DC, Schmalstieg FC, Finegold MJ et al. (1985) The severe and moderate phenotypes of heritable Mac-1, LFA-1 deficiency; their quantitative definition and relation to leukocyte dysfunction and clinical features. *J Infect Dis* **152**: 668–89.

Anderson DC, Springer TA (1987) Leukocyte adhesion deficiency: an inherited defect in the Mac-1, IFA-1 and p150,95 glycoproteins. *Annu Rev Med* **38**: 175–94.

Arnaout MA, Dana N, Gupta SK et al. (1990) Point mutations impairing cell surface expression of the common beta subunit (CD18) in a patient with leukocyte adhesion molecule (Leu-CAM) deficiency. *J Clin Invest* **85**: 977–81.

Arno A, Schei O, Lovdal A, Waerhaug J (1959) Alveolar bone loss as a function of tobacco consumption. *Acta Odontol Scand* **17**: 3–10.

Axtelius B, Soderfeldt B, Nilsson A et al. (1998) Therapy-resistant periodontitis. Psychosocial characteristics. *J Clin Periodontol* **25**: 482–91.

Baab DA, Page RC, Ebersole JL et al. (1986) Laboratory studies of a family manifesting premature exfoliation of deciduous teeth. *J Clin Periodontol* **13**: 677–83.

Baehni PC, Payot P, Tsai CC, Cimasoni G (1983) Periodontal status associated with chronic neutropenia. *J Clin Periodontol* **10**: 222–30.

Baer PN, Benjamin S (1974) *Periodontal Diseases in Children and Adolescents.* Philadelphia: JP Lippincott.

Baer PN, Brown NC, Hammer JE (1964) Hypophosphatasia: report of two cases with dental findings. *Periodontics* **2**: 209–15.

Ballieux RE (1991) Impact of mental stress on the immune response. *J Clin Periodontol* **18**: 427–30.

Barkin RM, Weston WL, Humbert JR, Sunada K (1980a) Phagocytic function in Down's syndrome. I. Chemotaxis. *J Ment Defic Res* **24**: 243–9.

Barkin RM, Weston WL, Humbert JR, Sunada K (1980b) Phagocytic function in Down's syndrome. II. Bacteriocidal activity and phagocytosis. *J Ment Defic Res* **24**: 252–6.

Barr-Agholme M, Dahllof G, Linder L, Modeer T (1992) *Actinobacillus actinomycetemcomitans, Capnocytophaga* and *Porphyromonas gingivalis* in subgingival plaque of adolescents with Down's syndrome. *Oral Microbiol Immunol* **7**: 244–8.

Bauer WH (1946) The supporting tissues of the tooth in acute secondary agranulocytosis (arsphenamine neutropenia). *J Dent Res* **25**: 501–8.

Beck JD, Garcia R, Heiss G et al. (1996) Periodontal disease and cardiovascular disease. *J Periodontol* **67**(10 suppl.): 1123–37.

Beck JD, Elter J, Southerland JH, Champagne CME (1999) Periodontal status of cardiovascular disease subjects. IADR Abstr. 2190.

Beck JD, Pankow J, Tyroler HA, Offenbacher S (2000) Dental infections and atherosclerosis. *Am Heart J* **138**: 528–33.

Bergstrom J, Preber H (1994) Tobacco use as a risk factor. *J Periodontol* **65**: 545–50.

Berkovitz BKB, Moxham BJ, Newman HN (1982) *The Periodontal Ligament in Health and Disease.* Oxford: Pergamon.

Beumer J, Trowbridge HO, Silverman S, Eisenberg E (1973) Childhood hypophosphatasia and the premature loss of teeth. *Oral Surg Oral Med Oral Pathol* **35**: 631–40.

Bimstein E, Lustman J, Sela MN et al. (1990) Periodontitis associated with Papillon Lefèvre syndrome. *J Periodontol* **61**: 373–7.

Bixler D (1976) Heritable disorders affecting cementum and the periodontal structure. In: Stewart RE, Prescott GH (eds) *Oral Facial Genetics.* St Louis: CV Mosby.

Bixler D, Porland CP, Brandt IK, Nicholas NJ (1974) Autosomal dominant hypophosphatasia without skeletal disease. *Am J Hum Genet* **26**: 14A.

Black PH (1985) HTLV-III, AIDS and the brain. *New Engl J Med* **313**: 1538–40.

Blume RS, Wolff SM (1972) The Chediak–Higashi syndrome: studies in four patients and a review of the literature. *Medicine* **51**: 247.

Breivik T, Thrane PS, Murison R, Gjermo P (1996) Review. Emotional stress effects on immunity, gingivitis and periodontitis. *Eur J Oral Sci* **104**: 327–34.

Brown RH (1973) Necrotizing ulcerative gingivitis in mongoloid and non-mongoloid retarded individuals. *J Periodont Res* **8**: 290–5.

Brown LR, Roth GD, Hoover D et al. (1969) Alveolar bone loss in leukemic and non-leukemic mice. *J Periodontol* **40**: 725–30.

Brownstein MH, Skolnik P (1972) Papillon–Lefèvre syndrome. *Arch Dermatol* **106**: 533–4.

Bruckner RJ, Rickles NH, Porter DR (1962) Hypophosphatasia with premature shedding of teeth and aplasia of cementum. *Oral Surg Oral Med Oral Pathol* **15**: 1351–69.

Byers PH, Holbrook KA, Barsh GS (1983) Ehlers–Danlos syndrome. In: Emery AEH, Rimoin DL (eds) *Principles and Practice of Medical Genetics.* New York: Churchill Livingstone.

Carranza FA, Gravian O, Cabrini RL (1965) Periodontal and pulpal pathosis in leukemic mice. *Oral Surg* **20**: 374.

Carrassi A, Abati S, Santarelli G, Vogel G (1989) Periodontitis in a patient with chronic neutropenia. *J Periodontol* **60**: 352–7.

Carroll GC, Sebor RJ (1980) Dental flossing and its relationship to transient bacteremia. *J Periodontol* **51**(12): 691–2.

Carvel RI (1969) Palmar-plantar hyperkeratosis and premature periodontal destruction. *J Oral Med* **24**: 73–82.

Casson M (1969) Oral manifestations of primary hypophosphatasia. *Br Dent J* **127**: 561–6.

Chadwick BL, Crawford PJM, Alfred MJ (1989) Massive giant cell epulis in a child with familial cyclic neutropenia. *Br Dent J* **167**: 279–81.

Chapple ILC (1993) Hypophosphatasia: dental aspects and mode of inheritance. *J Clin Periodontol* **20**: 615–22.

Chapple ILC, Thorpe GHG, Smith GM et al. (1992) Hypophosphatasia: a family study involving a case diagnosed from gingival crevicular fluid. *J Oral Pathol Med* **21**: 426–31.

Chen HA, Johnson BD, Sims TJ (1991) Humoral immune response to *Porphyromonas gingivalis* before and following therapy in rapidly progressive periodontitis patients. *J Periodontol* **62**: 781-91.

Cheung WS (1987) A mild form of hypophosphatasia as a cause of premature exfoliation of primary teeth: report of two cases. *Pediatr Dent* **9**: 49–52.

Chiu B (1998) Multiple infections in carotid atherosclerotic plaques. In: *International Symposium in Infection and Atherosclerosis.* INSEM Abstr. p. 95.

Chodirker BN, Evan JA, Seargeant LE et al. (1990) Hyperphosphatemia in infantile hypophosphatemia: implications for carrier diagnosis and screening. *Am J Hum Genet* **46**: 280–5.

Christen AG, Armstrong WR, McDaniel RK (1979) Intraoral leukoplakia, abrasion, periodontal breakdown and tooth loss in a snuff dipper. *J Am Dent Assoc* **98**: 584–6.

Chrousos GP, Gold PW (1992) The concepts of stress and stress system disorders. Overview of physical and behavioral homeostasis. *JAMA* **267**: 1244–52.

Cianciola LJ, Genco RJ, Patters MR et al. (1977) Defective polymorphonuclear leukocyte function in human periodontal disease. *Nature* **265**: 445–7.

Cianciola LJ, Park BH, Bruck E et al. (1982) Prevalence of periodontal disease in insulin-dependent diabetes mellitus (juvenile diabetes). *J Am Dent Assoc* **104**(5): 653–60.

Cichon L, Crawford L, Grimm WD (1998) Early-onset periodontitis associated with Down's Syndrome—a clinical intervention study. *Ann Periodontol* **3**: 370–80.

Clark RA, Kimball HR (1971) Defective neutrophil chemotaxis in the Chediak–Higashi syndrome. *J Clin Invest* **50**: 2645–52.

Clinton SK, Fleet JC, Loppnow H et al. (1991) Interleukin-1 gene expression in rabbit vascular tissue in vivo. *Am J Pathol* **138**(4): 1005–14.

Cohen DW, Goldman HM (1960) Clinical observations on the modification of human oral tissue metabolism by local intraoral factors. *Ann NY Acad Sci* **85**: 68–95.

Cohen DW, Morris AL (1961) Periodontal manifestations of cyclic neutropenia. *J Periodontol* **32**: 159–68.

Cohen MM, Winer RA, Schwartz S, Shklar G (1961) Oral aspects of mongolism. Part 1. Periodontal disease in Mongolism. *J Oral Surg* **14**: 92–107.

Collin HL, Uusitupa M, Niskanen L et al. (1998) Periodontal findings in elderly patients with non-insulin dependent diabetes mellitus. *J Periodontol* **69**(9): 962–6.

Collins JG, Smith MA, Arnold RR, Offenbacher S (1994) Effects of *Escherichia coli* and *Porphyromonas gingivalis* lipopolysaccharide on pregnancy outcome in the golden hamster. *Infect Immun* **62**(10): 4652–5.

Connolly GN, Winn DM, Heght SS et al. (1986) The reemergence of smokeless tobacco. *New Engl J Med* **314**: 1020–7.

Corbi AL, Vera A, Ursa A et al. (1992) Molecular basis for a severe case of leukocyte adhesion deficiency. *Eur J Immunol* **22**: 1877–81.

Cortellini P, Pini Prato GP, Tonetti MS (1996) Long-term stability of clinical attachment following guided tissue regeneration and conventional therapy. *J Clin Periodontol* **23**: 106–11.

Cranin AN, Rockman R (1981) Oral symptoms in histiocytosis X. *J Am Dent Assoc* **103**: 412–16.

Creath CJ, Cutter G, Bradley DH, Wright JT (1991) Oral leukoplakia and adolescent smokeless tobacco use. *Oral Surg Oral Med Oral Pathol* **72**: 35–41.

Crowley CA, Curnutte JT, Rosin RE et al. (1980) An inherited abnormality of neutrophil adhesion: its genetic transmission and its association with a missing protein. *New Engl J Med* **302**: 1163–8.

Cullen JW, Blot JS, Henninfield J et al. (1986) Health consequences of using smokeless tobacco: summary of the Advisory Committee's Report to the Surgeon General. *Publ Health Rep* **101**: 355–72.

Curtis AB (1971) Childhood leukemias: initial oral manifestations. *J Am Dent Assoc* **83**: 159–64.

Cutress TW (1971) Periodontal disease and oral hygiene in trisomy 21. *Arch Oral Biol* **16**: 1345–55.

Damare SM, Wells S, Offenbacher S (1997) Eicosanoids in periodontal diseases: potential for systemic involvement. *Adv Exp Med Biol* **433**: 23–35.

da Silva AM, Newman HN, Oakley DA (1995) Psychosocial factors in inflammatory periodontal diseases. A review. *J Clin Periodontol* **22**: 516–26.

Danlos M (1908) Un cas de cutis laxa avec tumeurs par contusion chronique des coudes et dex genoux (xanthome juvenile pseudo-diabetique de MM Hallopeau et Mace de Lepinay). *Bull Soc Franc Derm Syph* **19**: 70–2.

Darling MR, Arendorf TM (1992) Review of the effects of cannabis smoking on oral health. *Int Dent J* **42**: 19–22.

Darveau RP, Tanner A, Page RC (1997) The microbial challenge in periodontitis. *Periodontol 2000* **14**: 12–32.

Davis WC, Douglas SD (1972) Defective granule formation in the Chédiak–Higashi syndrome in man and animals. *Semin Hematol* **9**: 431–50.

Dello Russo NM, Temple HV (1982) Cocaine effects on gingiva. *Am J Dent Assoc* **104**: 13.

Desphande RG, Kahn MB, Genco CA (1998) Invasion of aortic and heart endothelial cells by *Porphyromonas gingivalis*. *Infect Immun* **66**: 5337–43.

DeStefano F, Anda RF, Kahn HS et al. (1993) Dental disease and risk of coronary heart disease and mortality. *Br Med J* **306**(6879): 688–91.

Dixon NG, Ebright D, Defrancesco MA, Hawkins RE (1994) Orogenital contact: a cause of chorioamnionitis? *Obstet Gynec* **84**(4 Pt 2): 654–5.

Djawari D (1978) Deficient phagocytic function in Papillon–Lefèvre syndrome. *J Clin Periodontol* **156**: 189–92.

Dow RS (1951) A preliminary study of periodontoclasia in Mongolian children at Polk State School. *Am J Ment Defic* **55**: 535–8.

Eastman JR, Bixler D (1982) Lethal and mild hypophosphatasia in two half-sibs. *J Craniofac Genet Devel Bio* **2**: 35–44.

Eastman JR, Bixler D (1983) Clinical, laboratory and genetic investigations of hypophosphatasia: support for autosomal dominant inheritance with homozygous lethality. *J Craniofac Genet* **3**: 213–34.

Ebersole JL, Machen RL, Steffen MJ, Willmann DE (1997) Systemic acute-phase reactants, C-reactive protein and haptoglobin, in adult periodontitis. *Clin Exp Immunol* **107**(2): 347–52.

[EEC] EEC Clearinghouse on Oral Problems Related to HIV Infection and WHO Collaborating Centre on Oral Manifestations for the Immunodeficiency Virus (1990) An update of the classification and diagnostic criteria of the oral lesions in HIV infection. *J Oral Pathol Med* **20**: 97–100.

[EEC] EEC Clearinghouse on Oral Problems Related to HIV Infection and WHO Collaborating Centre on Oral Manifestations for the Immunodeficiency Virus (1993)

Classification and diagnostic criteria for oral lesions in HIV infection. *J Oral Pathol Med* **22**: 289–91.

Ehlers E (1901) Cutis laxa, neigung zu haemorrhagien in der haut, lockerung mehrerer artikulationen. *Der Zschr* **8**: 173–5.

Elter J, Beck J, Offenbacher S (1999) Mortality following periodontal attachment loss. IADR Abstr. 3581.

Epstein LG, Sharer LR, Joshi VV et al. (1985) Progressive encephalopathy in children with acquired immune deficiency syndrome. *Ann Neurol* **17**: 488–96.

Etzioni A (1994) Adhesion molecules deficiencies and their clinical significance. *Cell Adhes Commun* **2**: 257–60.

Etzioni A (1996) Adhesion molecules: their role in health and disease. *Pediatr Res* **39**: 191–8.

Felig PJ, Baxter JD, Frohman LA (1995) *Endocrinology and Metabolism.* New York: McGraw Hill.

Filocoma D, Needleman HL, Arceci R et al. (1993) Pediatric histiocytosis. Characterization, prognosis, and oral involvement. *Am J Pediatr Hematol Oncol* **15**: 226–30.

Firatli E (1997) The relationship between clinical periodontal status and insulin-dependent diabetes mellitus. Results after 5 years. *J Periodontol* **68**(2): 136–40.

Fischer A, Descamps-Latascha B, Gerita I et al. (1983) Bone marrow transplantation for inborn error of phagocytic cells associated with defective adherence, chemotaxis, and oxidative response during opsonized particle phagocytosis. *Lancet* **ii**: 473–6.

Fonseca RO (1996) *Frequency of oral manifestations in HIV-infected children*. Dissertation, Federal University of Rio de Janeiro School of Dentistry.

Foster P, Jackson M (1993) Distribution of lipoprotein phenotypes, cholesterol, and lipids in inner-city blacks. *J Natl Med Assoc* **85**: 211–15.

Fraser D (1957) Hypophosphatasia. *Am J Med* **22**: 730–46.

Freeman R, Goss S (1993) Stress measurements as predictors of periodontal disease—a preliminary communication. *Commun Dent Oral Epidemiol* **21**: 176–7.

Gallin JI, Klimerman JA, Padgett GM, Wolff SM (1975) Defective mononuclear leukocyte chemotaxis in the Chédiak–Higashi syndrome of human, mink, and cattle. *Blood* **45**: 863–70.

Garcia RI, Krall EA, Vokonas PS (1998) Periodontal disease and mortality from all causes in the VA Dental Longitudinal Study. *Ann Periodontol* **3**(1): 339–49.

Gargiulo AV Jr, Toto PD, Gargiulo AW (1985) Cocaine induced gingival necrosis. *Periodont Case Rep* **7**: 44–5.

Genco RJ (1992) Host responses in periodontal diseases: current concepts. *J Periodontol* **63**: 338–55.

Genco RJ, Ho AW, Kopman J et al. (1998) Models to evaluate the role of stress in periodontal disease. *Ann Periodontol* **3**: 288–302.

Genco RJ, Ho AW, Grossi SG et al. (1999) Relationship of stress, distress, and inadequate coping behaviors to periodontal disease. *J Periodontol* **70**: 711–23.

Giansanti JS, Hrabak RP, Waldron CA (1973) Palmar-plantar hyperkeratosis and concomitant periodontal destruction. (Papillon–Lefèvre syndrome). *Oral Surg Oral Med Oral Pathol* **36**: 40–8.

Glenwright HD, Rock WP (1990) Papillon–Lefèvre syndrome. *Br Dent J* **168**: 27–9.

Gorlin RJ, Sedano H, Anderson VE (1964) The syndrome of palmar-plantar hyperkeratosis and premature periodontal destruction of the teeth. *J Pediatr* **65**: 895–908.

Grau AJ, Buggle F, Ziegler C et al. (1997) Association between acute cerebrovascular ischemia and chronic and recurrent infection. *Stroke* **28**(9): 1724–9.

Green LN, Tryon NW, Merks B, Huryn J (1986) Periodontal disease as a function of life events stress. *J Hum Stress* **12**: 32–6.

Greenberg CR, Evans JA, McKendry-Smith S et al. (1990) Infantile hypophosphatasia: localization within chromosome region 1p36.1–34 and prenatal diagnosis using linked DNA markers. *Am J Hum Genet* **46**: 286–92.

Greenberger J, Crocker A, Bawter G et al. (1981) Results of treatment of 127 patients with systemic histiocytosis. *Medicine* **60**: 311–38.

Grossi SG, Genco RJ (1998) Periodontal disease and diabetes mellitus: a two-way relationship. *Ann Periodontol* **3**(1): 51–61.

Grossi SG, Zambon JJ, Ho AW et al. (1994) Assessment of risk for periodontal disease. I. Risk indicators for attachment loss. *J Periodontol* **65**: 260–7.

Gustke CJ (1999) Treatment of periodontitis in the diabetic patient. A critical review. *J Clin Periodontol* **26**(3): 133–7.

Haffajee AD, Socransky SS (1994) Microbial agents of destructive periodontal diseases. *Periodontol 2000* **5**: 78–111.

Hamilton RE, Giansanti JS (1974) The Chediak–Higashi syndrome. *Oral Surg* **37**: 754–61.

Haneke E (1971) The Papillon–Lefèvre syndrome: keratosis palmoplantaris with periodontopathy. *Hum Genet* **51**: 1–35.

Haneke E, Narnstein OP, Lex C (1975) Increased susceptibility to infections in the Papillon–Lefèvre syndrome. *Dermatologica* **150**: 283–6.

Haraszthy VI, Zambon JJ, Zeid M, Genco RJ (1998) Identification of pathogens in atheromatous plaques. Program and Abstracts Annual Session IADR, Vancouver, 1998 [Abstr. 273].

Harlan JM (1993) Leukocyte adhesion deficiency syndrome: insights into the molecular basis of leukocyte emigration. *Clin Immunol Immunopathol* **67**: S16–S24.

Hart TC, Shapira L, Van Dyke TE (1994) Neutrophil defects as risk factors for periodontal diseases. *J Periodontol* **65**: 521–9.

Hartman K (1980) Histiocytosis X: a review of 114 cases with oral involvement. *Oral Surg* **49**: 38–54.

Hartsfield JK Jr, Kousseff BG (1990) Phenotypic overlap of Ehlers–Danlos syndrome Types IV and VIII. *Am J Genet* **37**: 465–70.

Hemler ME (1990) VLA proteins in the integrin family: structures, functions, and their role on leukocytes. *Ann Rev Immunol* **8**: 365–400.

Hernichel-Gorbach E, Kornman KS, Holt SC et al. (1994) Host responses in patients with generalized refractory periodontitis. *J Periodontol* **65**(1): 8–16.

Herzberg MC, Meyer MW (1996) Effects of oral flora on platelets: possible consequences in cardiovascular disease. *J Periodontol* **67**(10 suppl.): 1138–42.

Herzberg MC, Meyer MW (1998) Dental plaque, platelets, and cardiovascular diseases. *Ann Periodontol* **3**(1): 151–60.

Hill GB (1998) Preterm birth: associations with genital and possibly oral microflora. *Ann Periodontol* **3**(1): 222–32.

Ho DD, Rota T, Schooley RT et al. (1985) Isolation of HTLV from cerebrospinal fluid and the neural tissues of patients with neurologic syndromes related to the acquired immunodeficiency syndrome. *New Engl J Med* **313**: 1493–7.

Hoge HW, Kirkham DB (1983) Clinical management and soft tissue reconstruction of periodontal damage resulting from habitual use of snuff. *J Am Dent Assoc* **107**: 744–5.

Hormand J, Frandsen A (1979) Juvenile periodontitis localization of bone loss in relationship to age, sex and teeth. *J Clin Periodontol* **6**: 407–16.

Iughetti L, Marino R, Bertolani MF, Bernasconi S (1999) Oral health in children and adolescents with IDDM—a review. *J Ped Endocrinol Metab* **12**(5): 603–10.

Izumi Y, Sugiyama S, Shinozuka O et al. (1989) Defective neutrophil chemotaxis in Down's syndrome

patients and its relationship to periodontal destruction. *J Periodontol* **60**: 238–42.

Jambou D, Dejour N, Bayer P et al. (1993) Effect of human native low-density and high-density lipoproteins on prostaglandin production by mouse macrophage cell line P388D1: possible implications in pathogenesis of atherosclerosis. *Biochim Biophys Acta* **1168**(1): 115–21.

Jedrychowski JR, Duperon D (1979) Childhood hypophosphatasia with oral manifestations. *J Oral Med* **35**: 18–22.

Johansson IP, Tidehag P, Lundberg V, Hallmans G (1994) Dental status, diet and cardiovascular risk factors in middle-aged people in northern Sweden. *Commun Dent Oral Epidemiol* **22**(6): 431–6.

Johnson NP, Young MA (1963) Periodontal disease in mongols. *J Periodontol* **34**: 41–7.

Jones KL (1988) Down Syndrome. In: *Smith's Recognizable Patterns of Human Malformation*, 4th edn. Philadelphia: WB Saunders.

Joshipura KJ, Douglass CW, Willett WC (1998) Possible explanations for the tooth loss and cardiovascular disease relationship. *Ann Periodontol* **3**(1): 175–83.

Kahn AJ, Evans HE, Glass L et al. (1975) Defective neutrophil chemotaxis in patients with Down's syndrome. *J Pediatr* **87**: 87–9.

Kaldahl WB, Johnson GK, Patil KD, Kalkwarf KL (1996) Levels of cigarette consumption and response to periodontal therapy. *J Periodontol* **67**: 675–81.

Kannel WB, Anderson K, Wilson PW (1992) White blood cell count and cardiovascular disease. Insights from the Framingham Study. *JAMA* **267**(9): 1253–6.

Karfalainen KM, Knuuttila MLE (1996) The onset of diabetes and poor metabolic control increases gingival bleeding in children and adolescents with insulin dependent diabetes mellitus. *J Clin Periodontol* **23**: 1060-7.

Katz MH, Mastrucci M, Leggott PJ et al. (1993) Prognostic significance of oral lesions in children with perinatally acquired immunodeficiency virus infection. *Am J Dis Child* **147**: 45–8.

Ketchem L, Berkowitz RJ, McIlveen L et al. (1990) Oral findings in HIV-seropositive children. *Pediatr Dent* **12**: 143–6.

Kishimoto TK, Hollander N, Roberts TM et al. (1987) Heterogeneous mutations in the b subunit common to the LFA-a, Mac-1, and p150,95 glycoproteins cause leukocyte adhesion deficiency. *Cell* **50**: 193–202.

Kisling E, Krebs G (1963) Periodontal conditions in adult patients with Mongolism (Down's Syndrome). *Acta Odont Scand* **21**: 401–5.

Kjellman M, Oldfelt V, Nordenram A, Olow-Nordenram M (1973) Five cases of hypophosphatasia with dental findings. *Int J Oral Surg* **2**: 152–8.

Kornman S, Crane A, Wang HY et al. (1997) The interleukin genotype as a severity factor in adult periodontal disease. *J Clin Periodont* **24**: 72–7.

Kweider M, Lowe GD, Murray GD et al. (1993) Dental disease, fibrinogen and white cell count; links with myocardial infarction? *Scott Med J* **38**(3): 73–4.

Lahey ME (1962) Prognosis in reticuloendotheliosis in children. *J Pediatr* **60**: 664.

Lahey ME (1975) Histiocytosis: an analysis of prognostic factors. *J Pediatr* **87**: 184–9.

Lahey ME (1981) Prognostic factors in histiocytosis X. *Am J Pediatr Hom/Oncol* **3**: 57–60.

Lalla E, Lamster IB, Schmidt AM (1998) Enhanced interaction of advanced glycation end products with their cellular receptor RAGE: implications for the pathogenesis of accelerated periodontal disease in diabetes. *Ann Periodontol* **3**(1): 13–9.

Lamster IB, Ostrain RL, Harper DS (1987) Infantile agranulocytosis with survival into adolescence: periodontal manifestations and laboratory findings. A case report. *J Periodontol* **42**: 516–19.

Lapiere CM, Nusgens BV (1981) Ehlers–Danlos type VII skin has a reduced proportion of collagen type III. *J Invest Dermatol* **76**: 422–9.

Lavine WS, Page RC, Padgett GA (1976) Host response in chronic periodontal disease. V. The dental and periodontal status of mink and mice affected by Chediak–Higashi syndrome. *J Periodontol* **47**: 621–35.

Leggott PJ (1992) Oral manifestations of HIV infection in children. *Oral Surg Oral Med Oral Pathol* **73**: 192–7.

LeJeunne J, Gautier M, Turpin R (1959) Etude des chromosomes somatique de neuf enfants Mongolien. *Comp Rend Acad Sci* **248**: 1721–22.

Lewit EM, Baker LS, Cornman H, Shiono PH (1995) The direct cost of low birth weight. *Future Child* **5**(1): 35–56.

Lichtenstein L (1953) Integration of eosinophilic granuloma of bone, "Letterer–Siwe Disease", and "Schuller–Christian Disease" as related manifestations of a single nosologic entity. *AMA Arch Pathol* **56**: 84–102.

Linch DC, Acton CHC (1979) Ehlers–Danlos syndrome presenting with juvenile destructive periodontitis. *Br Dent J* **147**: 95–6.

Linden GJ, Mullally BH, Freeman R (1996) Stress and the progression of periodontal disease. *J Clin Periodontol* **23**: 675–80.

Lipton JM (1983) The pathogenesis, diagnosis and treatment of histiocytosis syndromes. *Pediatr Dermatol* **1**: 112–120.

Listgarten MA, Houpt M (1969) Ultrastructural features of the root surface of deciduous teeth in patients with hypophosphatasia. *J Periodont Res* **4**(suppl.): 34–5.

Locker D, Leake JL (1992) Risk indicators and risk markers for periodontal disease experience in older adults living independently in Ontario, Canada. *J Dent Res* **72**: 9–17.

Löe H (1993) Periodontal disease: the sixth complication of diabetes mellitus, *Diabet Care* **16**(suppl.): 329–34.

Loesche WJ, Schork A, Terpenning MS et al. (1998) The relationship between dental disease and cerebral vascular accident in elderly United States veterans. *Ann Periodontol* **3**(1): 161–74.

Lopatin DE, Taylor GW, Loesche WJ et al. (1999) Periodontal pathogens and congestive heart failure. IADR Abstr. 3580.

Lopes-Virella MF, Virella G (1985) Immunological and microbiological factors in the pathogenesis of atherosclerosis. *Clin Immunol Immunopathol* **37**(3): 377–86.

Lundgren T, Westphal O, Bolme P et al. (1991) Retrospective study of children with hypophosphatasia with reference to dental changes. *Scand J Dent Res* **99**: 357–64.

Lyberg T (1982) Immunological and metabolic studies in two siblings with Papillon–Lefèvre syndrome. *J Periodont Res* **17**: 563–8.

Lynch MA, Ship II (1967) Initial oral manifestations of leukemia. *J Am Dent Assoc* **75**: 932–40.

Mackay CR, Imhof BA (1993) Cell adhesion in the immune system. *Immunol Today* **14**: 99–102.

Madigan A, Murray PA, Houpt M et al. (1996) Caries experience and cariogenic markers in HIV-positive children and their siblings. *Pediatr Dent* **18**: 129–35.

Majorana A, Notarangelo LD, Savoldi E et al. (1999) Leukocyte adhesion deficiency in a child with severe oral involvement. *Oral Surg Oral Med Oral Pathol Oral Radiol Endod* **87**: 691–4.

Marcus AJ, Hajjar DP (1993) Vascular transcellular signaling. *J Lipid Res* **34**(12): 2017–31.

Marion RW, Wiznia AA, Hutcheon G, Rubinstein A (1986) Human T-cell lymphotropic virus III (HTLV-III) embryopathy. A new dysmorphic syndrome associated with HTLV-III infection. *Am J Dis Child* **140**: 638–40.

Martin-Iverson NA, Phatouros A, Tennant M (1999) A brief review of indigenous Australian health as it impacts on oral health. *Aust Dent J* **44**(2): 88–92.

Matsuura S, Kishi F, Tsukahara M et al. (1992) Leukocyte adhesion deficiency: identification of novel mutations in two Japanese patients with a severe form. *Biochem Biophys Res Commun* **184**: 1460–7.

Mattila KJ (1993) Dental infections as a risk factor for acute myocardial infarction. *Eur Heart J* **14**(suppl. K): 51–3.

Mattila KJ, Nieminen MS, Valtonen VV et al. (1989) Association between dental health and acute myocardial infarction [see comments], *Br Med J* **298**(6676): 779–81.

Mattila KJ, Valle MS, Nieminen MS et al. (1993) Dental infections and coronary atherosclerosis. *Atherosclerosis* **103**(2): 205–11.

McCarty MF (1999) Interleukin-6 as a central mediator of cardiovascular risk associated with chronic inflammation, smoking, diabetes, and visceral obesity: downregulation with essential fatty acids, ethanol and pentoxifylline. *Med Hypoth* **52**(5): 465–77.

McEver RP (1992) Leukocyte-endothelial cell interactions. *J Cell Biol* **4**: 840–9.

McGregor JA, French JI, Jones W et al. (1994) Bacterial vaginosis is associated with prematurity and vaginal fluid mucinase and sialidase: results of a controlled trial of topical clindamycin cream. *Am J Obstet Gynecol* **170**(4): 1048–59 [discussion 1059–60].

McKusick VA (1972) *Heritable Disorders of Connective Tissue*, 4th edn. St Louis: CV Mosby.

Meskin LH, Farsht EM, Anderson DL (1968) Prevalence of *Bacteroides melaninogenicus* in the gingival crevice area of institutionalized trisomy 21 and cerebral palsy and normal children. *J Periodontol* **39**: 326–8.

Michalowicz B (1994) Genetic and heritable risk factors in periodontal disease. *J Periodont* **65**: 479–88.

Michaud M, Baehner RL, Bixler D, Kafrawy AH (1977) Oral manifestations of acute leukemia in children. *J Am Dent Assoc* **95**: 1145–50.

Moniaci D, Calvallari M, Greco D et al. (1993) Oral lesions in children born to HIV-1 positive women. *J Oral Pathol Med* **22**: 8–12.

Morinushi T, Lopatin DE, van Poperin N (1997) The relationship between gingivitis and the serum antibodies to the microbiota associated with periodontal disease in children with Down's syndrome. *J Periodontol* **68**: 626–31.

Morrison HI, Ellison LF, Taylor GW (1999) Periodontal disease and risk of fatal coronary heart and cerebrovascular diseases. *J Cardiovasc Risk* **6**(1): 7–11.

Murray PA (1994) Periodontal diseases in patients infected by human immunodeficiency virus. *Periodontol 2000* **6**: 50–67.

Murray M, Moonsnick F (1941) Incidence of bacteremia in patients with dental plaque. *J Lab Clin Med* **26**: 801–2.

Narayanan AS, Page RC (1983) Connective tissues of the periodontium: a summary of current work. *Collag Rel Res* **3**: 33–64.

National Center for Health Statistics (1993) *Monthly Vital Statistics Report, 1991*, vol 42, no. 3 (suppl.). Hyattsville: Public Health Service.

Nazzaro V, Blachet-Bardon C, Mimoz C et al. (1988) Papillon–Lefèvre syndrome: ultrastructural study and successful treatment with acitretin. *Arch Dermatol* **124**: 533–9.

Nelson RG, Shlossman M, Budding LM et al. (1990) Periodontal disease and NIDDM in Pima Indians. *Diabet Care* **13**(8): 836–40.

Nezelof D, Basset F, Rousseau MF (1973) Histiocytosis X: histogenetic arguments for a Langerhans cell origin. *Biomedicine* **18**: 365–71.

Obura CW (1965) Pink disease. Report of a case. *Br Dent J* **119**: 273–4.

Offenbacher S (1996) Periodontal diseases: pathogenesis. *Ann Periodontol* **1**(1): 821–78.

Offenbacher S, Salvi GE (1999) Induction of prostaglandin release from macrophages by bacterial endotoxin. *Clin Infect Dis* **28**(3): 505–13.

Offenbacher S, Weathers DR (1985) Effects of smokeless tobacco on the periodontal, mucosal, and caries status of adolescent males. *J Oral Pathol* **14**: 169–81.

Offenbacher S, Katz V, Fertik G et al. (1996) Periodontal infection as a possible risk factor for preterm low birth weight. *J Periodontol* **67**(10 suppl.): 1103–13.

Offenbacher S, Jared HL, O'Reilly PG et al. (1998) Potential pathogenic mechanisms of periodontitis associated pregnancy complications. *Ann Periodontol* **3**(1): 233–50.

Offenbacher S, Beck JD, Elter J et al. (1999a) Periodontal status of cardiovascular disease subjects. IADR Abstr. 2190. UNC Center for Oral and Systemic Diseases, University of North Carolina, Chapel Hill, NC, USA.

Offenbacher S, Madianos PN, Suttle M et al. (1999b) Elevated human fetal IgM suggests in utero exposure to periodontal pathogens. IADR Abstr. 2191.

Oleske J, Minnefor A, Cooper R et al. (1983) Immune deficiency syndrome in children. *JAMA* **249**: 2345–9.

Oliver RC, Tervonen T (1993) Periodontitis and tooth loss: comparing diabetics with the general population. *J Am Dent Assoc* **124**: 71-6.

Orner G (1976) Periodontal disease among children with Down's syndrome and their siblings. *J Dent Res* **55**: 778–82.

Page RC (1998) The pathobiology of periodontal diseases may affect systemic diseases: inversion of a paradigm. *Ann Periodontol* **3**: 108–20.

Page RC, Kornman KS (1997) Pathogenesis of human periodontitis: an introduction. *Periodontol 2000* **14**: 9–11.

Page RC, Altman L, Ebersole J et al. (1983) Rapidly progressive periodontitis—a distinct clinical condition. *J Periodontol* **54**: 197–209.

Paller AS, Nanda V, Spates C, O'Gorman M (1994) Leukocyte adhesion deficiency: recurrent childhood skin infections. *J Am Acad Dermatol* **31**: 316–19.

Papillon MM, Lefèvre P (1924) Deux cas de kératodermie palmaire et plantaire symétrique familiale (Maladie de Meléda) chez le frère et la soeur. Coexistence de les deux cas d'altérations dentaires grabes. *Bull Soc Fr Dermatol Syph* **31**: 82–7.

Parry J, Porter S, Scully C et al. (1996) Mucosal lesions due to oral cocaine use. *Br Dent J* **180**: 462–4.

Paunio K, Impivaara O, Tiekso J, Maki J (1993) Missing teeth and ischaemic heart disease in men aged 45–64 years. *Eur Heart J* **14** (suppl. K): 54–6.

Pearce WH, Sweis I, Yao JS et al. (1992) Interleukin-1 beta and tumor necrosis factor-alpha release in normal and diseased human infrarenal aortas. *J Vasc Surg* **16**(5): 784–9.

Phillips AN, Neaton JD, Cook DG et al. (1992) Leukocyte count and risk of major coronary heart disease events. *Am J Epidemiol* **136**(1): 59–70.

Pimstone B, Eisenberg E, Silverman S (1966) Hypophosphatasia: genetic and dental studies. *Ann Intern Med* **65**: 722–9.

Pizzo PA (1990) Pediatric AIDS: problems within problems. *J Infect Dis* **16**: 316–25.

Preus H, Gjermo P (1987) Clinical management of prepubertal periodontitis in 2 siblings with Papillon–Lefèvre syndrome. *J Clin Periodontol* **14**: 156–60.

Price TH, Ochs HD, Gershoni-Baruch R et al. (1994) In vivo neutrophil and lymphocyte function studies with leukocyte adhesion deficiency Type II. *Blood* **84**: 1635–9.

Prichard JF, Ferguson DM, Windmiller J, Hurt WC (1984) Prepubertal periodontitis affecting the deciduous and permanent dentition in a patient with cyclic neutropenia: a case report and discussion. *J Periodontol* **55**: 114–22.

Pritchard J, Broadbent V (1994) Histiocytosis—an introduction. *Br J Cancer* **70**(suppl. 23): S1–3.

Ramos-Gomez FJ, Hilton JF, Canchola AJ et al. (1996) Risk factors for HIV-related orofacial soft-tissue manifestations in children. *Pediatr Dent* **18**: 121–6.

Rathbun JC (1948) "Hypophosphatasia". A new developmental anomaly. *Am J Dis Child* **75**: 822–31.

Reuland-Bosma W, van Dijk J (1986) Periodontal disease in Down's syndrome: a review. *J Clin Periodontol* **13**: 64–73.

Reuland-Bosma W, van Dijk LJ, van der Weele L (1986) Experimental gingivitis around deciduous teeth in children with Down's syndrome. *J Clin Periodontol* **13**: 294–300.

Reynolds JJ, Meikle MC (1997) Mechanisms of connective tissue matrix destruction in periodontitis. *Periodontol 2000* **14**: 144–57.

Ridker PM, Cushman M, Stampfer MJ et al. (1997) Inflammation, aspirin, and the risk of cardiovascular disease in apparently healthy men. *New Engl J Med* **336**(14): 973–9.

Ridker PM, Cushman M, Stampfer MJ et al. (1998) Plasma concentration of C-reactive protein and risk of developing peripheral vascular disease. *Circulation* **97**(5): 425–8.

Robbins SL, Cotran RS, Kumar V (1989) *Pathologic Basis of Disease*, 4th edn. Philadelphia: WB Saunders.

Roberts MW, Atkinson JC (1990) Oral manifestations associated with leukocyte adhesion deficiency: a five year case study. *Pediatr Dent* **2**: 107–11.

Robertson PB, Walsh M, Greene J et al. (1990) Periodontal effects associated with the use of smokeless tobacco. *J Periodontol* **61**: 438–43.

Roistacher SL (1973) Numbness: a significant finding. *Oral Surg* **36**: 22–7.

Root RK, Rosenthal AS, Balestra DJ (1972) Abnormal bactericidal, metabolic and lysosomal functions of Chediak–Higashi syndrome leukocytes. *J Clin Invest* **51**: 649–65.

Salbach PB, Specht E, von Hodenberg E et al. (1992) Differential low density lipoprotein receptor-dependent formation of eicosanoids in human blood-derived monocytes. *Proc Natl Acad Sci USA* **89**(6): 2439–43.

San Martin T, Jadinski JJ, Palumbo P et al. (1992) Periodontal diseases in children infected with HIV. *J Dent Res* **71**: 366.

Santos R, Shanfeld J, Casamassimo P (1996) Serum antibody response to *Actinobacillus actinomycetemcomitans*. *Spec Care Dent* **16**: 80–3.

Saxen L, Aula S (1982) Periodontal bone loss in patients with Down's syndrome: a follow up study. *J Periodontol* **53**: 158–62.

Saxen L, Aula S, Westermarck T (1977) Periodontal disease associated with Down's syndrome: an orthopantomographic evaluation. *J Periodontol* **48**: 337–40.

Schoen D, Murray P, Jadinski J et al. (1995) Periodontal status of HIV-positive vs. HIV-negative children. *J Dent Res* **74**: 127.

Schroeder HE, Seger RA, Keller HV, Rateitschak-Pluss EM (1988) Behavior of neutrophilic granulocytes in a case of Papillon–Lefevre syndrome (PLS). *J Clin Periodontol* **15**: 17–26.

Schwartz Z, Goultschin J, Dean DD, Boyan BD (1997) Mechanisms of alveolar bone destruction in periodontitis. *Periodontol 2000* **14**: 158–72.

Sconyers JR, Crawford JJ, Moriarty JD (1973) Relationship of bacteremia to toothbrushing in patients with periodontitis. *J Am Dent Assoc* **87**(3): 616–22.

Selter P (1903) *Arch Kinderheilk* **37**: 468.

Seymour RA, Steele JG (1998) Is there a link between periodontal disease and coronary heart disease? *Br Dent J* **184**(1): 33–8.

Seymour GJ, Gemmell E, Reinhardt R et al. (1993) Immunopathogenesis of chronic inflammatory periodontal disease: cellular and molecular mechanisms. *J Periodont Res* **28**: 478–86.

Shannon KM, Ammann AJ (1985) Acquired immune deficiency syndrome in childhood. *J Pediatr* **106**: 332–42.

Shapira LB, Gordon B, Warbington M, VanDyke T (1994) Priming effect of *Porphyromonas gingivalis* lipopolysaccharide on superoxide production by neutrophils from healthy and rapidly progressive periodontitis subjects. *J Periodontol* **65**(2): 129–33.

Shlossman M, Knowler WC, Pettitt DJ (1990) Type 2 diabetes mellitus and periodontal disease. *J Am Dent Assoc* **121**: 532–36.

Sigala JL, Silverman S, Brody HA, Kushner JH (1972) Dental involvement in histiocytosis. *Oral Surg* **33**: 42–8.

Silver JG, Martin AW, McBride BC (1980) Experimental transient bacteremia in human subjects with varying degrees of plaque accumulation and gingival inflammation. *J Clin Periodontol* **4**: 92–9.

Silverman JL (1962) Apparent dominant inheritance of hypophosphatasia. *Arch Intern Med* **110**: 191–8.

Sjöstrom K, Ou JG, Whitney C (1994) Effect of treatment in patients with rapidly progressive periodontitis. *Infect Immun* **62**: 145–51.

Slade GD, Offenbacher S, Beck JD et al. (2000) Acute-phase inflammatory response to periodontal disease in the US population. *J Dent Res* **79**: 49–57.

Sligh JE, Hurwitz MY, Zhu C et al. (1992) An initiation codon mutation in CD18 in association with the moderate phenotype of leukocyte adhesion deficiency. *J Biol Chem* **267**: 714–18.

Snajder N, Carrarro JJ, Otero E, Carranza FA (1968) Clinical periodontal findings in trisomy 21 (mongolism). *J Periodontol Res* **3**: 1–5.

Sobel EH, Clark LC, Fox RP, Robinow M (1958) Rickets, deficiency of "alkaline" phosphatase activity and premature loss of teeth in childhood. *Pediatrics* **11**: 309–21.

Sofaer JA (1990) Genetic approaches to the study of periodontal disease. *J Clin Periodontol* **7**: 401-8.

Sohol PD, Johannessen AC, Kritofferson T et al. (1992) In situ characterization of mononuclear cells in marginal periodontitis of patients with Down's syndrome. *Acta Odontol Scand* **60**: 238–42.

Soskolne WA (1998) Epidemiological and clinical aspects of periodontal diseases in diabetics. *Ann Periodontol* **3**(1): 3–12.

Soubry R, Taelman H, Banyangiliki V et al. (1995) Necrotizing periodontal disease in HIV-1 infected patients; a 4-year study in Kigali, Rwanda. In: Greenspan JS, Greenspan D (eds) *Oral Manifestations of HIV Infection.* Carol Stream: Quintessence.

Springer TA (1990) Adhesion receptors of the immune system. *Nature* **246**: 425–34.

Stabholz A, Soskolne V, Machtei E et al. (1990) Effect of benign familial neutropenia on the periodontium of Yemenite Jews. *J Periodontol* **61**: 51.

Stewart RE, Holliste DW, Rimoin DL (1977) A new variant of Ehlers–Danlos syndrome: an autosomal disorder of fragile skin, abnormal scarring, and generalized periodontitis. *Birth Def* **13**: 85–93.

Sutton PR (1989) Is faulty collagen formation the cause of the exfoliation of the teeth in the Papillon–Lefèvre syndrome? *Med Hypoth* **29**: 43–4.

Svatum B, Gjermo P (1978) Oral hygiene, periodontal health and need for periodontal treatment among institutionalized mentally subnormal persons in Norway. *Acta Odontol Scand* **36**: 89–95.

Swallow JN (1964) Dental disease in children with Down's syndrome. *J Ment Defic Res* **8**: 102–18.

Syrjanen J, Peltola J, Valtonen V et al. (1989) Dental infections in association with cerebral infarction in young and middle-aged men. *J Intern Med* **225**(3): 179–84.

Tempel TR, Kimball HR, Kakehashi S, Amen CR (1973) Host factors in periodontal disease: periodontal manifestations of Chediak–Higashi syndrome. *J Periodont Res* **7**: 26–7.

Terheggen HG, Wischermann A (1984) Congenital hypophosphatasia. *Monatsschr Kinderheilkd* **132**: 512–22.

Thorstensson H (1995) Periodontal disease in adult insulin-dependent diabetics. *Swed Dent J* (suppl.) **107**: 1–68.

Thorstensson HJ, Kuylenstierna J, Hugoson A (1996) Medical status and complications in relation to periodontal disease experience in insulin-dependent diabetics. *J Clin Periodontol* **23**(3.1): 194–202.

Tinanoff N, Tanzer JM, Kornman KS, Maderazo EG (1986) Treatment of the periodontal component of Papillon–Lefèvre syndrome. *J Clin Periodontol* **13**: 6–10.

Todd RF, Freyer DR (1988) The CD11/CD18 leukocyte glycoprotein deficiency. *Hematol/Oncol Clin North Am* **2**: 13–31.

Tovo PA, De Martino M, Gabiano C (1992) Prognostic factors and survival in children with perinatal HIV-1 infection. *Lancet* **339**: 1249–53.

Ulseth LO, Hestness A, Stovner LJ, Storhaug K (1991) Dental caries and periodontitis in persons with Down's syndrome. *Spec Care Dent* **11**: 71–3.

Valdez IH, Pizzo PA, Atkinson JC (1994) Oral health of pediatric AIDS patients. A hospital-based study. *ASDC J Dent Child* **61**: 114–18.

Valtonen VV (1991) Infection as a risk factor for infarction and atherosclerosis. *Ann Med* **23**(5): 539–43.

Valtonen VA, Kuikka A, Syrjanen J (1993) Thrombo-embolic complications in bacteraemic infections. *Eur Heart J* **14**(suppl. K): 20–3.

Van Dyke TE, Hoop GA (1990) Neutrophil function and oral disease. *Crit Rev Oral Biol Med* **1**: 117–33.

Van Dyke TE, Taubman MA, Ebersole JL et al. (1984) The Papillon–Lefèvre syndrome: neutrophil dysfunction with severe periodontal disease. *Clin Immunol Immunopath* **31**: 419–29.

Vaughn AG, Vrahopolous TP, Joachim F et al. (1990) A case report of chronic neutropenia: clinical and ultra-structural findings. *J Clin Periodontol* **17**: 435–45.

Vieira R, Ribeiro de Souza IP, Modesto A et al. (1998) Gingival status of HIV+ children and the correlation with caries incidence and immunologic profile. *Pediatr Dent* **20**: 169–72.

Waldrop TC, Anderson DC, Hallmon WC et al. (1987) Periodontal manifestations of the heritable MAC-1, LFA-1 deficiency syndrome–clinical, histopathologic, and molecular characteristics. *J Periodontol* **58**: 400–16.

Warkany J, Hubbard DM (1948) *Lancet* **i**: 829.

Watanabe K, Umeda M, Seki T, Ishikawa I (1993) Clinical and laboratory studies of severe periodontal disease in an adolescent associated with hypophos-phatasia. A case report. *J Periodontol* **64**: 174.

Watanabe H, Goseki-Sone M, Limura T et al. (1999) Molecular diagnosis of hypophosphatasia with severe periodontitis. *J Periodontol* **70**: 688–91.

Whyte MP (1989) Hypophosphatasia. In: Scriver CR, Beaud, Sly WS et al. (eds) *The Metabolic Basis of Inherited Disease*, 6th edn. New York: McGraw–Hill.

Worth HM (1966) Some significant abnormal radio-graphic appearances in young jaws. *Oral Surg* **21**: 609–17.

Wray A, McGuirt F (1993) Smokeless tobacco usage associated with oral carcinoma. *Arch Otolaryngol Head Neck Surg* **119**: 929–33.

Young M, Engebretson S, Desvarieux M et al. (1999) Periodontal disease in ischemic stroke patients and controls. IADR Abstr. 2812.

Yukna RA (1991) Cocaine periodontitis. *Int J Periodontol Restor Dent* **11**: 73–9.

Zambon JJ, Reynolds H, Genco RJ (1990) Studies of the subgingival microflora in patients with acquired immunodeficiency syndrome. *J Periodontol* **61**: 699–704.

Zancharski LR, Elveback KR, Linman JV (1971) Leukocyte counts in healthy adults. *Am J Clin Pathol* **56**: 148–50.

Zubery Y, Moses O, Kozlovsky A (1991) Agranulocytosis: periodontal manifestations and treat-ment of the acute phase: a case report. *Clin Prevent Dent* **13**: 5–8.

PART IV

Etiology of periodontal disease

7
Pathogenesis of aggressive periodontitis

Harvey A. Schenkein

It is accepted dogma that all forms of periodontitis have a bacterial cause (Haffajee and Socransky, 1994). Thus, the expression of the disease is not expected to be seen in the absence of pathogenic bacterial agents. However, carriage of an etiological bacterial agent—even in large quantities—does not necessarily translate into disease expression. Part of the explanation is that members of a bacterial species are not all alike and do not necessarily contain all the elements necessary to cause disease; thus, strain or biotype variability may influence the pathogenic potential of bacteria. Just as pertinent, however, is the fact that people vary in their susceptibility to disease, owing to innate acquired or inherited host factors or other environmental influences.

The pathogenic mechanisms responsible for aggressive periodontitis (AP) can be placed into two interdependent categories. The first is the direct effect of bacterial pathogens on the periodontal tissues. For example, bacteria may produce enzymes that directly degrade the connective tissues of the periodontal ligament. The second category comprises the indirect effects of bacterial pathogens. An example of this would be the secretion by bacteria of a substance that reacts with a host cell, inducing it to release an enzyme that degrades connective tissue components.

The pathology of AP appears to be associated with unique host characteristics that increase susceptibility of certain individuals to disease, with unique components of bacterial plaque, and with pathways in common with other forms of periodontitis leading to loss of connective tissue and bone. In many cases, these unique host characteristics and the disease itself appear to be familial, indicating that host susceptibility may also be familial and possibly inherited (Hart 1996). Alternatively, the familial expression of disease could be due to the passage of an infectious agent within the household.

Protective host responses in aggressive periodontitis

In order to understand the pathological processes leading to lesions characteristic of AP, it is essential to understand the mechanisms that protect the periodontium against disease. It is only when these protective processes are overcome or subverted that disease is initiated or disease progression occurs.

Chemotaxis

Typically, healthy periodontal tissues are characterized by a paucity of inflammatory cells within the connective tissue. However, polymorphonuclear leukocytes, or neutrophils, are commonly found lining the junctional epithelium and separating bacterial plaque from the tissues. Thus, neutrophils are considered to be the first line of defense against plaque. The appearance of neutrophils in areas of bacterial accumulation is mediated by a process called *chemotaxis*, or induction of movement of cells towards the origin of a chemical signal. Many bacteria produce compounds that are recognized by specific neutrophil membrane receptors; these receptors are proteins that can specifically bind to chemical agents, which in turn activate biochemical processes within the cell, resulting in biological functions. Additionally, chemical mediators of chemotaxis are produced by cells as a result of contact with bacteria or bacterial products. These mediators will also bind to their specific receptors to induce neutrophil functional activities such as chemotaxis.

In order for leukocytes to leave the bloodstream, chemical signals from the tissues adjacent to the bacteria must reach the local vasculature, where they induce the vessels to cause the cells to slow down, leave the bloodstream, and enter the tissues. Additional chemical signals induce changes in the blood vessel walls. Thus, the neutrophils slow within the local capillaries, marginate along the vessel walls, squeeze between the endothelial cells lining the vessels, and move towards the source of the chemical signal (the bacteria or the tissues surrounding the bacteria) all as a result of chemical signaling induced by the infecting agent. Some of the unique pathogenic mechanisms that increase risk for AP are thought to entail aberrations in neutrophil migration.

Recognition of bacteria by neutrophils

Neutrophils are endowed with the ability to consume, or phagocytose, most bacteria to which they have been summoned. However, additional chemical interactions are usually necessary for this process to be efficient. The immune system participates in this process by making the bacteria more readily recognized and more easily attached to the surface of the neutrophil. This process is called opsonization, and the chemicals that coat the bacteria and make them more easily recognized are called opsonins.

Complement, antibodies, and bacterial recognition

An important component of innate immunity is the complement system (Figure 7.1). It is "innate" in that it can be activated by many bacteria to which it has never previously been exposed. This contrasts with "acquired immunity", which only develops following an initial exposure to bacteria or other foreign substances (antigens). The complement system is activated either by mechanisms involving specific immunity (that is, following binding of antibodies to the bacterial surface) or by non-specific means.

Upon exposure of bacteria to the proteins of the complement system (in plasma or in inflammatory exudates), a chemical reaction cascade is initiated that results in the coating of bacteria with complement-derived opsonins and, for some bacteria, death. This alternative complement pathway can be activated by certain bacteria, including all Gram-negative bacteria, without the need for specific antibody. These bacteria have molecules, most importantly lipopolysaccharide (LPS), which provide a suitable chemical environment for the assembly of an enzyme that catalyzes the formation of the complement-derived opsonin C3b, which coats the bacterial surface. The physiological degradation product of C3b, called iC3b, is also an opsonin. Phagocytes have surface receptors for both C3b and iC3b, and so the coating of bacteria with these proteins promotes recognition of bacteria by neutrophils. These receptors are called CR1, CR2, and CR3.

When specific antibodies to bacteria of the immunoglobulin (Ig) G or IgM classes have been induced by prior exposure to the organism, the binding of these antibodies to bacterial antigens can activate the classical complement pathway. Although a different series of reactions occur at the bacteria surface to initiate the formation of C3-degrading enzymes, the outcome is similar, in that C3b and iC3b coat the bacterial surface, and promote bacterial recognition. Furthermore, the antibodies themselves promote both recognition and ingestion (phagocytosis) of bacteria because phagocytes have a series of receptors on their surfaces that recognize bound antibodies. These phagocyte membrane proteins are called Fc receptors; they bind to the Fc portion of antibody molecules which are bound in antigen–antibody complexes.

A further outcome of the activation of complement by either activation pathway is the assembly of additional complement proteins in the bacterial surface which promote formation of pores through the membranes and can lead to osmotic lysis or

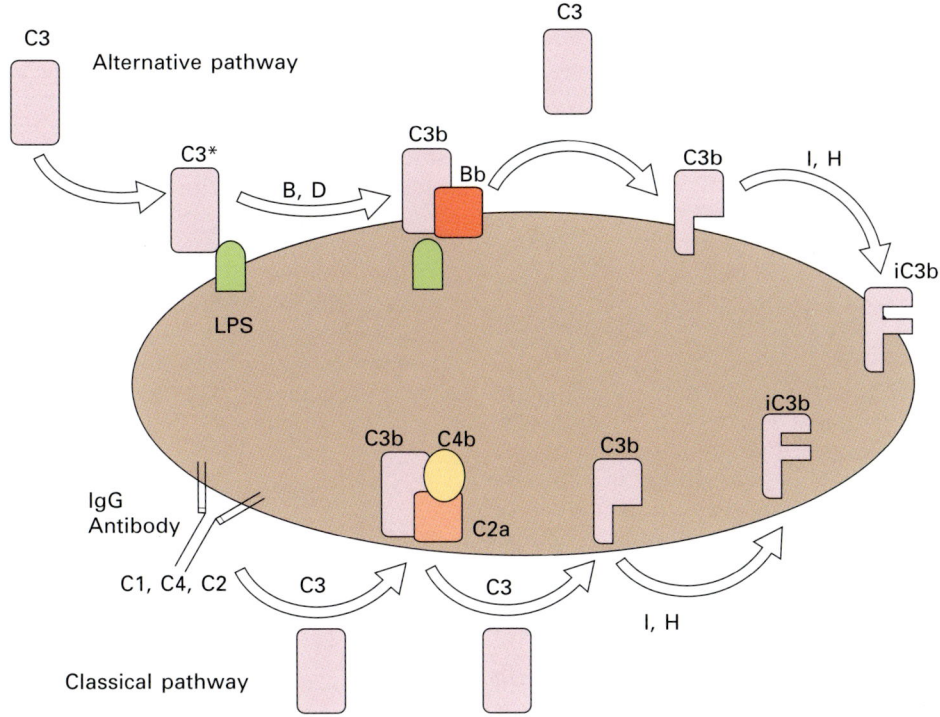

Figure 7.1

Complement activation by Gram-negative bacteria. The two major complement activation pathways are illustrated. The upper part of the figure depicts the *alternative pathway*: C3 molecules transiently acquire the ability to bind to LPS, where-upon factor B binds to C3 and is fragmented by factor D. The factor B fragment Bb then splits the C3 molecule into C3a and C3b. The C3b on the bacterial cell associates with more factor B, leading to formation of more C3b. The enzyme factor I, in the presence of its cofactor H, converts C3b to iC3b. The *classical pathway* is activated by specific antibody, which initiates a cascade of enzymatic cleavages: C1, C4, and C2 in turn are cleaved and incorporated into a C3-cleaving enzyme that splits C3 into C3a and C3b; iC3b is formed as described above. C4b, C3b, and iC3b are opsonins, as is IgG antibody.

killing of the bacteria. This complex of complement proteins is called the membrane attack complex (MAC). Not all bacteria, however, are susceptible to killing by the MAC; those that are, are described as being "serum sensitive". Some of the unique pathogenic mechanisms that increase risk for AP may entail variations in the function of Fc receptors.

Phagocytosis and killing

Antibody molecules and engagement of the Fc receptors are generally required for the next step in the phagocytic process. Complement-derived opsonins, which enhance recognition of bacteria by phagocytes, also greatly increase phagocytosis of bacteria in the sense that fewer antibody molecules are required for ingestion to occur if complement is also present. Once bacteria are recognized and bound to neutrophils, engulfment and ingestion of bacteria occur.

Neutrophils possess a variety of means of killing bacteria or impeding their replication. Within the neutrophil, bacteria may be exposed to bactericidal compounds within phagolysosomes, the organelles formed consequent to ingestion of the bacteria. Amongst these compounds are lysozyme, lactoferrin, defensins, cathepsin G, and elastase, which are released into the phagolysosome during a process known as degranulation. Additionally, oxidative mechanisms kill many bacteria by production of hydrogen peroxide, hydroxyl radicals, and other compounds. Many of the bactericidal and bacteriostatic compounds can also be released into the surrounding environment following phagocytosis and degranulation.

Interactions of bacteria with monocytes, lymphocytes, and fibroblasts

The interaction of bacterial antigens with inflammatory cells, cells participating in immune responses, and connective tissue cells such as fibroblasts results in the production of mediators by these cells. These mediators are responsible both for maintenance of homeostasis and for pathological reactions. In particular, cytokines are proteins produced by cells as part of a communications network between cells. The purpose of this network is the production of biological responses protective against attacks by foreign substances. The particular cytokines produced, and their concentrations, control the nature and intensity of the biological response. For example, a series of cytokine mediators is known to be necessary for the maturation and differentiation of B lymphocytes, the interaction of T lymphocytes with B lymphocytes, and eventually the production of antibodies by plasma cells. Inflammatory mediators such as prostaglandins and other lipid mediators also carry out normal physiological functions but can behave as tissue-destructive substances.

The monocyte/macrophage series of cells is particularly important in connective tissue homeostasis and remodeling. They are functionally heterogeneous, in that subsets of these cells produce differing biological effects. These cells are phagocytic and also secretory, producing a wide variety of enzymes, cytokines, and inflammatory mediators following encounters with bacteria. The major cytokines produced by monocytes are the interleukins IL-1 and IL-6, and tumor necrosis factor alpha (TNF-α). Secretion of IL-1 can stimulate other cells to release tissue-destroying enzymes called matrix metalloproteinases (MMPs), such as collagenase. Many

other substances can also be stimulated by these cytokines which both regulate MMPs (tissue inhibitors of MMPs) and promote angiogenesis, fibroblast growth, and nerve regeneration. The tissue destruction seen in periodontal lesions is thought to be a result of dysregulation of this system of catabolic and anabolic processes, resulting in overstimulation of tissue catabolism in the presence of bacterial pathogens.

The number of cytokines and inflammatory substances is too great for a full review, but the key mediators and their likely role in periodontal tissue destruction are summarized below.

Protective immune responses against aggressive periodontitis pathogens

Clues that specific pathogens are involved as etiologic agents in AP came from serologic studies of the antibodies present in serum from affected patients. The results of such studies have indicated that many AP patients produce high levels of antibody reactive with antigens of *Actinobacillus actinomycetemcomitans*, *Porphyromonas gingivalis*, or both (Genco et al., 1980; Ebersole et al., 1982; Gooss et al., 1986). Furthermore, AP patients in general produce very high levels of IgG2 subclass immunoglobulins (Califano et al., 1991, 1992; Wilson and Hamilton 1992, 1995; Lu et al., 1993).

Antibody reactive with *A. actinomycetemcomitans*

Patients with AP can produce remarkably high serum concentrations of antibody against *Actinobacillus actinomycetemcomitans*. Levels of such antibody can be greater than 1 mg/ml (g/l), a remarkable concentration when one considers that total IgG concentrations in serum reach around 10–14 mg/ml (g/l). In addition, AP patients produce antibody against *A. actinomycetemcomitans* locally in the gingival tissues, as evidenced by its elevated concentration in gingival crevicular fluid (GCF) (Ebersole et al., 1985; Genco et al., 1985; Tew et al., 1985). It has been found that the immunodominant antigen of *A. actinomycetemcomitans* (i.e., the antigen against which the majority of antibody is being produced) is a carbohydrate side-chain on its LPS (Califano et al., 1989, 1991, 1992; Wilson and Schifferle, 1991). This is the same antigen that determines the serotype specificity of a given strain of *A. actinomycetemcomitans*. Antibodies have also been found that react with a number of other important antigens, including antibodies against the *A. actinomycetemcomitans* leukotoxin (Tsai et al., 1981; Ebersole et al., 1995; Califano et al., 1997). These antibodies are opsonic, that is, they can mediate complement activation and complement-mediated phagocytosis of *A. actinomycetemcomitans* in patients with appropriate variants of genetically determined Fc receptors (Baker and Wilson, 1989; Underwood et al., 1993; Wilson et al., 1995; Wilson and Bronson, 1997) (see below).

Production of IgG2

An additional immunologic characteristic unique to AP patients is the production of high overall levels of IgG2 in serum (Wilson and Hamilton, 1992; Lu et al., 1994; Zhang et al., 1996). These patients' sera contain approximately 1 mg/ml (1 g/l) more IgG2 protein than do sera from healthy subjects or patients with adult periodontitis. It appears that monocytes from AP blood secrete a factor or factors that stimulate high levels of IgG2 production. Since some of the cytokines and inflammatory mediators thought to be in imbalance in AP patients (e.g., IL-1, PGE$_2$) are involved in IgG2 production, it is possible that these high immunoglobulin levels are a reflection of such mediator production.

Function of antibodies to periodontal pathogens in aggressive periodontitis

The interaction between neutrophils, antibody, and complement provides primary protection against the deleterious effects of periodontal pathogens (Figure 7.2). In general, high levels of

antibody do not appear in patients' serum or GCF until some time after the disease process has begun. High levels of antibodies reactive with bacterial virulence factors such as *A. actinomycetemcomitans* leukotoxin, LPS, or *P. gingivalis* proteases, or with whole bacterial antigen preparations, do not occur until later in the disease process and probably do not play an important role in prevention of disease initiation. However, it appears that in the case of the antibody response to *A. actinomycetemcomitans* and *P. gingivalis* in AP patients, the extent and severity of disease is the least in patients with the highest titers (Ranney et al., 1982; Gunsolley et al., 1987; Califano et al., 1997). Thus, some antibody responses to periodontal disease pathogens may ultimately prevent or delay progression of existing disease.

Bacterial pathogenic characteristics associated with aggressive periodontitis

Characteristics of bacteria that permit organisms to persist in the host and cause disease are called *virulence factors*. These are usually bacterial constituents or metabolites that can disrupt homeostatic or protective host mechanisms. Under appropriate conditions, they can promote survival and growth of bacteria in the host and induce progression or initiation of the disease. The pathogenesis of periodontitis lesions is dependent upon the virulence of the bacteria in the flora as well as on their concentration.

Characteristics of pathogenic oral bacteria include the capacity to colonize the subgingival domain, the ability to evade antibacterial host defense mechanisms, and the presence or production of substances that can directly initiate tissue destruction.

Evasion of host defenses

An important feature of nearly all pathogenic microorganisms is their ability to evade the host defense mechanisms that would ordinarily prevent disease. Foremost among these defense

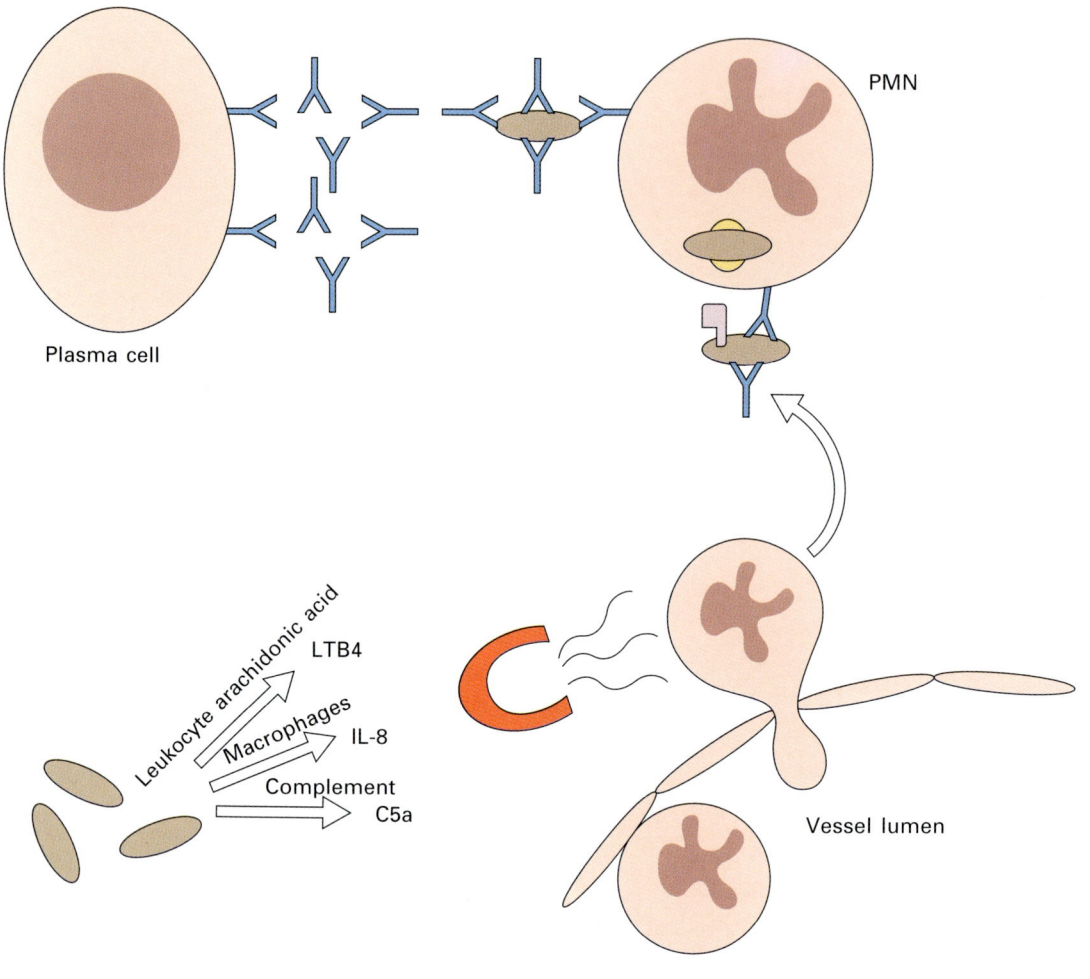

Figure 7.2

Protective antibacterial responses. Exposure to bacteria induces production of specific antibodies by plasma cells. Infection with bacteria leads to production of chemotactic factors which recruit PMNs from the blood. Antibodies coat bacteria, which are then recognized by PMN Fc receptors; complement-derived opsonins also coat bacteria, which are recognized by PMN complement receptors. The PMNs phagocytose bacteria and kill them through a variety of antibacterial mechanisms.

mechanisms in the periodontium is clearance of bacteria by neutrophils with the assistance of antibodies and complement proteins. The local repository of such antibody molecules is the GCF, a modified inflammatory exudate which flows through the junctional and sulcular epithelium into the gingival crevice or pocket. The GCF contains serum antibody molecules, locally produced antibody molecules, and other substances such as neutrophil granule constituents and cytokines, which reflect local immunologic and inflammatory processes. Antibacterial antibodies have many protective functions, including promotion of phagocytosis via interactions with phagocyte Fc receptors, activation of the complement system, neutraliza-

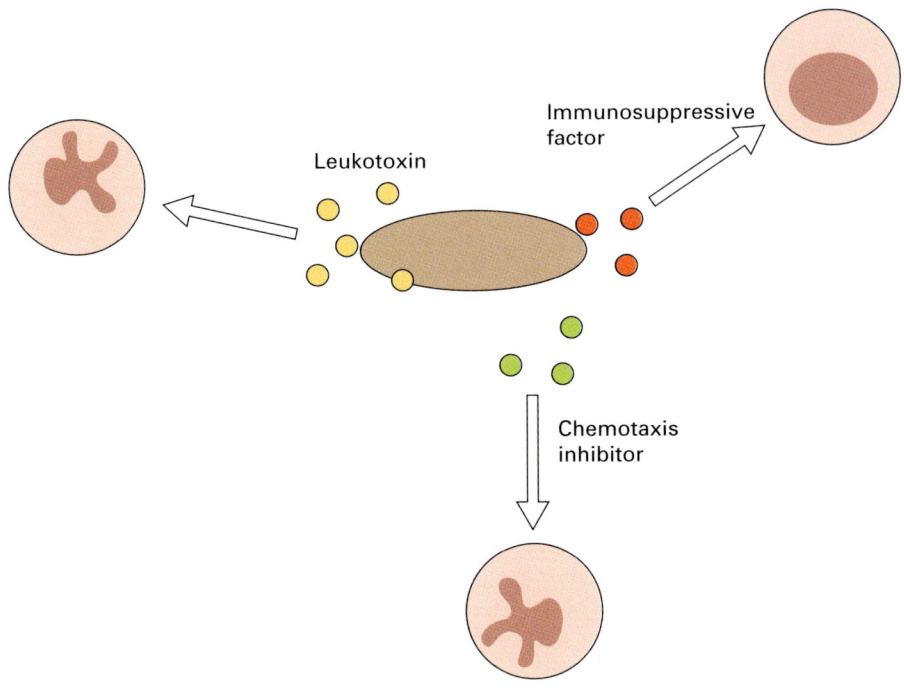

Figure 7.3

Actinobacillus actinomycetemcomitans evades protective immunological and inflammatory responses in a number of ways. For example, it produces an inhibitor of PMN chemotaxis, as well as a leukotoxin that kills PMNs. Additionally, it produces immunosuppressive factors that dampen specific production of antibody as well as cell-mediated immune responses by lymphoid cells.

tion of bacterial toxins and enzymes, and disruption of bacterial colonization by preventing adherence to the tooth or epithelial surface or to other bacteria. These defense mechanisms can be subverted by pathogenic bacteria in the following ways (Figure 7.3).

Toxin production

Some strains of *Actinobacillus actinomycetemcomitans* produce a leukotoxin, a protein that is capable of killing the primary host defensive cell, the polymorphonuclear leukocyte (PMN) (Tsai et al., 1979; Taichman et al., 1980). This property is thought to be an important pathogenic factor in cases of AP associated with this species. Although all strains of *A. actinomycetemcomitans* have the gene necessary for production of

this leukotoxin, only certain strains are capable of producing it at high levels (Haubek et al., 1996). Such strains have been shown to have a deletion in the promoter region of the gene which permits enhanced gene transcription. Several interesting studies have characterized this gene in different patient populations. The highly toxic strains are found almost exclusively in populations of African origin; Europeans with AP rarely if ever have strains of *A. actinomycetemcomitans* demonstrating the deletion in the promoter region of this gene. Furthermore, it appears that patients of African origin who undergo initiation of tissue loss characteristic of AP also have this type of strain, while older patients with a history of AP do not (Haubek et al., 1997; Bueno et al., 1998). It is possible to interpret these findings as indicating that there is a strong association of this toxin (and strains of

A. actinomycetemcomitans capable of producing it) with onset of AP in patients of African origin, but that AP can probably occur in the absence of such bacterial strains. This indicates that there is heterogeneity in the pathogenesis of AP—or perhaps more than one form of AP. (Similar conclusions can be drawn from data on PMN chemotaxis defects, discussed below.)

Immunosuppressive factors

Actinobacillus actinomycetemcomitans produces an immunosuppressive factor that depresses immunologic responses by inhibiting activities of T cells (DNA, RNA, and protein synthesis) and B cells (IgG and IgM production). The secretion of this factor is likely to result in a dampening of protective immune responses in the periodontal lesion to a variety of bacterial antigens and non-specific activators of lymphocyte function (Shenker et al., 1982a, 1990).

Proteolytic enzymes

The ability to destroy host proteins that have antibacterial properties would be an effective virulence mechanism for bacteria. *Porphyromonas gingivalis* produces a series of potent proteases called gingipains, plus a number of other protein-degrading enzymes. Antibody molecules and complement proteins are readily digested by these enzymes and probably contribute to the ability of *P. gingivalis* to survive in fluids (such as GCF) known to have such host proteins. Additionally, opsonins that are able to bind to the surface of *P. gingivalis* are rapidly removed by these enzymes. In proteolytically degrading proteins such as complement components *P. gingivalis* may also cause production of fragments of these proteins with biological activity. For example, degradation of complement protein C3 and C5 by certain proteases produces fragments C3a and C5a, which have biological functions. Both are termed *anaphylatoxins*, and are capable of reacting with mast cells and basophils to induce mediator release. Also, C5a is a chemotactic agent which will enhance the inflammatory response. When certain cytokines that are central to the inflammatory response are exposed to *P. gingivalis* proteases, they too are inactivated. Finally, these proteases may also react with the coagulation and kinin-generating systems to further promote inflammation (Maeda and Molla, 1989; Schenkein, 1989; Fishburn et al., 1991; Cutler et al., 1993).

Invasion of host tissues

Both *P. gingivalis* and *A. actinomycetemcomitans* have been shown to invade host tissues (Sreenivasan et al., 1993; Fives-Taylor et al., 1995; Lamont et al., 1995; Wilson and Henderson 1995). *Actinobacillus actinomycetemcomitans* can pass through epithelial cells into the underlying connective tissues (Figure 7.4), while *P. gingivalis* can invade and persist in epithelial cells. The tissue invasiveness of these organisms may explain the difficulty of eradicating *A. actinomycetemcomitans* by mechanical root debridement, and could also explain the higher concentrations of serum antibody reactive with these two species in comparison with other bacteria in dental plaque. Furthermore, their intracellular invasion may sequester these bacteria in a manner that makes their detection by the immune system more difficult.

Destruction of host tissues

Other virulence characteristics have the property of potentially destroying host tissues or impairing their repair. Bacteria associated with AP lesions produce the following factors.

Lipopolysaccharide

All Gram-negative bacteria have LPS in their outer membranes. Lipopolysaccharides from AP pathogens share their properties with other forms of LPS, though it should be noted that LPS from different bacteria may have quite different biological activities, particularly with respect to potency. Lipopolysaccharide from *A. actinomycetemcomitans* and *P. gingivalis* stimulates bone resorption. Importantly, LPS stimulates macrophages to produce cytokines and inflammatory mediators such as IL-1, TNF, and prostaglandin E_2 (PGE_2), which themselves

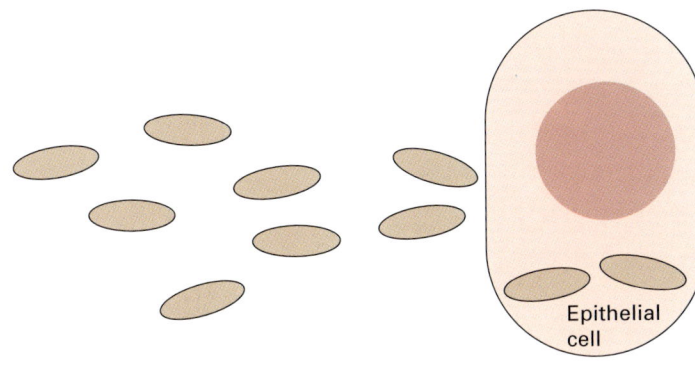

Figure 7.4

Actinobacillus actinomycetemcomitans has the unique property of invading and transmigrating epithelial cells. This capacity to exist intracellularly confers several important pathological properties to the microorganism, including evading detection by the immune system and evading eradication by conservative mechanical periodontal therapy.

Epithelial cell

participate in tissue-destructive biological reactions (Koga et al., 1987; Tamura et al., 1992; Shapira et al., 1994a, b) (see below).

Cytotoxic factors

Actinobacillus actinomycetemcomitans produces a distinct factor that inhibits the growth of fibroblasts, by decreasing DNA and RNA synthesis (Shenker et al., 1982b). This is likely to inhibit repair of periodontitis lesions, by impairing collagen production.

Proteolytic enzymes

Proteolytic enzymes, some of which are capable of contributing to evasion of host defenses, also can directly degrade host tissues. Both *A. actinomycetemcomitans* and *P. gingivalis* produce a collagenase that could degrade collagenous connective tissues (Zambon 1985; Takahashi et al., 1991).

Clonality and bacterial virulence

It is now apparent that within a given pathogenic species such as *Actinobacillus actinomycetemcomitans* or *Porphyromonas gingivalis* only a subset of bacterial types or clonal or genetic subtypes may be pathogenic (Haffajee and Socransky, 1994; Zambon et al., 1996). Thus the presence of a pathogenic bacterial species in the

subgingival plaque may not by itself imply that a pathogen is present with virulence characteristics necessary to initiate or propagate periodontitis lesions. For example, strains of *A. actinomycetemcomitans* in young patients with aggressive periodontitis differ from those in older patients with previously active disease in their ability to produce leukotoxin. Not all *P. gingivalis* strains behave identically in assays of bacterial virulence: some strains produce dissecting lesions and death following inoculation into mice, while others produce only local lesions which heal (Chen et al., 1987). The differences in virulence may be due to factors such as possession of a carbohydrate capsule or differential ability to produce large amounts of proteolytic enzymes.

Destructive mechanisms common to all forms of periodontitis

Although AP is a disease phenotype with unique characteristics with respect to age of onset and the distribution and appearance of associated periodontal lesions, it is likely that the mechanisms responsible for destruction of periodontal tissues are similar to those in other forms of periodontitis. There is increasing evidence that tissue destruction in established periodontitis lesions is a result of the mobilization of host tissues via activation of monocytes, lymphocytes, fibroblasts, and other host cells. Bacterial

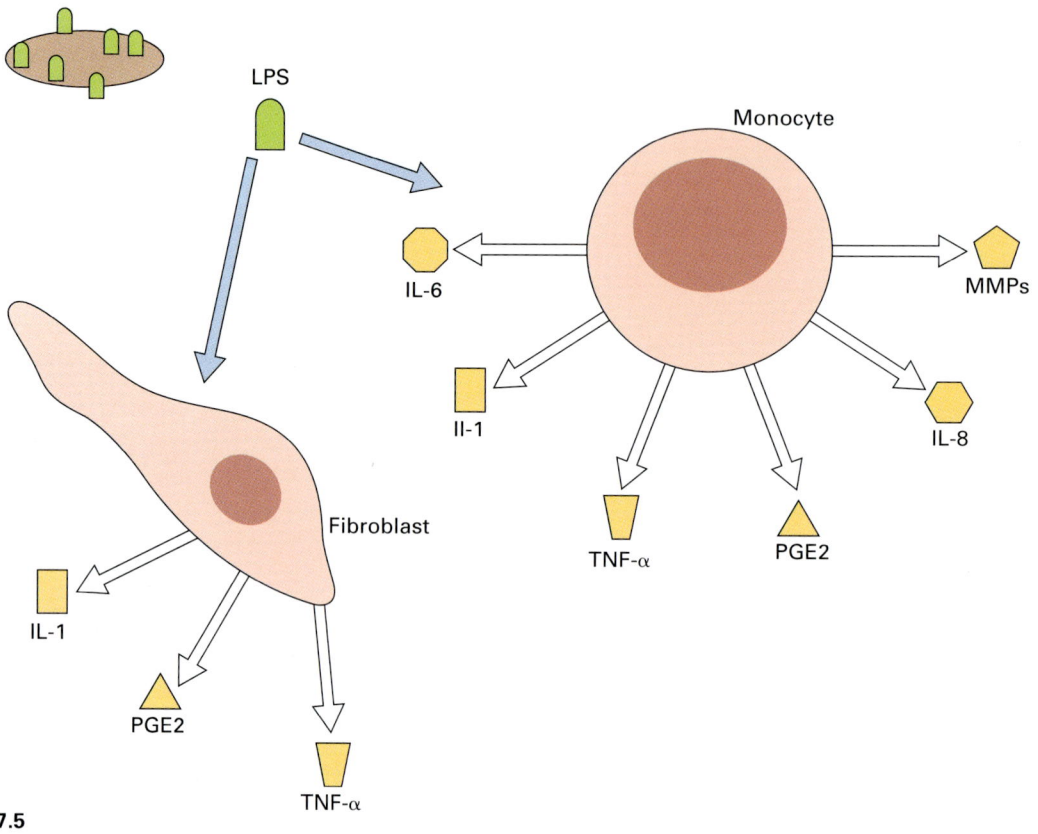

Figure 7.5

Stimulation of host cells to produce mediators of tissue destruction: *A. actinomycetemcomitans*, by virtue of its LPS and other cellular constituents, stimulates host cells to produce several mediators that contribute to periodontal tissue destruction and attachment loss. These mediators include cytokines, prostaglandins, and enzymes, which directly or indirectly cause destruction of connective tissue and bone.

components such as LPS are capable of activating host cells to produce catabolic (tissue-destructive) compounds that themselves either directly induce tissue destruction or promote release of additional mediators or enzymes that destroy the periodontal tissues (Figure 7.5). It is noteworthy that the specific pathways for tissue destruction in AP—if there are any that are unique—are not known.

Stimulation of tissues and cells present in the periodontium by LPS is an excellent model for explaining how periodontitis lesions are likely to occur. All forms of periodontitis, including AP, are associated with Gram-negative "pathogens" that are likely to be etiologic agents. These pathogens have unique mechanisms for surviv-

ing and initiating inflammation in the oral cavity (as outlined above), and once they overwhelm host defenses their constituents have access to the host. It should be kept in mind that AP patients appear to have unique susceptibility factors that increase risk for such infections (see below). Once defensive mechanisms have been averted, the subgingival bacterial microflora becomes established as a predominantly anaerobic, Gram-negative infection. The pathologic appearance of the periodontitis lesion and the mediators, mediator precursors, and mRNA protein templates recognizable either in the GCF or within cellular elements of the gingival tissues are consistent with the expected outcome of a local infection with Gram-negative bacteria.

Cytokines, molecules released by host cells into the local environment, provide molecular signals to other cells thereby affecting their function. Inflammatory mediators such as prostaglandins have similar properties. Many cytokines and inflammatory mediators are produced by cells in periodontitis lesions in response to bacterial LPS; the most important are described below.

Interleukin-1

Interleukin-1 is a proinflammatory, multifunctional cytokine (Tatakis, 1993). There are two forms: IL-1α and IL-1β. The predominant form in the periodontal tissues is IL-1β, which is produced primarily by macrophages (Matsuki et al., 1991, 1992). Both forms have similar biological activities. Amongst these activities are promotion of ingress of inflammatory cells into sites of infection, promotion of bone resorption, stimulation of eicosanoid production (specifically PGE$_2$) and release by monocytes and fibroblasts, stimulation of production of matrix metalloproteinases (e.g., collagenase), and participation in many aspects of the immune response (such as antibody production). Studies have demonstrated that IL-1 levels in general are elevated in both tissues and GCF from diseased, inflamed periodontal tissues compared with healthier sites (Jandinski et al., 1991; Stashenko et al., 1991; Wilton et al., 1992; Preiss and Meyle, 1994; Hou et al., 1995; Yavuzyilmaz et al., 1995). Furthermore, elevated levels of IL-1 have been shown to be associated with active periodontal disease in animal models (Smith et al., 1993).

Interleukin-6

Interleukin-6 (Lotz, 1995) is produced by lymphocytes, monocytes, and fibroblasts (Matsuki et al., 1992); it stimulates plasma cell proliferation and therefore promotes antibody production. This cytokine has also been shown to stimulate osteoclast formation, and thus its production is associated with resorption of bone. Like IL-1, IL-6 is associated with periodontal disease lesions. Levels of IL-6 have been shown to be elevated in inflamed periodontal tissues, are higher in

periodontitis than in gingivitis tissues, and are higher in GCF from "refractory periodontitis" patients (Geivelis et al., 1993; Reinhardt et al., 1993; Yamazaki et al., 1994). Thus, this cytokine may in large part account for both the predominance of plasma cells in periodontitis lesions as well as bone resorption.

Interleukin-8

Interleukin-8 (Bickel, 1993) is a chemoattractant mainly produced by monocytes. It is produced in response to contact with LPS or other cytokines such as IL-1 or TNF-α. In addition to serving as a chemoattractant for neutrophils, it selectively stimulates MMP activity from these cells, and thus may account for a portion of the collagen destruction within periodontitis lesions. It is found to be present at high concentrations in periodontitis lesions, mainly associated with the junctional epithelium and macrophages (Tonetti et al., 1994; Fitzgerald and Kreutzer, 1995). Furthermore, its levels in GCF are higher in periodontitis patients than in healthy controls (Tsai et al., 1995).

Tumor necrosis factor

Tumor necrosis factor alpha (Moldawer, 1994; Rink and Kirchner 1996) shares many of its biological activities (proinflammatory properties, matrix metalloproteinase stimulation, eicosanoid production, and bone resorption) with IL-1. In addition, its secretion by monocytes and fibroblasts is stimulated by bacterial LPS.

Prostaglandin E$_2$

Prostaglandin E$_2$ (Offenbacher et al., 1993a, b) is an eicosanoid (a product of arachidonic acid metabolism through the cyclooxygenase system) produced by many cells including monocytes and fibroblasts. Its activities include induction of bone resorption and matrix metalloproteinase secretion. Many studies have demonstrated that elevated levels of PGE$_2$ in tissues and GCF are closely

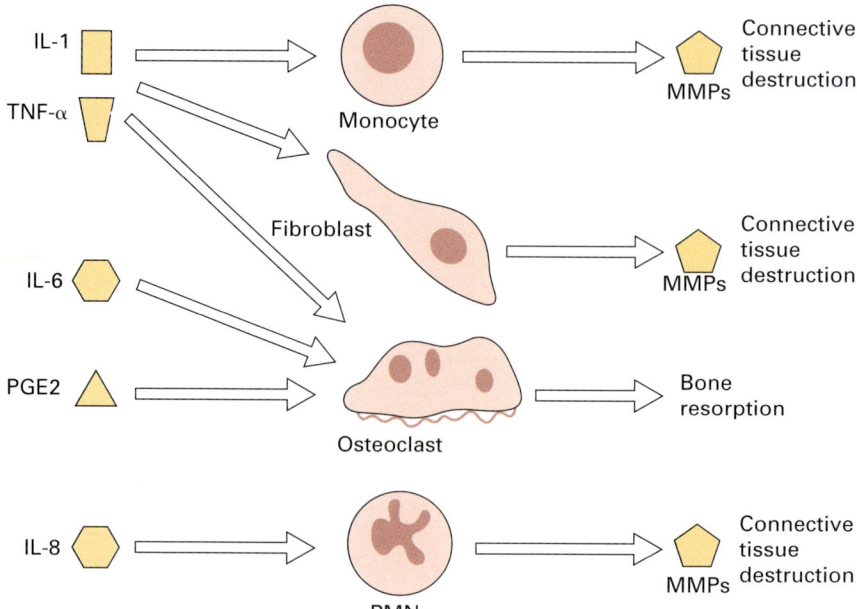

Figure 7.6

Stimulation of host cells by mediators induced by periodontal pathogens. The mediators produced in response to infection with *A. actinomycetemcomitans* stimulate production of matrix metalloproteinases by monocytes/ macrophages, fibroblasts, and PMNs. They also stimulate induction of osteoclasts. The overstimulation of the catabolic processes that would otherwise contribute to connective tissue homeostasis lead to net loss of periodontal tissues.

associated with periodontal tissue inflammation, progressive periodontitis, and patients at high risk of periodontitis (e.g., EOP, refractory periodontitis, diabetes mellitus) (Goodson et al., 1974; Offenbacher et al., 1981, 1984, 1986; Ohm et al., 1984; Sengupta et al., 1990; Heasman et al., 1993; Zhou et al., 1994). The likely importance of eicosanoids in periodontal disease pathogenesis is underscored in several studies demonstrating the beneficial effects of both systemic and topical non-steroidal anti-inflammatory drugs on periodontitis in animal models and also in humans (Heasman and Seymour 1989; Williams et al., 1989; Offenbacher et al., 1992, 1993a, 1993b; Paquette 1992; Howell and Williams 1993).

The pathogenesis scenario

Periodontal lesions may develop in the following way. Virulent microorganisms capable of initiating or propagating periodontal attachment loss must be present in the local lesion at a minimal infective dose. In susceptible individuals—or at susceptible periodontal sites—protective mechanisms are breached by the virulence factors possessed by most pathogens. Some bacteria can not only evade the defenses provided by antibodies, complement-derived opsonins, and PMNs, but can also disarm the immune system by killing phagocytes and producing substances that interfere with protective cellular immune responses. The enhanced survival of these bacteria results in increased exposure of the underlying tissues and cells to bacterial constituents. Bacterial components themselves, or host cells stimulated to release chemotactic agents such as IL-8, attract phagocytes such as PMNs and monocytes to the infected site. These cells may be overwhelmed by bacteria such as *A. actinomycetemcomitans*, which are armed with toxins that kill some PMNs and cause others to release tissue-destroying enzymes. Additionally, LPS from Gram-negative bacteria induces monocytes and macrophages to secrete these enzymes. These events lead to destruction of gingival connective tissues and of the periodontal ligament. Simultaneously, LPS stimulates production of cytokines such as IL-1, TNF-α, and IL-6, as well as eicosanoids such as PGE$_2$, which can act in concert to stimulate resorption of bone (Figure 7.6).

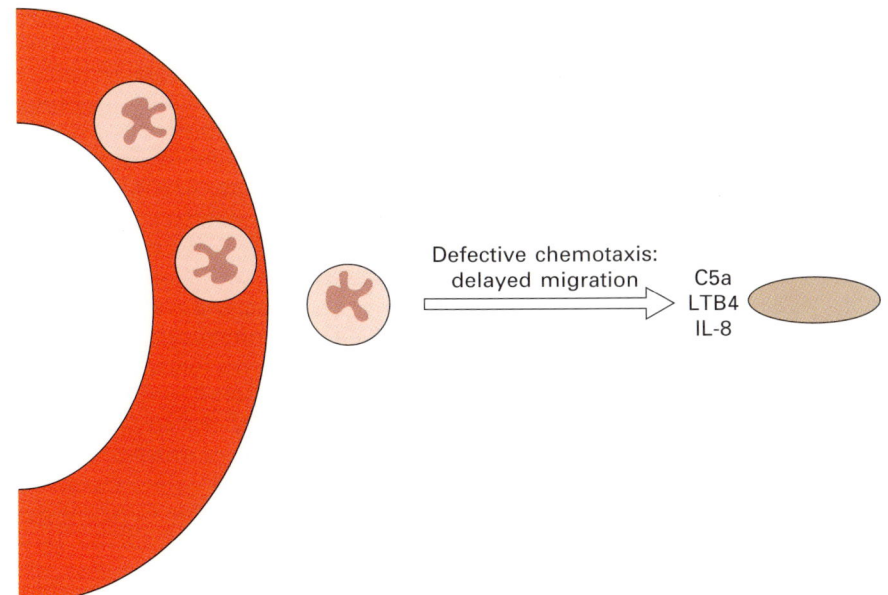

Defective chemotaxis:
delayed migration

C5a
LTB4
IL-8

Figure 7.7

Bacteria stimulate host cells to release chemotactic factors such as IL-8 and leukotriene B4 (LTB4), and activate the complement system to produce C5a. These recruit PMNs from the blood. However, in aggressive periodontitis PMNs demonstrate defective chemotaxis and are slow to respond to such stimuli.

Host response characteristics that increase risk of aggressive periodontitis

Although bacteria are considered to be the etiologic agents of AP, certain host characteristics may enhance the risk of developing this disease: these include characteristically aberrant inflammatory or immunologic responses to challenge with bacteria, or genetically determined traits that are more common in AP populations than in healthy populations. It is noteworthy that none of these characteristics is known to be a true risk factor for AP, rather they are correlates of the disease phenotype which are thought to explain a portion of the increased susceptibility to periodontal infections.

Defective chemotactic responses of PMNs

In the mid-1970s, investigators in several laboratories noted that PMNs purified from the peripheral blood of patients with AP performed poorly in chemotaxis assays when compared with PMNs from subjects without periodontitis (Cianciola et al., 1977; Clark et al., 1977; Lavine et al., 1979).

These experiments were generally carried out in a Boyden chamber, in which two liquid-filled compartments (one containing a chemotactic agent, the other containing PMNs) separated by a filter were used to measure the number of cells that migrated through the filter towards the chemotactic agent. Over a given period, fewer PMNs from AP patients moved a given distance through the filters than did PMNs from healthy individuals (Figure 7.7). These experiments were repeated many times in many different laboratories, and demonstrated that some but not all (about 70%) AP patients demonstrated a chemotaxis "defect". This defect is not complete, since the PMNs from AP patients do move towards a chemotactic agent, but do so more slowly than cells from healthy patients. In studies in which chemotaxis was actually measured in vivo, by placing a chemotactic substance at the gingival margin and collecting and enumerating PMNs in gingival fluid, it was found that a substantial proportion of the AP patients' PMNs entered the gingival fluid more slowly than cells from healthy patients (Singh et al., 1984).

The nature of this defect has been the subject of considerable study. It appears that the defect persists even after the disease no longer appears to be active, indicating that the defect is intrinsic as opposed to being induced by the disease (Van Dyke et al., 1980). Furthermore, a study of AP families indicated that chemotaxis defect, when present in a family member with AP, was also present in all other family members with AP and absent in those without AP; conversely, if the proband with AP had no chemotaxis defect then neither did the siblings with AP. The pattern of chemotaxis defects within the families were consistent with an inherited trait that is autosomal dominant (Van Dyke et al., 1985). Thus it is hypothesized that both the chemotaxis defect and the disease itself may be heritable.

It has been found that defective PMN chemotactic responsiveness is seen with nearly all types of chemotactic agents (Van Dyke et al., 1983; Lester et al., 1992). This indicates that the lesion responsible for the defect is likely to lie in the biochemical pathways common to induction of chemotaxis by a variety of agents. Data indicate possible defects in the "second messengers" that mediate the signal induced by the chemotactic agent through its receptor and result in directional locomotion (Agarwal et al., 1989; Daniel et al., 1993; Hurttia et al., 1997).

Since the first line of defense against periodontal microorganisms is thought to be the PMN, it is thought that the defect in chemotaxis noted in AP patients is likely to be a host factor that would increase the risk for infections with certain periodontal microorganisms. A combination of defective PMN chemotactic function and the presence of toxic strains of *Actinobacillus actinomycetemcomitans*, for example, would be a combination likely to favor the defeat of an important host-protective mechanism.

It is important to keep in mind, however, that not all patients with AP can be shown to have defective chemotaxis. Two ways to interpret this observation are that (a) having a chemotaxis defect is just one of several factors that can lead to development of AP, or (b) AP comprises more than one disease with different pathologic processes resulting in the same disease phenotype.

Phagocytic defects: polymorphisms of PMN Fc receptors

Individuals inherit structurally and genetically different (polymorphic) forms of proteins. These variants are found in the population at different frequencies and may confer different functional properties on the proteins. One such protein is the FcγRII (or CD32) molecule: this is a receptor molecule on PMNs that binds to the Fc region of IgG antibody molecules (mainly those of the IgG2 subclass) after the IgG antibody has bound to an antigen. Once this occurs, and a bacterial cell has adhered to the PMN surface via the antibody molecule, the PMN proceeds to engulf or phagocytose the bacteria. Most bacteria are killed inside PMNs subsequent to their phagocytosis.

It was thought for many years that IgG2 antibodies were not very good opsonins, since measurements of phagocytosis of IgG2-coated particles by human PMNs was so variable. However, it is now known that not all FcγRII receptors are the same, because people inherit polymorphic forms of this molecule. Two basic forms (alleles) of the gene coding for this receptor exist, called *H* and *R*; cells with receptors of the *H* variety (where the individual inherits an *H* allele from each parent resulting in an *H/H* genotype) have PMNs with high phagocytic capacity for antigens coated with IgG2 antibodies. Individuals with the *R/R* genotype have low phagocytic capacity, and those with the *H/R* genotype have intermediate phagocytic capacity (Figure 7.8).

The major antibody subclass produced in response to some important bacterial antigens such as the LPS from *A. actinomycetemcomitans* is IgG2; extremely high levels of this antibody are frequently found in sera from AP patients. The manner in which phagocytes handle the resulting IgG2-coated bacteria depends upon the genetically determined characteristics of the FcγRII receptor. It has been proposed that PMNs from AP patients are predominately of the *R/R* genotype, resulting in poor phagocytosis of *A. actinomycetemcomitans* despite the very high levels of antibody. This would increase the risk of infection with this bacteria and therefore increase the risk of AP (Wilson and Hamilton 1992, 1995; Wilson and Kalmar, 1996; Wilson and Bronson, 1997).

Associations with major histocompatibility complex antigens

The major histocompatibility antigens are proteins present on most cells. These are

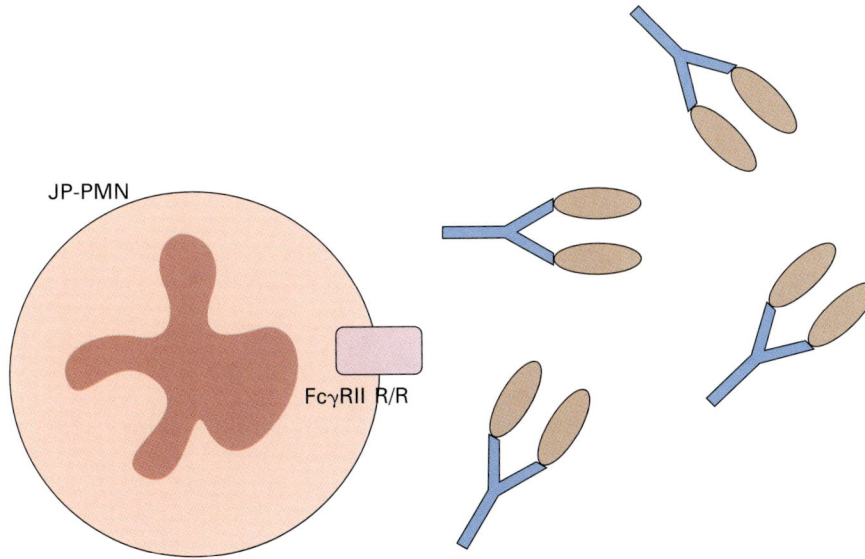

JP-PMN

FcγRII R/R

Figure 7.8

Impaired phagocytosis by PMNs in aggressive periodontitis. Polymorphic forms of the Fc receptor for IgG2 have different capacities for recognizing and binding IgG2 antibodies. A preponderance of AP patients may have an inherited form of the Fc receptor (*R/R*) which binds poorly to IgG2–bacteria complexes, impairing recognition of bacteria.

alloantigens—antigens that differentiate individuals from each other. These proteins are found on cell surfaces and are major transplantation antigens. Furthermore, genes located in the region of those genes coding for HLA as well as the HLA antigens themselves, have a substantial impact on immunologic responses, and have been shown to be associated with many diseases which have aberrant immunity as a pathological feature. A number of studies examined associations between early onset periodontitis (EOP) and the HLA antigens. Unfortunately, studies of EOP and other forms of periodontitis have not been of sufficient size to establish or refute an association between HLA and periodontitis. Reports have indicated a negative correlation between HLA-A2 and localized aggressive periodontitis (LAP) (Kaslick et al., 1975; Terasaki et al., 1975), as well as increased frequencies of HLA-A9, HLA-A28, and HLA-Bw15 in LAP subjects (Reinholdt et al., 1977). Other investigators found no significant associations or linkage between AP and HLA antigens (Cullinan et al., 1980; Saxen and Koskimies, 1984). A number of other studies also failed to conclusively demonstrate an association with HLA antigens. Data from several studies were compiled by Sofaer (1990) who concluded that the strongest negative associations with EOP are

with HLA-A2 and that subjects with HLA-A9 or HLA-B15 may have increased risk of localized AP.

Racial variables influencing pathogenesis of aggressive periodontitis

In the USA, AP is far more common in African-Americans than in Americans of European ancestry (Löe and Brown, 1991). Epidemiological surveys of other populations, and in other countries, confirm that this disease is more common in some patient groups, including those of African background (Waerhaug, 1967; Rao and Tweani, 1968; Saxen, 1980; Ben Yehouda et al., 1991; Lopez et al., 1991; Melvin et al., 1991). These patients seem to display biological characteristics that could either place them at higher risk for AP, or could modify the expression of early onset periodontitis to favor AP.

Association of race with virulent bacterial phenotypes

Strains of *Actinobacillus actinomycetemcomitans* are heterogeneous with regard to their ability to produce high levels of leukotoxin (Haubek et al., 1996, 1997; Bueno et al., 1998). A high proportion of AP patients of African origin have strains bearing the deletion in the promoter region of the gene for leukotoxin, while most Europeans and European-Americans with AP lack this type of strain.

PMN chemotaxis and race

Examination of PMN chemotactic function has revealed racial differences. Comparisons of chemotaxis in vitro between African-American and white subjects revealed significantly lower, but not necessarily defective, levels of chemotactic function in the former group (Schenkein et al., 1991). Since chemotactic function may be an important protective mechanism in AP, lower innate chemotactic activity in African-Americans may place them at higher risk of this condition.

Antibody and immunoglobulin production and race

Serum immunoglobulin levels, including IgG subclass (e.g., IgG2) levels, are also influenced by race. In general, African-Americans have higher concentrations of IgG2 than do white Americans. Examination of the IgG2 response to *A. actinomycetemcomitans* revealed that African-American patients with EOP have significantly higher concentrations of such antibody than white Americans, despite a comparable prevalence of *A. actinomycetemcomitans* colonization (Gunsolley et al., 1988, 1990, 1991). Such data may seem incongruous since high levels of antibody to *A. actinomycetemcomitans* appear to be associated with lower extent and severity of EOP. However, in *A. actinomycetemcomitans*-related EOP it is possible that the ability of a patient group to mount a protective response against this bacterium may limit the extent and severity of clinical disease. This may explain why the localized form of AP is disproportionately more common in African-Americans—the antibody prevents progression to more generalized forms. In patients who cannot mount a protec-tive response against *A. actinomycetemcomitans* (e.g., white subjects), the AP can become more generalized.

Conclusion

Aggressive periodontitis, which encompasses a number of clinical entities, probably results from the mobilization of tissue-destructive mechanisms which are common to most forms of periodontal disease. The unique attributes of the disease process are due to the virulence of the pathogens and the host susceptibility of patients with these diseases. Such host susceptibility may be due to heritable or acquired susceptibility factors which permit expression of periodontitis at a relatively young age. Since most of the host susceptibility factors appear to be intrinsic, that is, they exist prior to and following disease episodes (e.g., PMN chemotaxis defects, phago-cytic defects), these diseases probably occur in children as a result of defective resistance to infection with oral pathogens. However, the reasons for the expression of these diseases at or around puberty are unknown, as are the reasons for the unusual clinical presentation of the localized form of AP. It has been proposed that the affected teeth (first molars and incisors) have been at risk the longest because they are the first teeth to erupt. Nevertheless, the patho-logical processes occurring at the time of puberty leading to severe loss of bone and connective tissue have yet to be elucidated.

References

Agarwal S, Reynolds MA, Duckett LD, Suzuki JB (1989) Altered free cytosolic calcium changes and neutrophil chemotaxis in patients with juvenile periodontitis. *J Periodont Res* **24**: 149–54.

Baker P, Wilson M (1989) Opsonic IgG antibody against *Actinobacillus actinomycetemcomitans* in localized juvenile periodontitis. *Oral Microbiol Immunol* **4**: 98–105.

Ben Yehouda A, Shifer A, Katz J et al. (1991) Prevalence of juvenile periodontitis in Israeli military recruits as determined by panoramic radiographs. *Commun Dent Oral Epidemiol* **19**: 359–60.

Bickel M (1993) The role of interleukin-8 in inflammation and mechanisms of regulation. *J Periodontol* **64**(suppl 5): 456–60.

Bueno LC, Mayer MP, DiRienzo JM (1998) Relationship between conversion of localized juvenile periodontitis—susceptible children from health to disease and Actinobacillus actinomycetemcomitans leukotoxin promoter structure [see comments]. *J Periodontol* **69**(9): 998–1007.

Califano JV, Schenkein HA, Tew JG (1989) Immunodominant antigen of *Actinobacillus actinomycetemcomitans* strain Y4 (AaY4) in high responder patients. *Infect Immun* **57**: 1582–9.

Califano JV, Schenkein HA, Tew JG (1991) Immunodominant antigens of *Actinobacillus actinomycetemcomitans* serotypes a and c in high responder patients. *Oral Microbiol Immunol* **6**: 228–35.

Califano JV, Schenkein HA, Tew JG (1992) Immunodominant antigens of Actinobacillus actinomycetemcomitans serotype b in early-onset periodontitis patients. *Oral Microbiol Immunol* **7**(2): 65–70.

Califano JV, Gunsolley JC, Nakashima K et al. (1996) Influence of Anti-*Actinobacillus actinomycetemcomitans* Y4 (serotype b) LPS on severity of generalized early-onset periodontitis. *Infect Immun* **64**: 3908–10.

Califano JV, Pace BE, Gunsolley JC et al. (1997) Antibody reactive with Actinobacillus actinomycetemcomitans leukotoxin in early-onset periodontitis patients. *Oral Microbiol Immunol* **12**(1): 20–6.

Chen PB, Neiders ME, Millar SJ et al. (1987) Effect of immunization on experimental *Bacteroides gingivalis* infection in a murine model. *Infect Immun* **55**: 2534–7.

Cianciola LJ, Genco RJ, Patters MR et al. (1977) Defective polymorphonuclear leukocyte function in a human periodontal disease. *Nature* (London) **265**: 445–7.

Clark R, Page RC, Wilde G (1977) Defective neutrophil chemotaxis in juvenile periodontitis. *Infect Immun* **18**: 694–700.

Cullinan MP, Sachs J, Wolf E, Seymour GJ (1980) The distribution of HLA-A and -B antigens in patients and their families with periodontosis. *J Periodont Res* **15**: 177–84.

Cutler C, Arnold R, Schenkein H (1993) Inhibition of C3 and IgG proteolysis enhances phagocytosis of Porphyromonas gingivalis. *J Immunol* **151**(12): 7016–29.

Daniel MA, McDonald G, Offenbacher S, Van Dyke TE (1993) Defective chemotaxis and calcium response in localized juvenile periodontitis neutrophils. *J Periodontol* **64**: 617–21.

Ebersole JL, Cappelli D, Sandoval MN, Steffen MJ (1995) Antigen specificity of serum antibody in A. actinomycetemcomitans-infected periodontitis patients. *J Dent Res* **74**(2): 658–66.

Ebersole JL, Taubman MA, Smith JA et al. (1982) Human immune responses to oral micro-organisms I. Association of localized juvenile periodontitis (LJP) with serum antibody responses to *Actinobacillus actinomycetemcomitans*. *Clin Exp Immunol* **47**: 43–52.

Ebersole JL, Taubman MA, Smith DJ (1985) Gingival crevicular fluid antibody to oral microorganisms. II. Distribution and specificity of local antibody responses. *J Periodont Res* **20**: 349–56.

Fishburn CS, Slaney JM, Carman RJ, Curtis MA (1991) Degradation of plasma proteins by the trypsin-like enzyme of *Porphyromonas gingivalis* and inhibition of protease activity by a serine protease inhibitor of human plasma. *Oral Microbiol Immunol* **6**: 209–15.

Fitzgerald J, Kreutzer D (1995) Localization of interleukin-8 in human gingival tissues. *Oral Microbiol Immunol* **10**(5): 297–303.

Fives-Taylor P, Meyer D, Mintz K (1995) Characteristics of Actinobacillus actinomycetemcomitans invasion of and adhesion to cultured epithelial cells. *Adv Dent Res* **9**(1): 55–62.

Geivelis M, Turner D, Pederson E, Lamberts B (1993) Measurements of interleukin-6 in gingival crevicular fluid from adults with destructive periodontal disease. *J Periodontol* **64**(10): 980–3.

Genco RJ, Taichman NA, Sadowski CA (1980) Precipitating antibodies to *Actinobacillus actinomycetemcomitans* in localized juvenile periodontitis. *J Dent Res* **59**: 329.

Genco RJ, Zambon JJ, Murray PA (1985) Serum and gingival fluid antibodies as adjuncts in the diagnosis of *Actinobacillus actinomycetemcomitans*–associated periodontal disease. *J Periodontol* **56** (special issue): 41–50.

Goodson J, Dewhirst F, Brunetti A (1974) Prostaglandin E_2 levels and human periodontal disease. *Prostaglandins* **6**(1): 81–5.

Gooss CM, Ranney RR, Sarbin AG, Tew JG (1986) Serum antibody reactive with *Actinobacillus actinomycetemcomitans* and *B. gingivalis* in juvenile periodontitis families. *J Dent Res* **65**: 929 [abstract].

Gunsolley JC, Burmeister JA, Tew JG et al. (1987) Relationship of serum antibody to attachment level patterns in young adults with juvenile periodontitis or generalized severe periodontitis. *J Periodontol* **58**: 314–19.

Gunsolley JC, Tew JG, Gooss CM et al. (1988) Effects of race and periodontal status on antibody reactive with *Actinobacillus actinomycetemcomitans* strain Y4. *J Periodont Res* **23**: 303–7.

Gunsolley JC, Tew JG, Gooss C et al. (1990) Serum antibodies to periodontal bacteria. *J Periodontol* **61**: 412–19.

Gunsolley JC, Tew JG, Conner T et al. (1991) Relationship between race and antibody reactive with periodontitis-associated bacteria. *J Periodont Res* **26**: 59–63.

Haffajee AD, Socransky SS (1994) Microbial etiological agents of destructive periodontal diseases. *Periodontology 2000* **5**: 78–111.

Hart TC (1996) Genetic risk factors for early-onset periodontitis. *J Periodontol* **67**: 355–66.

Haubek D, Poulsen K, Westergaard J et al. (1996) Highly toxic clone of Actinobacillus actinomycetemcomitans in geographically widespread cases of juvenile periodontitis in adolescents of African origin. *J Clin Microbiol* **34**(6): 1576–8.

Haubek D, Dirienzo JM, Tinoco EM et al. (1997) Racial tropism of a highly toxic clone of Actinobacillus actinomycetemcomitans associated with juvenile periodontitis. *J Clin Microbiol* **35**(12): 3037–42.

Heasman P, Seymour R (1989) The effect of a systemically-administered non-steroidal anti-inflammatory drug (flurbiprofen) on experimental gingivitis in humans. *J Clin Periodontol* **16**(9): 551–6.

Heasman P, Collins J, Offenbacher S (1993) Changes in crevicular fluid levels of interleukin-1 beta, leukotriene B4, prostaglandin E2, thromboxane B2 and tumor necrosis factor alpha in experimental gingivitis in humans. *J Periodont Res* **28**(4): 241–7.

Hou L, Liu C, Rossomando E (1995) Crevicular interleukin-1 beta in moderate and severe periodontitis patients and the effect of phase I periodontal treatment. *J Clin Periodontol* **22**(2): 162–7.

Howell T, Williams R (1993) Nonsteroidal anti-inflammatory drugs as inhibitors of periodontal disease progression. *Crit Rev Oral Biol Med* **4**(2): 177–96.

Hurttia HM, Pelto LM, Leino L (1997) Evidence of an association between functional abnormalities and defective diacylglycerol kinase activity in peripheral blood neutrophils from patients with localized juvenile periodontitis. *J Periodont Res* **32**(4): 401–7.

Jandinski J, Stashenko P, Feder L et al. (1991) Localization of interleukin-1 beta in human periodontal tissue. *J Periodontol* **62**(1): 36–43.

Kaslick RS, West TL, Chasens AI et al. (1975) Association between HL-A2 antigen and various periodontal diseases in young adults. *J Dent Res* **54**: 424.

Koga T, Odaka C, Moro I et al. (1987) Local Shwartzman activity of lipopolysaccharides from several selected strains of suspected periodontopathic bacteria. *J Periodont Res* **22**(2): 103–7.

Lamont R, Chan A, Belton C et al. (1995) Porphyromonas gingivalis invasion of gingival epithelial cells. *Infect Immun* **63**(10): 3878–85.

Lavine WS, Maderazo EG, Stolman J et al. (1979) Impaired neutrophil chemotaxis in patients with juvenile and rapidly progressing periodontitis. *J Periodont Res* **14**: 10–19.

Lester M, Schneider A, Warbington M, Van Dyke TE (1992) Defective neutrophil chemotaxis to interleukin-8 in localized juvenile periodontitis patients. *J Dent Res* **72**: 653 [abstract].

Löe H, Brown LJ (1991) Juvenile periodontitis in the United States of America. *J Periodontol* **62**: 608–16.

Lopez NJ, Rios V, Pareja MA, Fernandez O (1991) Prevalence of juvenile periodontitis in Chile. *J Clin Periodontol* **18**: 529–33.

Lotz M (1995) Interleukin-6: a comprehensive review. *Cancer Treat Res* **80**: 209–33.

Lu H, Califano JV, Schenkein HA, Tew JG (1993) Immunoglobulin class and subclass distribution of antibodies reactive with the immunodominant antigen of *Actinobacillus actinomycetemcomitans* serotype b. *Infect Immun* **61**: 2400–7.

Lu H, Wang M, Gunsolley JC et al. (1994) Serum immunoglobulin G subclass concentrations in periodontally healthy and diseased individuals. *Infect Immun* **62**: 1677–82.

Maeda H, Molla A (1989) Pathogenic potentials of bacterial proteases. *Clin Chim Acta* **185**: 357–68.

Matsuki Y, Yamamoto T, Hara K (1991) Interleukin-1 mRNA-expressing macrophages in human chronically inflamed gingival tissues. *Am J Pathol* **138**(6): 1299–305.

Matsuki Y, Yamamoto T, Hara K (1992) Detection of inflammatory cytokine messenger RNA (mRNA)-expressing cells in human inflamed gingiva by combined in situ hybridization and immunohistochemistry. *Immunology* **76**(1): 42–7.

Melvin WL, Sandifer JB, Gray JL (1991) The prevalence and sex ratio of juvenile periodontitis in a young racially mixed population. *J Periodontol* **62**: 330–4.

Moldawer L (1994) Biology of proinflammatory cytokines and their antagonists. *Crit Care Med* **22**(7): S3–7.

Offenbacher S, Farr D, Goodson J (1981) Measurement of prostaglandin E in crevicular fluid. *J Clin Periodontol* **8**(4): 359–67.

Offenbacher S, Odle B, Gray R, Van Dyke TE (1984) Crevicular fluid prostaglandin E levels as a measure of the periodontal disease status of adult and juvenile periodontitis patients. *J Periodont Res* **19**(1): 1–13.

Offenbacher S, Odle B, Van Dyke TE (1986) The use of crevicular fluid prostaglandin E2 levels as a predictor of periodontal attachment loss. *J Periodont Res* **21**(2): 101–12.

Offenbacher S, Williams R, Jeffcoat M et al. (1992) Effects of NSAIDs on beagle crevicular cyclooxygenase metabolites and periodontal bone loss. *J Periodont Res* **27**(3): 207–13.

Offenbacher S, Collins J, Heasman P (1993a) Diagnostic potential of host response mediators. *Adv Dent Res* **7**(2): 175–81.

Offenbacher S, Heasman P, Collins J (1993b) Modulation of host PGE2 secretion as a determinant of periodontal disease expression. *J Periodontol* **64**(suppl 5): 432–44.

Ohm K, Albers H, Lisboa B (1984) Measurement of eight prostaglandins in human gingival and periodontal disease using high pressure liquid chromatography and radioimmunoassay. *J Periodont Res* **19**(5): 501–11.

Paquette D (1992) Potential role of nonsteroidal anti-inflammatory drugs in the treatment of periodontitis. *Compendium* **13**(12): 1174–9.

Preiss D, Meyle J (1994) Interleukin-1 beta concentration of gingival crevicular fluid. *J Periodontol* **65**(5): 423–8.

Ranney RR, Yanni NR, Burmeister JA, Tew JG (1982) Relationship between attachment loss and precipitating serum antibody to *Actinobacillus actinomycetemcomitans* in adolescents and young adults having severe periodontal destruction. *J Periodontol* **53**: 1–7.

Rao SS, Tweani SV (1968) Prevalence of periodontosis among Indians. *J Periodontol* **39**: 27–34.

Reinhardt R, Masada M, Kaldahl W et al. (1993) Gingival fluid IL-1 and IL-6 levels in refractory periodontitis. *J Clin Periodontol* **20**(3): 225–31.

Reinholdt J, Bay I, Svejgaard A (1977) Association between HLA-antigens and periodontal disease. *J Dent Res* **56**: 1261–3.

Rink L, Kirchner H (1996) Recent progress in the tumor necrosis factor-alpha field. *Int Arch Allerg Immunol* **111**(3): 199–209.

Saxen L (1980) Prevalence of juvenile periodontitis in Finland. *J Clin Periodontol* **7**: 165–76.

Saxen L, Koskimies S (1984) Juvenile periodontitis—no linkage with HLA-antigens. *J Periodont Res* **19**: 441–4.

Schenkein H (1989) Failure of Bacteroides gingivalis W83 to accumulate bound C3 following opsonization with serum. *J Periodont Res* **24**(1): 20–7.

Schenkein HA, Best AM, Gunsolley JC (1991) The influence of race and periodontal clinical status on neutrophil chemotactic responses. *J Periodont Res* **26**: 272–5.

Sengupta S, Fine J, Wu-Wang C et al. (1990) The relationship of prostaglandins to cAMP, IgG, IgM and alpha-2–macroglobulin in gingival crevicular fluid in chronic adult periodontitis. *Arch Oral Biol* **35**(8): 593–6.

Shapira L, Soskolne W, Sela M et al. (1994a) The secretion of PGE2, IL-1 beta, IL-6, and TNF alpha by adherent mononuclear cells from early onset periodontitis patients. *J Periodontol* **65**(2): 139–46.

Shapira L, Takashiba S, Amar S, Van Dyke TE (1994b) Porphyromonas gingivalis lipopolysaccharide stimulation of human monocytes: dependence on serum and CD14 receptor. *Oral Microbiol Immunol* **9**: 112–17.

Shenker B, Tsai C, Taichman N (1982a) Suppression of lymphocyte responses by Actinobacillus actinomycetemcomitans. *J Periodont Res* **17**(5): 462–5.

Shenker BJ, Kushner ME, Tsai CC (1982b) Inhibition of fibroblast proliferation by Actinobacillus actinomycetemcomitans. *Infect Immun* **38**(3): 986–92.

Shenker B, Vitale L, Welham D (1990) Immune suppression induced by Actinobacillus actinomycetemcomitans: effects on immunoglobulin production by human B cells. *Infect Immun* **58**(12): 3856–62.

Singh S, Golub LM, Iacono VJ et al. (1984) In vivo crevicular leukocyte response in humans to a chemotactic challenge. *J Periodontol* **55**: 1–8.

Smith M, Braswell L, Collins J et al. (1993) Changes in inflammatory mediators in experimental periodontitis in the rhesus monkey. *Infect Immun* **61**(4): 1453–9.

Sofaer JA (1990) Genetic approaches in the study of periodontal diseases. *J Clin Periodontol* **17**: 401–8.

Sreenivasan PK, Meyer DH, Fives-Taylor PM (1993) Requirements for invasion of epithelial cells by *Actinobacillus actinomycetemcomitans*. *Infect Immun* **61**: 1239–45.

Stashenko P, Fujiyoshi P, Obernesser M et al. (1991) Levels of interleukin 1 beta in tissue from sites of active periodontal disease. *J Clin Periodontol* **18**(7): 548–54.

Taichman NS, Dean RT, Sanderson CJ (1980) Biochemical and morphological characterization of the killing of human monocytes by a leukotoxin derived from *Actinobacillus actinomycetemcomitans*. *Infect Immun* **28**(1): 258–68.

Takahashi N, Kato T, Kuramitsu HK (1991) Isolation and preliminary characterization of the *Porphyromonas gingivalis prtC* gene expressing collagenase activity. *FEMS Microbiol Lett* **68**: 135–8.

Tamura M, Tokuda M, Nagaoka S, Takada H (1992) Lipopolysaccharides of *Bacteroides intermedius*, and *Bacteroides gingivalis* induce interleukin-8 expression in human gingival fibroblast cultures. *Infect Immun* **60**: 4932–7.

Tatakis D (1993) Interleukin-1 and bone metabolism: a review. *J Periodontol* **64**(suppl 5): 416–31.

Terasaki PI, Kaslick RS, West TL, Chasens AI (1975) Low HL-A-2 frequency and periodontitis. *Tiss Antigen* **5**: 286–8.

Tew J, Marshall D, Burmeister J, Ranney R (1985) Relationship between gingival crevicular fluid and serum antibody titers in young adults with generalized and localized periodontitis. *Infect Immun* **49**(3): 487–93.

Tonetti M, Imboden M, Gerber L et al. (1994) Localized expression of mRNA for phagocyte-specific chemotactic cytokines in human periodontal infections. *Infect Immun* **62**(9): 4005–14.

Tsai C, McArthur W, Baehni P et al. (1979) Extraction and partial characterization of a leukotoxin from a plaque-derived Gram-negative microorganism. *Infect Immun* **25**(1): 427–39.

Tsai CC, McArthur WP, Baehni PC et al. (1981) Serum neutralizing activity against Actinobacillus actinomycetemcomitans leukotoxin in juvenile periodontitis. *J Clin Periodontol* **8**(4): 338–48.

Tsai C, Ho Y, Chen C (1995) Levels of interleukin-1 beta and interleukin-8 in gingival crevicular fluids in adult periodontitis. *J Periodontol* **66**(10): 852–9.

Underwood K, Sjöström K, Darveau R et al. (1993) Serum antibody opsonic activity against *Actinobacillus actinomycetemcomitans* in human periodontal diseases. *J Infect Dis* **168**: 1436–43.

Van Dyke TE, Horoszewicz HV, Cianciola LJ, Genco RJ (1980) Neutrophil chemotaxis dysfunction in human periodontitis. *Infect Immun* **27**: 124–32.

Van Dyke TE, Levine MJ, Tabak LA, Genco RJ (1983) Juvenile periodontitis as a model for neutrophil function: reduced binding of complement chemotactic fragment, C5a. *J Dent Res* **62**: 870–2.

Van Dyke TE, Schweinbraten M, Ciancola LJ et al. (1985) Neutrophil chemotaxis in families with localized juvenile periodontitis. *J Periodont Res* **20**: 503–14.

Waerhaug J (1967) Prevalence of periodontal disease in Ceylon. *Acta Odont Scand* **25**: 205–31.

Williams R, Jeffcoat M, Howell T et al. (1989) Altering the progression of human alveolar bone loss with the non-steroidal anti-inflammatory drug flurbiprofen. *J Periodontol* **60**(9): 485–90.

Wilson ME, Bronson PM (1997) Opsonization of Actinobacillus actinomycetemcomitans by immunoglobulin G antibodies to the O polysaccharide of lipopolysaccharide. *Infect Immun* **65**(11): 4690–5.

Wilson ME, Hamilton RG (1992) Immunoglobulin G subclass response of localized juvenile periodontitis patients to *Actinobacillus actinomycetemcomitans* Y4 lipopolysaccharide. *Infect Immun* **60**: 1806–12.

Wilson ME, Hamilton RG (1995) Immunoglobulin G subclass response of juvenile periodontitis subjects to principal outer membrane proteins of Actinobacillus actinomycetemcomitans. *Infect Immun* **63**(3): 1062–9.

Wilson M, Henderson B (1995) Virulence factors of Actinobacillus actinomycetemcomitans relevant to the pathogenesis of inflammatory periodontal diseases. *FEMS Microbiol Rev* **17**(4): 365–79.

Wilson ME, Kalmar JR (1996) FcgammaRIIa (CD32): a potential marker defining susceptibility to localized juvenile periodontitis. *J Periodontol* **67**: 323–31.

Wilson ME, Schifferle RE (1991) Evidence that the serotype b antigenic determinant of *Actinobacillus actinomycetemcomitans* Y4 resides in the polysaccharide moiety of lipopolysaccharide. *Infect Immun* **59**: 1544–51.

Wilson ME, Bronson PM, Hamilton RG (1995) Immunoglobulin G2 antibodies promote neutrophil killing of Actinobacillus actinomycetemcomitans. *Infect Immun* **63**(3): 1070–5.

Wilton J, Bampton J, Griffiths G et al. (1992) Interleukin-1 beta (IL-1 beta) levels in gingival crevicular fluid from adults with previous evidence of destructive periodontitis. A cross sectional study. *J Clin Periodontol* **19**(1): 53–7.

Yamazaki K, Nakajima T, Gemmell E et al. (1994) IL-4- and IL-6-producing cells in human periodontal disease tissue. *J Oral Pathol Med* **23**(8): 347–53.

Yavuzyilmaz E, Yamalik N, Bulut S et al. (1995) The gingival crevicular fluid interleukin-1 beta and tumour necrosis factor-alpha levels in patients with rapidly progressive periodontitis. *Aust Dent J* **40**(1): 46–9.

Zambon JJ (1985) Actinobacillus actinomycetemcomitans in human periodontal disease. *J Clin Periodontol* **12**(1): 1–20.

Zambon JJ, Haraszthy VI, Hariharan G et al. (1996) The microbiology of early-onset periodontitis: association of highly toxic *Actinobacillus actinomycetemcomitans* strains with localized juvenile periodontitis. *J Periodontol* **67**: 282–90.

Zhang JB, Quinn SM, Rausch M et al. (1996) Hyper-immunoglobulin G2 production by B cells from patients with localized juvenile periodontitis and its regulation by monocytes. *Infect Immun* **64**(6): 2004–9.

Zhou J, Zou S, Zhao W, Zhao Y (1994) Prostaglandin E2 level in gingival crevicular fluid and its relation to the periodontal pocket depth in patients with periodontitis. *Chin Med Sci J* **9**(1): 52–5.

8

Microbiology of periodontal diseases

Miriam Ting and Jørgen Slots

Children and adolescents often experience only a minor degree of gingivitis and show little or no destructive periodontal disease even in the presence of copious amounts of dental plaque (Matsson, 1978; Matsson and Goldberg, 1985; Bimstein and Ebersole, 1989). However, periodontitis in young individuals does occur, may proceed rapidly, and can, in a few years, result in a significant loss of periodontal supportive tissue. Severe types of periodontitis are often associated with infections by specific bacterial species, and perhaps herpesviruses. Because of the aggressive nature of periodontal infections in young patients, it is crucial to establish an early diagnosis and initiate early therapy in order to preserve affected teeth. Knowledge of infecting microbial pathogens can be essential for the successful treatment of periodontitis in these individuals.

Historical overview

Some of the first bacteria described by Antonio van Leeuwenhoek in 1683 originated from dental plaque; he noted a large number of bacteria associated with poor oral hygiene. Microbiological studies from the 1950s and 1960s were not able to associate specific bacterial species with destructive periodontal disease (Slots and Rams, 1992), and dental plaque composition was therefore thought to be similar in all individuals and also in sites within an individual; periodontitis was thought to develop in individuals or sites with low host resistance (Löe et al., 1986). The non-specific plaque hypothesis was embraced to explain the initiation and progression of various types of periodontitis.

In the mid-1970s, studies in the USA and Scandinavia suggested that the microbiota of aggressive periodontitis (AP; formerly juvenile periodontitis and rapidly progressive periodontitis) was distinct from those associated with periodontal health and gingivitis (Newman et al., 1976; Slots, 1976). The term "specific plaque hypothesis" was adopted to describe the microbial etiology of advanced periodontitis (Slots and Rams, 1992).

In the mid-1980s, *Actinobacillus actinomycetemcomitans*, *Porphyromonas gingivalis*, *Prevotella intermedia*, *Bacteroides forsythus*, *Treponema denticola*, *Campylobacter rectus*, *Peptostreptococcus micros*, *Fusobacterium* species, *Eubacterium* species, beta-hemolytic streptococci, and some superinfecting enteric rods were implicated in the pathogenesis of advanced juvenile or adult periodontitis (Slots and Rams, 1992).

In the mid-1990s, human cytomegalovirus, Epstein–Barr virus type 1 and other herpesviruses were added to the list of putative periodontal pathogens (Contreras and Slots, 2000). Herpesviruses may impair key cells of the periodontal defense and set the stage for subgingival overgrowth of pathogenic bacteria (Contreras and Slots, 2000).

The specific plaque hypothesis suggested treatment strategies that focused upon suppression or elimination of selected periodontal pathogens. Scaling and root planing, periodontal surgery, and topical and systemic antimicrobial drug therapies differ in their ability to control subgingival pathogens and periodontal disease.

Major periodontal pathogens

Major periodontal pathogens belong to the genera *Actinobacillus*, *Porphyromonas*, *Prevotella*, *Bacteroides*, and *Treponema* (Table

Table 8.1 Subgingival microorganisms in periodontal health and disease.

Health	Gingivitis	Localized aggressive periodontitis	Aggressive periodontitis of young adults
Gram-positive organisms	Gram-positive organisms	Gram-negative organisms	Gram-negative organisms
Streptococcus mitis	Actinomyces naeslundii	Actinobacillus	Porphyromonas gingivalis
Streptococcus oralis	Lactobacillus spp.	actinomycetemcomitans	Bacteroides forsythus
Streptococcus sanguis	Peptostreptococcus micros	Porphyromonas gingivalis	Prevotella intermedia
Actinomyces gerencseriae	Streptococcus anginosus	Prevotella intermedia	Fusobacterium nucleatum
Actinomyces naeslundii		Campylobacter rectus	Streptococcus intermedius
	Gram-negative organisms	Fusobacterium nucleatum	Accutely aggressive
Gram-negative organisms	Fusobacterium nucleatum	Selenomonas sputigena	periodontitis
Fusobacterium spp.	Prevotella intermedia	Eikenella corrodens	
Prevotella nigrescens	Veillonella parvula	Capnocytophaga	
Veillonella spp.	Campylobacter spp.	Treponema denticola	
	Haemophilus spp.		
	Selenomonas spp.	Herpesviruses	
	Treponema spp.	Human cytomegalovirus	
		Epstein–Barr virus type 1	

8.1). Five major periodontopathic species are briefly described below.

Actinobacillus actinomycetemcomitans

Actinobacillus actinomycetemcomitans is a Gram-negative facultative rod. Its occurrence is limited to the human oral cavity. This species differs genetically from animal Actinobacillus species but is closely related to human Haemophilus aphrophilus and Haemophilus paraphrophilus. Actinobacillus actinomycetemcomitans colonies are 0.5–1.0 mm in diameter, translucent, and adherent, with a characteristic internal star-shaped structure. Cells of Actinobacillus actinomycetemcomitans are small, short (0.4 μm × 1 μm), straight or slightly curved rods with rounded ends. The species includes five serotypes (a to e) of which serotype b is the most virulent. Some Actinobacillus actinomycetemcomitans strains produce a leuko-toxin that is capable of killing polymorphonu-clear leukocytes and is considered to constitute an important pathogenic trait of the organism. This species has the ability to invade epithelial cells and periodontal connective tissue, a feature that can complicate its removal from infected sites (Saglie et al., 1982).

Porphyromonas gingivalis

The Porphyromonas genus was created to accom-modate asaccharolytic, anaerobic, Gram-negative rods that grow with greenish-black colonies on blood agar plates. Porphyromonas gingivalis is a resident of the human oral cavity. Its dominant cell type consists of non-motile short rods, but longer cell forms can occur. Its proteases hydrolyze a wide spectrum of host-derived proteins including collagen, antibodies, and complement compo-nents. Porphyromonas gingivalis elaborates trypsin-like benzoyl-DL-arginine-naphthylamide (BANA) activity. Lipopolysaccharide from this species shows relatively low endotoxicity, but functions as a significant cytotoxin and a potent inducer of several host-derived cytokines and chemokines (Holt et al., 1999).

Prevotella intermedia

The Prevotella genus accommodates saccha-rolytic, anaerobic, Gram-negative rods, many of which were previously classified as Bacteroides. The Prevotella genus includes both black-pigmented and non-pigmented species. Prevotella intermedia forms black colonies on blood agar. Cells are pleomorphic, filamentous rods. Prevotella intermedia colonizes oral as well as non-oral sites. *Prevotella nigrescens* is a newly named species that is closely related to *Prevotella intermedia* (Tanner et al., 1992).

Bacteroides forsythus

The genus *Bacteroides* comprises non-motile, Gram-negative, saccharolytic, anaerobic rods that resemble non-oral *Bacteroides fragilis*, the type species of the genus. The oral species *Bacteroides forsythus* was created in 1986 for isolates previously recognized as "fusiform *Bacteroides*." Cells of *Bacteroides forsythus* frequently appear with tapered ends and can be up to 30 μm in length. Colonies on blood agar plates are pale pink and 1–2 mm in diameter. *Bacteroides forsythus* demonstrates strong trypsin-like BANA activity (Loesche et al., 1990).

Treponema denticola

Treponema organisms are motile, helical rods with tight regular or irregular spirals. They have a characteristic spirochetal cell structure with periplasmic flagella inserted at each end of the protoplasmic cylinder. Oral *Treponema* species are strictly anaerobic, Gram-negative organisms. *Treponema denticola* grows slowly, forming white, diffuse colonies 0.3–1.0 mm in diameter. It is the third major oral species that produces a trypsin-like BANA protease (Loesche et al., 1990).

Periodontal pathogens according to age and ethnicity

There is a lack of longitudinal studies examining changes in the periodontal microbiota from childhood to adulthood. In individuals with periodontal disease, it is difficult to discern if the microbial composition is due mainly to aging or to disease. Ethically, longitudinal microbiological studies without treatment intervention cannot be performed in subjects developing periodontal disease. Cross-sectional studies have compared the periodontal microbiota in deciduous teeth and permanent teeth in children with mixed dentition. Available data suggest increasing occurrence of subgingival *Porphyromonas gingivalis*, *Bacteroides forsythus*, and *Campylobacter* species with increasing age, and concomitant decreases in some *Peptostreptococcus* species and *Actinomyces naeslundii* (Kamma et al., 2000).

Actinobacillus actinomycetemcomitans is a major periodontal pathogen of young people (Figure 8.1) (Slots and Ting, 1999). *Porphyromonas gingivalis* occurs with significantly higher prevalence and concentration in subjects aged 30 years and over compared with younger subjects (Figure 8.2) (Slots and Ting, 1999; Savitt and Kent, 1991). *Prevotella intermedia*, *Bacteroides forsythus* and *Treponema denticola* show no predilection for any particular age group.

Periodontal pathogens can be transmitted vertically (parents to children) or horizontally (among spouses and siblings) within a family. Saliva is the common vehicle for oral microbial transmission. Parent–child transmission of *Actinobacillus actinomycetemcomitans* may occur in about one-third of families with infected parents. *Porphyromonas gingivalis* is not easily transmitted from parents to young children (Asikainen et al., 1996).

Periodontitis is more common in some ethnic groups than in others; for example, localized aggressive periodontitis (LAP) in adolescents (formerly localized juvenile periodontitis) affects more African-Americans (1.5–2.1%) than white Americans (0.1–0.3%) (Löe and Brown, 1991; Cogen et al., 1992). Differences in occurrence of periodontal pathogens among ethnic groups may help explain differences in disease prevalence.

Actinobacillus actinomycetemcomitans is more common in Hispanic (odds ratio 12.2) and Asian-American subjects (odds ratio 6.6) than in white Americans (odds ratio 1.0) (Umeda et al., 1998). This species occurs in 78% of Vietnamese children compared with 13% of Finnish children. However, since Vietnamese children show low prevalence of the periodontopathic *A. actinomycetemcomitans* serotype b (27%) and high prevalence of the less pathogenic serotypes a (36%) and c (63%), they may not experience significantly more periodontitis than individuals of other populations (Höltta et al., 1994). *Actinobacillus actinomycetemcomitans* serotype b antibody level is higher in LAP patients in the

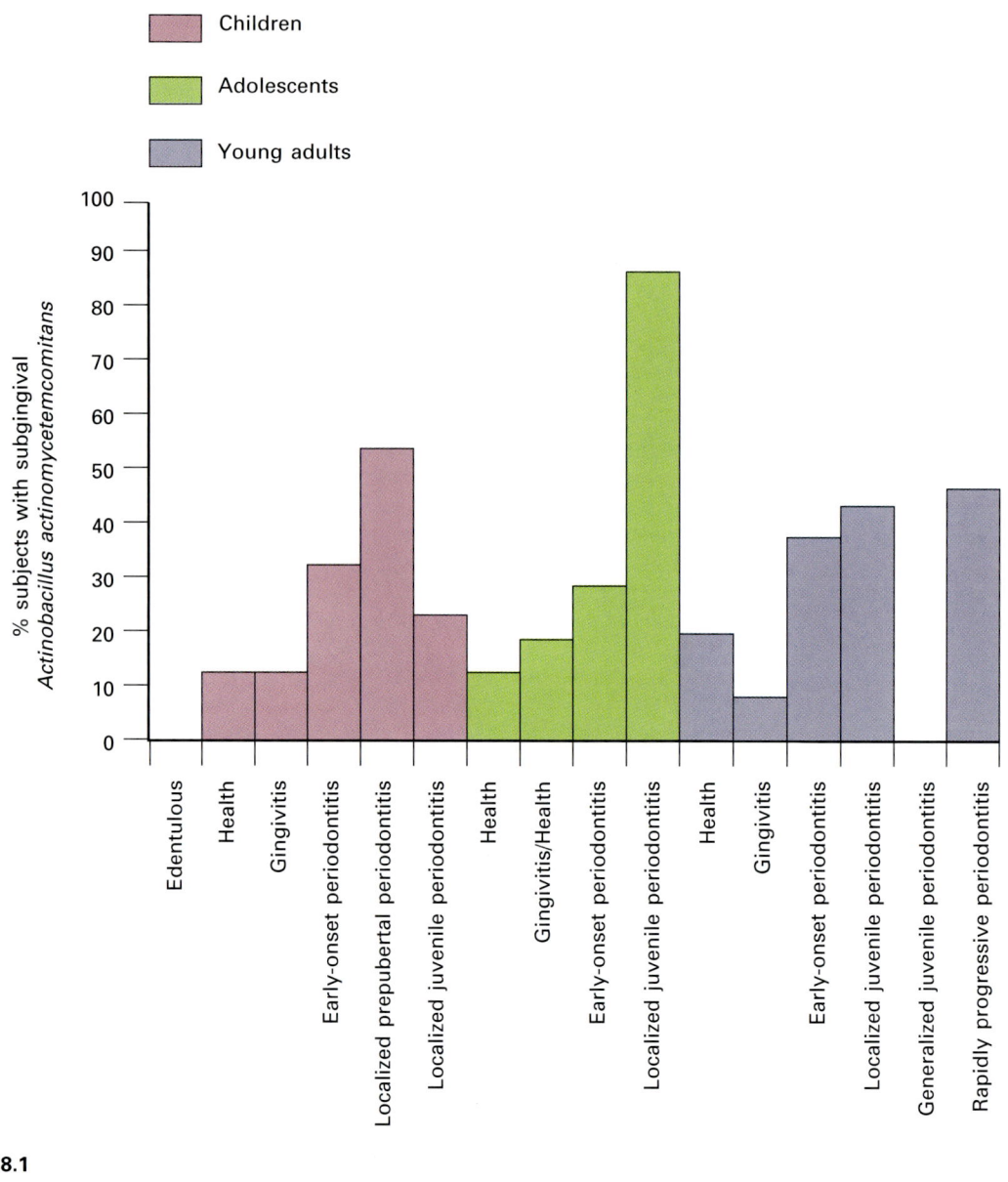

Figure 8.1

Subgingival *Actinobacillus actinomycetemcomitans* in periodontal health and disease (Slots and Ting, 1999).

USA than in Turkey. American patients of African descent may also contain more strains that produce high levels of leukotoxin compared with patients of European descent (Contreras et al., 2000).

Porphyromonas gingivalis is more prevalent in the subgingival microbiota of Hispanic (odds ratio 6.1), African-American (odds ratio 2.7), and Asian-American (odds ratio 5.4) subjects than in that of white Americans (odds ratio 1.0) (Umeda

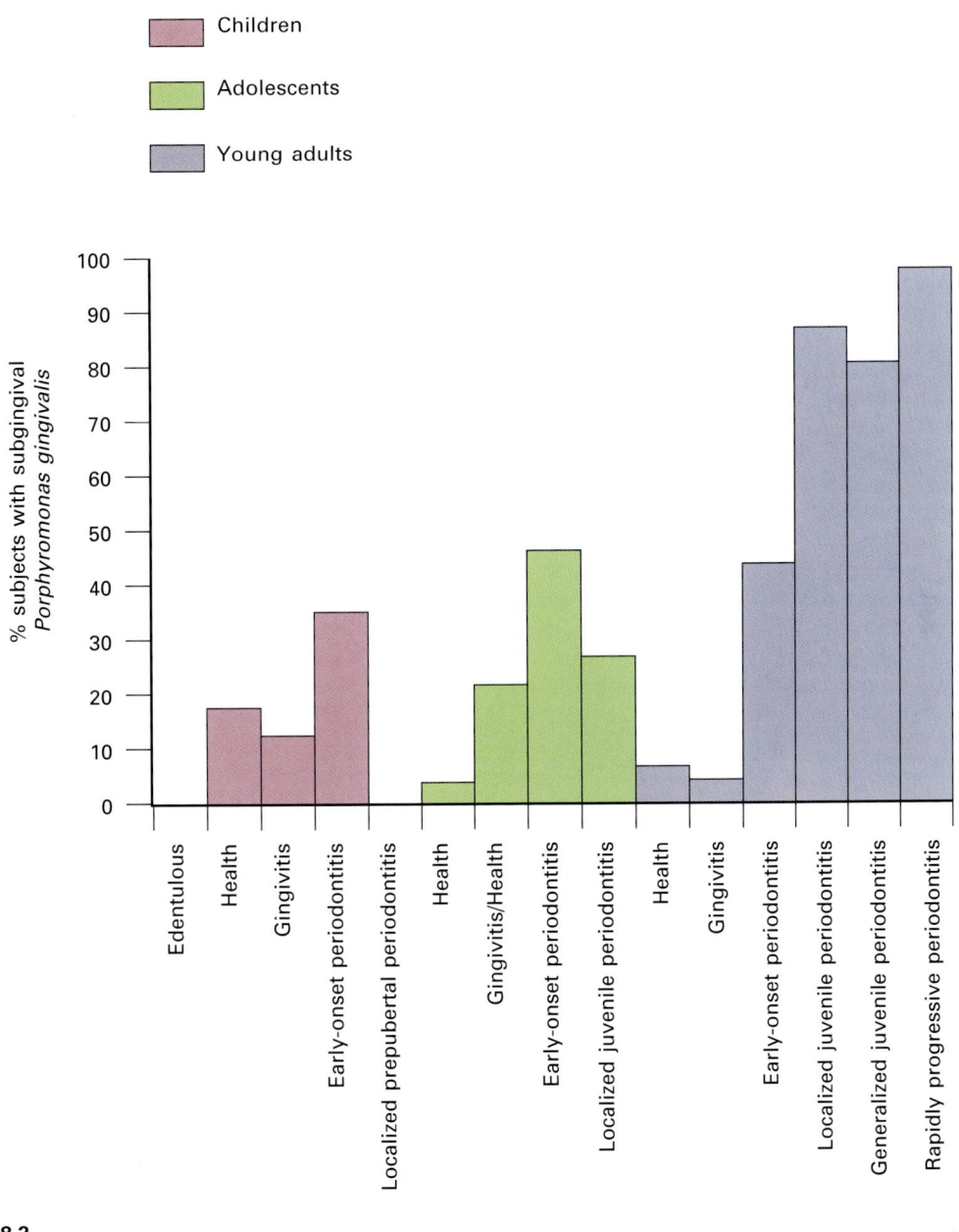

Figure 8.2

Subgingival *Porphyromonas gingivalis* in periodontal health and disease (Slots and Ting, 1999).

et al., 1998). *Porphyromonas gingivalis* appears to constitute the most common periodontal pathogen in the population of northern Cameroon and in indigenous Brazilians living in the Amazon region. It occurs 3–4 times more frequently in Indo-Pakistani children than in children of European descent. Localized aggressive periodontitis patients in Chile and Jamaica show high levels of *Porphyromonas gingivalis* (López et al., 1996; Michalowicz et al., 2000).

Periodontal microbiota in systemically healthy young individuals

Periodontal health

The subgingival microbiota in health protects against colonization by periodontal pathogens. Streptococci and other health-associated bacteria inhibit the growth of *Actinobacillus actinomycetemcomitans* and other pathogens (Hillman et al., 1985). Maintaining a health-associated microbiota, or changing the subgingival microbiota from one associated with periodontitis to one associated with periodontal health, is a major goal of modern therapy.

The healthy gingival sulcus harbors a scant microbiota dominated by Gram-positive organisms (85%) and facultatively anaerobic species (75%). *Actinomyces* and *Streptococcus* species each account for about 40% of total isolates. *Streptococcus oralis*, *Actinomyces gerencseriae* and *Actinomyces naeslundii* are the predominant species in periodontal health. Gram-negative isolates that belong to the genera *Fusobacterium*, *Prevotella*, and *Veillonella*. Black-pigmented anaerobic rods can be detected in low levels in about 70% of periodontally healthy subjects, the most common species being *Prevotella nigrescens*. Spirochetes and motile rods make up less than 5% of the healthy periodontal microbiota (Tanner et al., 1998).

Gingivitis

Chronic gingivitis

The experimental gingivitis model of Löe et al. (1965) examined the progression from periodontal health to gingivitis. In humans and animals, the withdrawal of oral hygiene results in dental plaque formation and the development of gingivitis within 10–21 days. Reinstatement of plaque removal quickly restores healthy gingival condition. Importantly, dental plaque develops prior to the occurrence of gingivitis and not secondary to gingival inflammation. In experimental gingivitis, the periodontal microbiota is initially dominated by Gram-positive cocci, Gram-positive rods, and Gram-negative cocci. With clinical inflammation, the microbiota becomes increasingly complex to include filaments, motile rods, and spirochetes. Experimental gingivitis in young adults is associated with *Actinomyces naeslundii*, *Actinomyces odontolyticus*, *Fusobacterium nucleatum*, *Lactobacillus* species, *Streptococcus anginosus*, *Veillonella parvula*, and *Treponema* species (Moore et al., 1982).

Chronic gingivitis can progress to loss of periodontal attachment; however, most young patients exhibit gingivitis for extended periods without experiencing periodontitis. Direct microscopic examination of chronic gingivitis microorganisms shows motile rods and spirochetes each making up about 20% of the total microbiota (Tanner et al., 1998). Culture studies show a predominance of Gram-positive facultative organisms (about 55%) but Gram-negative anaerobic organisms are almost as abundant (about 45%). Common Gram-positive organisms include *Actinomyces naeslundii*, *Streptococcus sanguis*, *Streptococcus mitis* and *Peptostreptococcus micros*. Gram-negative organisms include *Fusobacterium nucleatum*, *Prevotella intermedia*, *Veillonella parvula*, *Campylobacter* species, *Haemophilus* species, and *Treponema* species, (Tanner et al., 1998).

Mycoplasmas are the smallest free-living microorganisms bound by a pliable unit membrane and lacking a cell wall. In children aged 5–9 years, mycoplasmas were cultured from 93% of saliva samples and from 50% of plaque samples, and were detected in higher proportions with increasing levels of gingivitis (Wilson et al., 1992; Holt et al., 1995).

Gingivitis microbiota of children and adults may differ in microbial content. Compared with adults, children's gingivitis exhibits higher proportions of *Leptotrichia*, *Capnocytophaga*, *Selenomonas*, *Campylobacter*, and *Prevotella* species. On the other hand, children's gingivitis tends to show lower occurrence of *Actinobacillus actinomycetemcomitans*, *Bacteroides forsythus*, *Porphyromonas gingivalis*, *Prevotella intermedia*, *Prevotella nigrescens*, *Treponema denticola*, *Eikenella corrodens*, *Fusobacterium*, *Eubacterium*, and spirochetes (Ashimoto et al., 1996).

Orthodontic appliances can significantly interfere with plaque control. Teeth with fixed orthodontic appliances exhibit increased percentages of filaments, fusiforms, motile rods, and spirochetes, and a concomitant decrease in percentage of cocci. Also, children undergoing orthodontic treatment harbor more *Actinobacillus actinomycetemcomitans* than control subjects. However, with good oral hygiene, children with fixed orthodontic appliances can maintain gingival health despite increases in motile rods and spirochetes and a concurrent decrease in streptococci (Petti et al., 1997).

Pubertal gingivitis

Puberty is associated with increased incidence and severity of gingivitis which may not solely be due to increased amount of dental plaque. The microbiota of pubertal gingivitis is similar to that of young adults, and is predominated by *Prevotella intermedia*, spirochetes, motile rods, *Actinomyces* species, and *Capnocytophaga* species. Serum levels of testosterone in boys, and estradiol and progesterone in girls, are positively correlated with subgingival levels of *Prevotella intermedia* and *Prevotella nigrescens*. Sex hormones in gingival crevicular fluid can serve as growth factors for the two black-pigmented *Prevotella* species (Nakagawa et al., 1994).

Acute herpetic gingivostomatitis

Acute herpetic gingivostomatitis is caused by herpes simplex virus type 1 (HSV-1) and occasionally HSV-2. Herpetic gingivostomatitis manifests as painful vesicular lesions that burst to form shallow ulcers with smooth margins and a red halo. Lesions may affect attached gingiva and extend to the tongue, the oral mucosa, the lips and, occasionally, to extraoral sites. Treatment of acute herpetic gingivostomatitis is primarily supportive, but moderate to severe cases may require antiviral drugs such as acyclovir. Use of antibacterial drugs may be futile in treating the viral component of acute herpetic gingivostomatitis, but topical antiseptics can prevent bacterial superinfection (Scully et al., 1998).

Periodontitis

A limited number of bacterial species ("specific bacterial infection") may be responsible for the conversion of a gingivitis lesion to periodontitis.

Localized periodontitis in children (formerly localized prepubertal periodontitis)

Despite marked periodontal breakdown, localized periodontitis lesions in children often manifest minimal dental plaque and only minor gingival inflammation. The disease is associated with increased levels of subgingival Gram-negative anaerobic bacteria. Baab et al. (1986) recovered *Capnocytophaga ochracea*, *Fusobacterium nucleatum*, and *Prevotella intermedia*. Mishkin et al. (1986) detected *Actinobacillus actinomycetemcomitans*, *Porphyromonas gingivalis*, *Prevotella intermedia*, *Fusobacterium nucleatum*, and *Streptococcus sanguis*. Altman et al. (1985) detected *Fusobacterium nucleatum*, *Selenomonas*, *Campylobacter*, *Porphyromonas*, *Prevotella*, and *Capnocytophaga* species. D'Angelo et al. (1992) observed high proportions of spirochetes, black-pigmented anaerobic rods, and *Fusobacterium* species. Sweeney et al. (1987) reported black-pigmented anaerobic rods to constitute 11% of the total cultivable flora with a predominance of *Prevotella intermedia*.

Localized periodontitis in children can often be successfully treated with mechanical debridement alone. If systemic antibiotics are to be used, metronidazole–amoxicillin combination therapy (see below) may be considered. Tetracycline should not be prescribed to young patients because of the risk of tooth malformation and discoloration (Livingston and Dellinger, 1998).

Localized aggressive periodontitis (formerly localized juvenile periodontitis)

Actinobacillus actinomycetemcomitans is a major pathogen in LAP (Figure 8.3). Slots et al. (1980) detected *Actinobacillus actinomycetemcomitans* in 90% of patients with (LAP, in 79% of lesions. Mandell et al. (1987) recovered *Actinobacillus actinomycetemcomitans* from 100% of LAP patients with progressing sites and from 50% of patients with non-progressing sites. Other investigators identified *Actinobacillus actinomycetemcomitans* in 73–100% of LAP patients.

In longitudinal studies of LAP in children, Bogert et al. (1989) found a strong positive association between levels of *Actinobacillus*

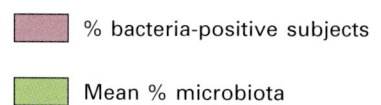

■ % bacteria-positive subjects

■ Mean % microbiota

Figure 8.3

Microorganisms in localized aggressive periodontitis (from studies described in Slots and Ting, 1999).

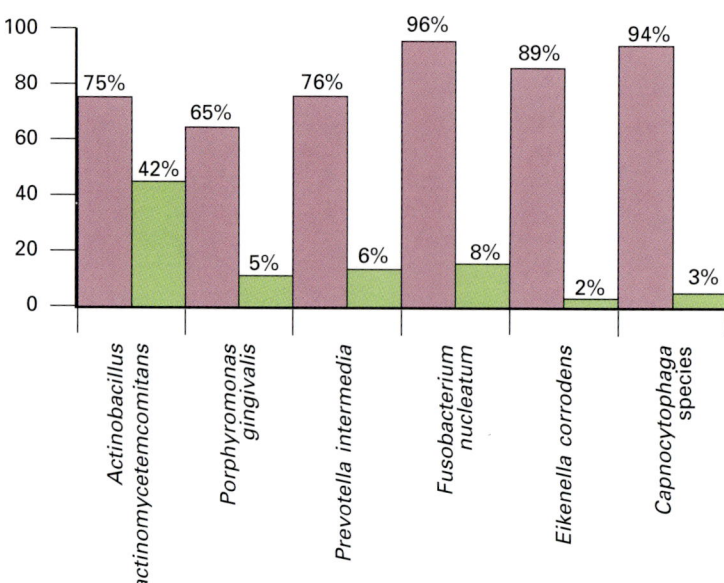

actinomycetemcomitans and disease activity. The high rate of occurrence of *Actinobacillus actinomycetemcomitans* in progressive lesions provides strong evidence for the etiological importance of the organism in the disease.

Subgingival *Actinobacillus actinomycetemcomitans* levels seem to peak at circumpubertal age. Asikainen (1985) recovered this microorganism from 85% of lesions in patients 14–16 years old, from 47% of lesions in patients 17–19 years old, and from 32% of lesions in patients 20–25 years old. Studies that reported *Actinobacillus actinomycetemcomitans* in only 23–40% of patients might have included older patients or atypical cases of LAP in children (Asikainen et al., 1991; López et al., 1996).

Actinobacillus actinomycetemcomitans produces several virulence factors of importance for oral colonization and persistence (e.g., fimbriae), interference with host's defenses (e.g., leukotoxin and immunosuppressive proteins), destruction of host tissues (e.g., cytotoxins, collagenase, and bone resorption agents), and inhibition of host tissue repair (e.g., fibroblast and bone inhibitors) (Fives-Taylor et al., 1999).

Bacteriocins produced by *Actinobacillus actinomycetemcomitans* may facilitate oral colonization of the organism by eliminating bacteria associated with periodontal health. Actinobacillin, a bacteriocin of *Actinobacillus actinomycetemcomitans*, inhibits the growth of *Streptococcus sanguis*, *Streptococcus uberis*, and *Actinomyces* species (Hammond et al., 1987; Stevens et al., 1987).

Actinobacillus actinomycetemcomitans can evade host defenses by a variety of mechanisms. By invading gingival epithelial cells, it may escape cellular and humoral host defenses, and its Fc-binding proteins inhibit opsonizing immunoglobulin G antibody binding and thereby phagocytosis by neutrophils. *Actinobacillus actinomycetemcomitans* secretes a low-molecular-weight leukotoxin capable of

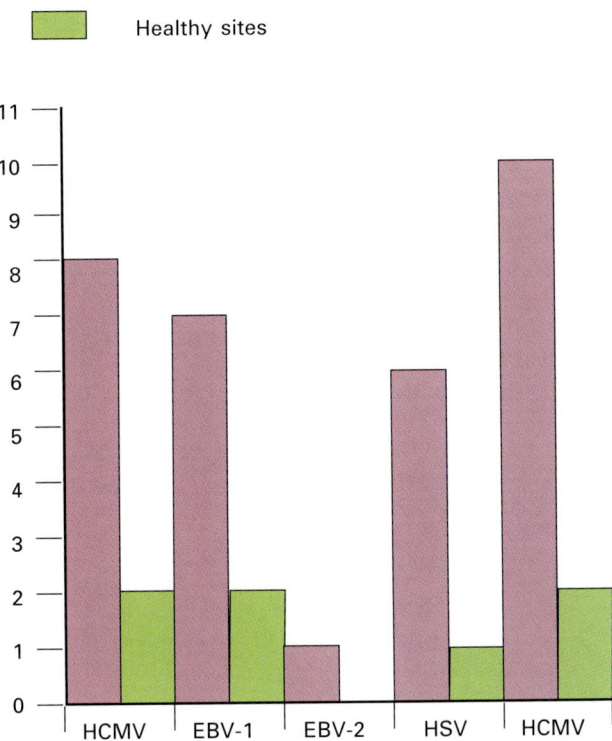

LJP sites

Healthy sites

Figure 8.4

Human herpesviruses in healthy and diseased sites in 11 patients with localized aggressive periodontitis (Ting et al., 2000). EBV, Epstein–Barr virus; HCMV, human cytomegalovirus; HSV, herpes simplex virus.

reducing neutrophil chemotaxis and inducing multiple membrane perforations in neutrophils, monocytes, and certain lymphocyte subsets (Taichman et al., 1987; Iwase et al., 1990).

Some strains of *Actinobacillus actinomycetemcomitans* contain a 530 base pair deletion in the promoter region of the leukotoxin gene operon, which makes them strong leukotoxin producers. Subjects harboring *Actinobacillus actinomycetemcomitans* strains with the 530 bp deletion are 22.5 times more likely to experience LAP than subjects colonized by strains containing the full-length leukotoxin promoter region (Bueno et al., 1998).

Actinobacillus actinomycetemcomitans possesses several tissue-destroying mechanisms: lipopolysaccharide and some surface proteins may serve as bone resorptive mediators, collagenase may reduce collagen fibers of the periodontal extracellular matrix, and fibroblast cytotoxin may inhibit fibroblast proliferation and interfere with collagen turnover (Shenker et al., 1982; Stevens et al., 1983; Kamin et al., 1986).

Notwithstanding the ample evidence that *Actinobacillus actinomycetemcomitans* is a cause of LAP in children, the presence of the organism in subgingival sites does not necessarily cause periodontal destruction. *Actinobacillus actinomycetemcomitans* strains have been recovered from 75% of periodontal sites with probing depths of 2–3 mm in patients aged 14–16 years. Also, if *Actinobacillus actinomycetemcomitans* were the sole cause of LAP in children, it is difficult to explain the limitation of periodontal destruction to first molars and incisors, and the lack of periodontal destruction of teeth in close proximity to affected sites. Most probably additional infectious agents or host factors as yet unidentified participate in the development of LAP in children (Ting et al., 2000).

Porphyromonas gingivalis is a rare organism in early LAP in children in Europe and North America but is found in 38–94% of established lesions. Other potentially pathogenic bacteria in this disease include *Prevotella intermedia*, *Campylobacter rectus*, *Fusobacterium nucleatum*, *Treponema denticola*, *Selenomonas sputigena*, *Eikenella corrodens*, and *Capnocytophaga* species (Eisenmann et al., 1983; Haffajee et al., 1984; Albandar et al., 1997).

A complex host–parasite relationship is responsible for the establishment and overgrowth of *Actinobacillus actinomycetemcomitans* in LAP lesions. Recent studies have pointed to the possible role of herpesviruses (cytomegalovirus and Epstein-Barr virus type 1) in development of LAP in adolescents (Michalowicz et al., 2000; Ting et al., 2000). Herpesviruses exert pathogenicity by decreasing host defenses. Viral inclusion bodies have been observed in inflammatory cells of AP lesions. Ting et al. (2000) detected subgingival cytomegalovirus or Epstein–Barr virus type 1 in 10 of 11 patients (Figure 8.4). Five of six patients aged 10–14 years with progressing periodontitis revealed *active* cytomegalovirus infection; such an infection may severely hamper important antimicrobial periodontal defenses and induce overgrowth of subgingival pathogenic bacteria, including *Actinobacillus actinomycetemcomitans* and *Porphyromonas gingivalis* (Ting et al., 2000).

Post-localized aggressive periodontitis in adolescents

Localized aggressive periodontitis in adolescents is self-limiting and the disease process can "burn out" in older teenagers. Predominant organisms in post-LAP include *Prevotella intermedia*, *Porphyromonas gingivalis*, *Bacteroides forsythus*, and *Actinobacillus actinomycetemcomitans*. *Treponema denticola* and other spirochetes are also frequently found in these lesions (Sasaki et al., 1989).

Atypical localized aggressive periodontitis in adolescents

Periodontal destruction around atypical teeth is less severe than that around first permanent molars and incisors, probably because it commences at the time that the disease would normally "burn out". *Actinobacillus actinomycetemcomitans* may also be responsible for periodontal breakdown around teeth usually not affected by LAP (Slots and Rams, 1992).

Generalized aggressive periodontitis (formerly generalized juvenile periodontitis)

Brown et al. (1996) found that 35% of patients with LAP develop generalized aggressive periodontitis within 6 years of the localized onset. However, many cases of generalized aggressive periodontitis begin with widespread periodontal destruction. *Porphyromonas gingivalis* and *Prevotella intermedia* have been isolated from patients with this condition (López et al., 1996).

Generalized aggressive periodontitis of young adults (formerly rapidly progressive periodontitis)

The clinical diagnosis of "generalized aggressive periodontitis of young adults" may constitute a variant of the type of generalized disease seen in adolescents (formerly generalized juvenile periodontitis) or a distinct clinical entity. Generalized aggressive periodontitis in young adults is associated with *Porphyromonas gingivalis* (92% of diseased sites), *Bacteroides forsythus* (53% of sites), *Prevotella intermedia* (88% of sites), *Fusobacterium nucleatum* (90% of sites), and *Streptococcus intermedius* (88% of sites) (Kamma et al., 1994).

Periodontal microbiota in medically compromised young individuals

Medically compromised patients experience more severe gingival and periodontal diseases than systemically healthy individuals; however, the periodontal microbiota of these patients has only been partially elucidated.

Drug-induced gingival overgrowth

Cyclosporine (an immunosuppressant agent), nifedipine (a calcium channel blocker), and phenytoin (an antiepileptic drug) can give rise to gingival overgrowth (Hallmon and Rossmann, 1999). Following transplantation, patients medicated with cyclosporine suffer from some degree of immune suppression. Little information is available about the microbiota of cyclosporine-induced gingival overgrowth. Candidal hyphae have been detected in superficial layers of the gingival epithelium of cyclosporine-associated overgrowth (Khocht and Schneider, 1997). Nifedipine medication for cardiovascular disorders can give rise to gingival overgrowth (especially in young patients) associated with *Fusobacterium* species, *Eubacterium alactolyticum*, *Campylobacter concisus*, *Propionibacterium acnes*, *Capnocytophaga* species, *Bacteroides gracilis*, and *Selenomonas sputigena* (Nakou et al., 1998). Children who receive phenytoin for epilepsy commonly manifest gingival overgrowth. Phenytoin therapy can lead to increased counts of subgingival Gram-negative anaerobic rods and suppression of subgingival streptococci, but a unique subgingival microbiota has not been identified (Smith et al., 1983). The subject of drug-influenced gingival enlargement is discussed in Chapter 3.

Gingivitis

Acute necrotizing ulcerative gingivitis

Young people under stress, having poor oral hygiene, or suffering from malnutrition, are at risk of acute necrotizing ulcerative gingivitis (ANUG). The disease starts with necrotic lesions at one or more interdental gingival papillae and progresses to its maximal extent within a few days. In some poorer countries, similar lesions, termed cancrum oris or noma, can expand considerably beyond the gingiva and cause life-threatening infections. The disease is associated with pain, bleeding, fetor ex ore and, occasionally, fever and malaise (Cogen, 1990).

The ANUG lesions consist of four zones (Listgarten, 1965). The outer surface of the lesion, the bacterial zone, contains a variety of bacteria and may resemble the subgingival microbiota of periodontal lesions. The neutrophil zone is rich in leukocytes and underscores the acute state of the disease. The necrotic zone contains cell debris as well as spirochetes and Gram-negative rods. The invasion zone exhibits infiltration of large and medium-sized spirochetes into apparently normal gingival connective tissue. Selective spirochetal invasion of underlying gingival connective tissue is unique to ANUG lesions.

Early direct microscopic examination of ANUG lesions identified high levels of fusobacteria and of intermediate and large spirochetes (Listgarten, 1965). However, using improved culture and immunofluorescence techniques, more recent studies found relatively small proportions of *Fusobacterium* and large proportions of *Prevotella intermedia*. The combined occurrence of *Treponema* species and *Prevotella intermedia* may be important for ANUG development (Chung et al., 1983). A recent study of young Nigerian children demonstrated a close association between periodontal cytomegalovirus and Epstein–Barr virus, malnutrition, and the occurrence of ANUG. Herpesviruses may set the stage for overgrowth of periodontal pathogens in ANUG patients (Contreras et al., 1997).

Treatment of ANUG involves mechanical debridement of the affected sites and institution of oral hygiene measures. Oral rinses with chlorhexidine may be beneficial. Patients with fever or other systemic manifestations may receive systemic metronidazole or other antimicrobial therapy effective against anaerobes (Murayama et al., 1994).

Generalized linear erythema (formerly HIV-associated gingivitis)

Generalized linear erythema may manifest as necrotizing ulcerative gingivitis or linear gingival erythema. *Candida albicans* can be recovered from human immunodeficiency virus-associated gingivitis and may play a role in petechiae and red lesion formation. *Porphyromonas gingivalis*, *Prevotella intermedia*, *Fusobacterium nucleatum*, and *Actinobacillus actinomycetemcomitans* occur significantly more frequently in HIV-associated gingivitis sites than in healthy periodontal sites of HIV-seropositive and HIV-negative patients (Murray, 1994). Human immunodeficiency virus-associated gingivitis and HIV-associated periodontitis show similar periodontal pathogens, suggesting that the gingivitis serves as a precursor to the periodontitis (Murray, 1994).

Treatment of generalized linear erythema involves oral hygiene measures, scaling, root planing, chlorhexidine rinses, and frequent maintenance therapy. However, diligent preventive therapy does not always prevent progression to HIV-associated periodontitis. Treatment with topical antifungal agents may help reduce gingival erythema and petechiae in HIV-associated gingivitis.

Periodontitis

Patients with various genetic syndromes or systemic diseases are susceptible to severe and precocious periodontal disease.

Generalized periodontitis in prepubertal patients

Neutropenia, acquired immune deficiency syndrome (AIDS), histiocytosis X, hypophosphatasia, leukocyte adhesion deficiency, and Papillon–Lefèvre syndrome are systemic diseases associated with severe and generalized periodontitis during prepuberty (Meyle, 1994).

Chronic or cyclical neutropenia of genetic origin is frequently associated with severe generalized periodontitis. Neutropenia may enhance subgingival microbial colonization. *Actinobacillus actinomycetemcomitans*, black Gram-negative anaerobic rods, *Fusobacterium* species, and spirochetes have been recovered from neutropenia-associated periodontitis. Bacteria do not invade the gingiva despite the weakened host response of neutropenic patients. Diligent oral hygiene and proper maintenance therapy may prevent further periodontal breakdown for years.

Children with Papillon–Lefèvre syndrome frequently lose teeth to periodontal disease within a few years of eruption (Bimstein et al., 1990; Hart and Shapira, 1994). Papillon–Lefèvre syndrome periodontitis is associated with *Actinobacillus actinomycetemcomitans* (Bimstein et al., 1990). Other potential pathogens include *Prevotella intermedia*, *Porphyromonas gingivalis*, *Fusobacterium nucleatum*, and *Eikenella corrodens* (Hart and Shapira, 1994). Cytomegalovirus and Epstein–Barr virus type 1 may also contribute to Papillon–Lefèvre syndrome periodontitis (Velazco et al., 1999). Treatment of the periodontal component of the syndrome may involve extractions of affected primary teeth in order to save the permanent dentition (Hart and Shapira, 1994). Systemic antibiotic therapy (amoxicillin–metronidazole combination) can be successful if implemented before eruption of the permanent teeth (Boutsi et al., 1997).

Down syndrome

Patients with Down syndrome have more periodontitis than the normal population (Barnett et al., 1986; Modeer et al., 1990). Adolescents with Down syndrome harbor relatively high levels of subgingival black-pigmented anaerobic rods, spirochetes (Meskin et al., 1968; Keyes et al., 1971) and *Actinobacillus actinomycetemcomitans* (Barr-Agholme et al., 1992). Scaling, root planing, and supragingival plaque control are often insufficient in controlling periodontal pathogens in these patients. Cichon et al. (1998) detected a 2-fold increase in *Prevotella intermedia* and a 2.5-fold increase in *Porphyromonas gingivalis* 4 weeks after initial therapy. Down syndrome periodontitis lesions show high prevalence of herpesviruses (Hanookai et al., 2000).

Insulin-dependent diabetes mellitus

Insulin-dependent diabetes mellitus (IDDM, type I diabetes) in young individuals is associated with a higher frequency of periodontitis than that in age-matched non-diabetic individuals. However, patients with well-controlled type I diabetes and good oral hygiene may not necessarily experience severe periodontitis (Yalda et al., 1994). *Capnocytophaga* species, *Actinobacillus actinomycetemcomitans*, *Campylobacter rectus*, and *Porphyromonas gingivalis* are present in diabetic periodontitis (Yalda et al., 1994). Patients with improved metabolic control show significant increases in subgingival streptococcal counts (Sastrowijoto et al., 1990).

HIV associated periodontitis

Infection with HIV in young individuals may be congenital or acquired. Associated periodontitis lesions can resemble early onset periodontitis (EOP), adult periodontitis, or (less frequently) necrotizing ulcerative periodontitis (Murray, 1994), and contain spirochetes, *Fusobacterium* species, *Actinobacillus actinomycetemcomitans*, *Campylobacter rectus*, *Peptostreptococcus micros*, and *Prevotella intermedia* (Rams et al., 1991). *Mycoplasma salivarium* can also occur in HIV periodontitis (Moore et al., 1993).

In addition to conventional periodontopathic bacteria, HIV periodontitis lesions may harbor more unusual microorganisms, including *Bacteroides fragilis, Fusobacterium necrophorum, Eubacterium aerofaciens, Clostridium* species, enterococci, *Pseudomonas aeruginosa*, various enteric rods, and *Candida albicans* (Murray, 1994). Patients experiencing a progression of HIV infection to AIDS show elevated levels of periodontal *Enterococcus avium, Entercoccus faecalis, Clostridium clostridiiforme, Clostridium difficile*, and *Klebsiella pneumoniae* (Zambon et al., 1990). Subgingival yeasts occur in 13% of HIV-positive subjects and comprise 0.05–0.0002% of total microbiota (Moore et al., 1993). In AIDS patients with periodontitis, 59% of subjects and 62% of periodontal sites harbored subgingival yeasts (Zambon et al., 1990).

Lesions of HIV-associated periodontitis also demonstrate a high frequency of several herpesviruses, including cytomegalovirus, Epstein–Barr virus type 1 and human herpesvirus 8. Human herpesvirus 8 is implicated in the development of Kaposi's sarcoma (Contreras et al., 2000).

Children infected with HIV are more susceptible to and more adversely affected by bacterial infections than are adults. Hence, HIV-associated periodontal lesions in children should be treated promptly. Necrotizing periodontitis can be managed for long periods by means of scaling, root planing, appropriate antimicrobial treatment, and adequate home care and maintenance therapy.

Effects of therapy on periodontal pathogens

Scaling and root planing are generally inefficient in removing subgingival *Actinobacillus actino-*

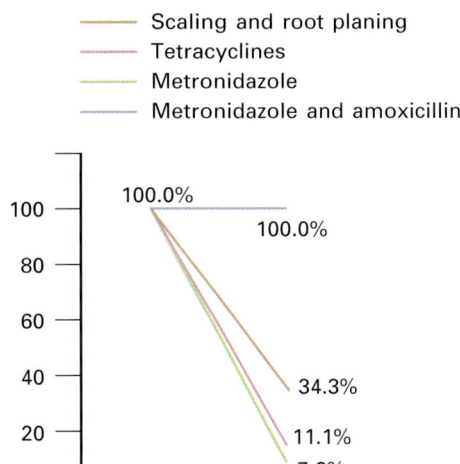

Figure 8.5

Effect of systemic antibiotic treatment on the percentage of *Actinobacillus actinomycetemcomitans*-infected subjects in localized aggressive periodontitis (Slots and Ting, 1999).

mycetemcomitans, especially in heavily infected periodontal sites. The inability of non-surgical therapy to control subgingival *Actinobacillus actinomycetemcomitans* may be related to the organism's ability to invade gingival tissue. Scaling and root planing are also unable to eradicate subgingival *Porphyromonas gingivalis* in most patients (Flemmig et al., 1998). *Porphyromonas gingivalis* residing in inaccessible areas, such as furcations or the base of periodontal pockets, may complicate attempts at mechanical removal.

Widman flap access surgery may suppress *Actinobacillus actinomycetemcomitans* to below detectable levels in only about 50% of AP lesions (Slots and Rosling, 1983). On the other hand, resective periodontal surgery is relatively effective in eradicating subgingival *Actinobacillus actinomycetemcomitans*, probably because of excision of infected gingival tissue and pocket depth reduction to a level permitting adequate cleaning by tooth brushing, flossing, and other oral hygiene measures (Ali et al., 1992; Tuan et al., 2000). Similarly, non-resective periodontal

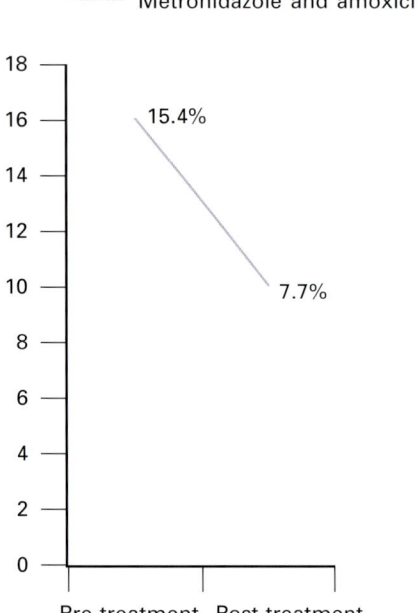

Figure 8.6

Effect of systemic metronidazole+amoxicillin treatment on the percentage of *Porphyromonas gingivalis*-infected subjects in localized aggressive periodontitis (Slots and Ting, 1999).

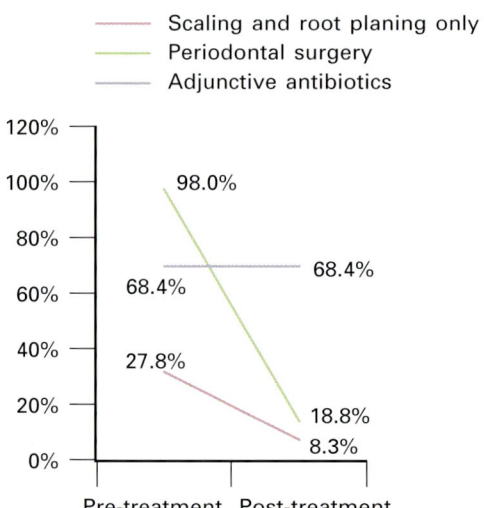

Figure 8.7

Effect of treatment on the percentage of *Actinobacillus actinomycetemcomitans*-infected subjects with early-onset periodontitis (Slots and Ting, 1999).

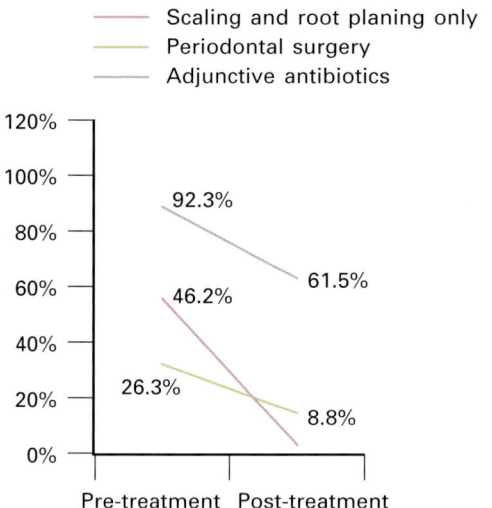

Figure 8.8

Effect of treatment on the percentage of *Porphyromonas gingivalis*-infected subjects with early-onset periodontitis (Slots and Ting, 1999).

surgery is ineffective in removing subgingival *Porphyromonas gingivalis*, but periodontal pocket reduction surgery may lead to a suppression of the organism (Rosenberg et al., 1993; Mombelli et al., 1995; Tuan et al., 2000).

Systemic antibiotic therapy has the potential to eradicate *Actinobacillus actinomycetemcomitans* residing in periodontal pockets and gingival tissue. Tetracycline was the first antibiotic to be used for this purpose (Slots et al., 1982; Slots and Rosling, 1983; Mandell et al., 1987). Tetracycline combined with scaling and root planing or with periodontal surgery can markedly suppress or eliminate *Actinobacillus actinomycetemcomitans* in some localized aggressive lesions in children but is ineffective in others (Slots and Rosling, 1983). Tetracycline is contraindicated in children younger than 6 years because of absorption of tetracycline into the developing tooth structure of permanent teeth, resulting in malformed and discolored teeth.

Systemic amoxicillin–metronidazole combination drug therapy has shown striking clinical results in the treatment of *Actinobacillus actinomycetemcomitans* in LAP (Figures 8.5 and 8.6) and in other forms of EOP (Figures 8.7 and 8.8) (van Winkelhoff et al., 1992; Bimstein et al., 1997). Amoxicillin increases the uptake of metronidazole by *Actinobacillus actinomycetemcomitans*. The present antibiotic recommendation for periodontal *A. actinomycetemcomitans* infection is a course of amoxicillin and metronidazole, 250 mg each, three times daily for 8 days (dosage for older children and adults). The amoxicillin–metronidazole combination therapy is also effective against other types of periodontal infections in young individuals. However, good clinical and microbiological outcomes are not guaranteed and partly depend on patient compliance, as demonstrated in a report that revealed persisting subgingival *Actinobacillus actinomycetemcomitans* after this therapy (Flemmig et al., 1998).

Subgingival topical antimicrobial agents often fail to reach microorganisms residing within gingival tissue or in the apical part of the periodontal pocket. Topical application of tetracyclines or metronidazole is usually unsuccessful in eradicating subgingival *Actinobacillus actinomycetemcomitans* and *Porphyromonas gingivalis*. In fact, studies have found elevated levels of *Actinobacillus actinomycetemcomitans* after topical tetracycline therapy. Topical antimicrobial agents may be useful in delaying subgingival recolonization of periodontal pathogens during the periodontal maintenance phase.

Conclusion

Destructive periodontal diseases in children and adolescents often exhibit a rapid course of progression. Medically compromised young individuals experience particularly severe periodontal disease, often associated with—and possibly caused by—the bacteria *Actinobacillus actinomycetemcomitans* and *Porphyromonas gingivalis;* and by the herpesviruses, cytomegalovirus and Epstein–Barr virus type 1.

Prevention of periodontal diseases in young individuals includes conventional plaque-reducing measures and possibly also periodontal treatment of relatives to interrupt intrafamilial transmission of periodontal pathogens.

Treatment includes scaling and root planing, antibiotic therapy, and occasionally surgery. Systemic amoxicillin–metronidazole combination drug therapy is effective in treating *Actinobacillus actinomycetemcomitans*-associated periodontitis, and other types of EOP.

As knowledge of the microorganisms involved in periodontal diseases of young individuals expands, dentists will be able to incorporate increasingly more effective antimicrobial therapies as part of their armamentarium.

References

Albandar JM, Brown LJ, Löe H (1997) Putative periodontal pathogens in subgingival plaque of young adults with and without early-onset periodontitis. *J Periodontol* **68**: 973–81.

Ali RW, Lie T, Skaug N (1992) Early effects of periodontal therapy on the detection frequency of four putative periodontal pathogens in adults. *J Periodontol* **63**: 540–7.

Altman LC, Page RC, Vandesteen GE et al. (1985) Abnormalities of leukocyte chemotaxis in patients with various forms of periodontitis. *J Periodont Res* **20**: 553–63.

Ashimoto A, Chen C, Bakker I, Slots J (1996) Polymerase chain reaction detection of 8 putative periodontal pathogens in subgingival plaque of gingivitis and advanced periodontitis lesions. *Oral Microbiol Immunol* **11**: 266–73.

Asikainen S (1985) Occurrence of *Actinobacillus actinomycetemcomitans* and spirochetes in relation to age in localized juvenile periodontitis. *J Periodontol* **56**: 537–41.

Asikainen S, Lai CH, Alaluusua S, Slots J (1991) Distribution of *Actinobacillus actinomycetemcomitans* serotypes in periodontal health and disease. *Oral Microbiol Immunol* **6**: 115–18.

Asikainen S, Chen C, Slots J (1996) Likelihood of transmitting *Actinobacillus actinomycetemcomitans* and *Porphyromonas gingivalis* in families with periodontitis. *Oral Microbiol Immunol* **11**: 387–94.

Baab DA, Page RC, Ebersole JL et al. (1986) Laboratory studies of a family manifesting premature exfoliation of deciduous teeth. *J Clin Periodontol* **13**: 677–83.

Barnett ML, Press KP, Friedman D, Sonnenberg EM (1986) The prevalence of periodontitis and dental caries in a Down's syndrome population. *J Periodontol* **57**: 288–93.

Barr-Agholme M, Dahllof G, Linder L, Modeer T (1992) *Actinobacillus actinomycetemcomitans, Capnocytophaga* and *Porphyromonas gingivalis* in subgingival plaque of adolescents with Down's syndrome. *Oral Microbiol Immunol* **7**: 244–8.

Bimstein E, Ebersole J (1989) The age-dependent reaction of the periodontal tissues to dental plaque. *ASDC J Dent Child* **56**: 358–62.

Bimstein E, Lustmann J, Sela MN et al. (1990) Periodontitis associated with Papillon-Lefèvre syndrome. *J Periodontol* **61**: 373–7.

Bimstein E, Sela MN, Shapira L (1997) Clinical and microbial considerations for the treatment of an extended kindred with seven cases of prepubertal periodontitis: a 2 year follow up. *Pediatr Dent* **19**: 396–403.

Bogert M, Bertold P, Brightman V et al. (1989) Longitudinal study of LJP families—two year surveillance. *J Dent Res* **68**: 312.

Boutsi EA, Umeda M, Nagasawa T et al. (1997) Follow-up of two cases of Papillon-Lefevre syndrome and presentation of two new cases. *Int J Periodont Rest Dent* **17**: 334–47.

Brown LJ, Albandar JM, Brunelle JA, Loe H (1996) Early-onset periodontitis: progression of attachment loss during 6 years. *J Periodontol* **67**: 968–75.

Bueno LC, Mayer PAM, DiRienzo JM (1998) Relationship between conversion of localized juvenile periodontitis-susceptible children from health and disease and *Actinobacillus actinomycetemcomitans* leukotoxin promotor structure. *J Periodontol* **69**: 998–1007.

Chung CP, Nisengard RJ, Slots J, Genco RJ (1983) Bacterial IgG and IgM antibody titers in acute necrotizing ulcerative gingivitis. *J Periodontol* **61**: 769–2.

Cichon P, Crawford L, Grimm WD (1998) Early-onset periodontitis associated with Down's syndrome—clinical interventional study. *Ann Periodontol* **3**: 370–80.

Cogen RB (1990) Acute necrotizing ulcerative gingivitis. In: Genco RJ, Goldman HM, Cohen DW (eds) *Contemporary Periodontics*. St Louis: Mosby, pp. 459–65.

Cogen RB, Wright JT, Tate AL (1992) Destructive periodontal disease in healthy children. *J Periodontol* **63**: 761–5.

Contreras A, Slots J (2000) Herpesviruses in human periodontal disease. *J Periodont Res* **35**: 3–16.

Contreras A, Falkler WA, Enwonwu CO et al. (1997) Human Herpesviridae in acute necrotizing ulcerative gingivitis in children in Nigeria. *Oral Microbiol Immunol* **12**: 259–65.

Contreras A, Mardirossian A, Slots J (2000) Herpesviruses in HIV-periodontitis. *J Clin Periodontol* (in press).

Contreras A, Rusitanonta T, Chen C et al. (2000) Frequency of 530–bp deletion in *Actinobacillus actinomycetemcomitans* leukotoxin promoter region. *Oral Microbiol Immunol* (in press).

D'Angelo M, Margiotta V, Ammatuma P, Sammartano F (1992) Treatment of prepubertal periodontitis. *J Clin Periodontol* **19**: 214–19.

Eisenmann AC, Eisenmann R, Sousa O, Slots J (1983) Microbiological study of localized juvenile periodontitis in Panama. *J Periodontol* **54**: 712–13.

Fives-Taylor PM, Meyer DH, Mintz KP, Brissette C (1999) Virulence factors of *Actinobacillus actinomycetemcomitans*. *Periodontol 2000* **20**: 136–67.

Flemmig TF, Milián E, Kopp C et al. (1998) Differential effects of systemic metronidazole and amoxillin on *Actinobacillus actinomycetemcomitans* and *Porphyromonas gingivalis* in intraoral habitats. *J Clin Periodontol* **25**: 1–10.

Haffajee AD, Socransky SS, Ebersole JL, Smith DJ (1984) Clinical, microbiological and immunological features associated with the treatment of active periodontosis lesions. *J Clin Periodontol* **11**: 600–18.

Hallmon WW, Rossmann JA (1999) The role of drugs in the pathogenesis of gingival overgrowth. A collective review of current concepts. *Periodontol 2000* **21**: 176–96.

Hammond BF, Lillard SE, Stevens RH (1987) A bacteriocin of *Actinobacillus actinomycetemcomitans*. *Infect Immun* **55**: 686–91.

Hanookai D, Nowzari H, Contreras A et al. (2000) Herpesviruses and periodontopathic bacteria in Trisomy 21 periodontitis. *J Periodontol* **71**: 376–84.

Hart TC, Shapira L (1994) Papillon–Lefèvre syndrome. *Periodontol 2000* **6**: 88–100.

Hillman JD, Socransky SS, Shivers M (1985) The relationships between streptococcal species and periodontopathic bacteria in human dental plaque. *Arch Oral Biol* **30**: 791–5.

Holt RD, Wilson M, Musa S (1995) Mycoplasmas in plaque and saliva of children and their relationship to gingivitis. *J Periodontol* **66**: 97–101.

Holt SC, Kesavalu L, Walker S, Genco AC (1999) Virulence factors of *Porphyromonas gingivalis*. *Periodontol 2000* **20**: 168–238.

Höltta P, Alaluusua S, Saarela M, Asikainen S (1994) Isolation frequency and serotype distribution of mutans streptococci and *Actinobacillus actinomycetemcomitans*, and clinical periodontal status in Finnish and Vietnamese children. *Scand J Dent Res* **102**: 113–19.

Iwase M, Lally ET, Berthold P et al. (1990) Effects of cations and osmotic protectants on cytolytic activity of *Actinobacillus actinomycetemcomitans* leukotoxin. *Infect Immun* **58**: 1782–8.

Kamin S, Harvey W, Wilson M, Scutt A (1986) Inhibition of fibroblast proliferation and collagen synthesis by capsular material from *Actinobacillus actinomycetemcomitans*. *J Med Microbiol* **22**: 245–9.

Kamma JJ, Nakou M, Manti FA (1994) Microbiota of rapidly progressive periodontitis lesions in association with clinical parameters. *J Periodontol* **65**: 1073–8.

Kamma JJ, Diamanti-Kipioti A, Nakou M, Mitsis FJ (2000) Profile of subgingival microbiota in children with mixed dentition. *Oral Microbiol Immunol* **15**: 103–11.

Keyes PH, Bellack S, Jordan HV (1971) Studies on the pathogenesis of destructive lesions of the gums and teeth in mentally retarded children. I. Dentobacterial plaque infection in children with Down's syndrome. *Clin Pediatr* **10**: 711–18.

Khocht A, Schneider LC (1997) Periodontal management of gingival overgrowth in the heart transplant patient: a case report. *J Periodontol* **68**: 1140–6.

Listgarten MA (1965) Electron microscopic observations on the bacterial flora of acute necrotizing ulcerative gingivitis. *J Periodontol* **36**: 328–38.

Livingston HM, Dellinger TM (1998) Intrinsic staining of teeth secondary to tetracycline. *Ann Pharmacother* **32**: 607.

Löe H, Brown LJ (1991) Early onset periodontitis in the United States of America. *J Periodontol* **62**: 608–16.

Löe H, Theilade E, Jensen SB (1965) Experimental gingivitis in man. *J Periodontol* **36**: 177–87.

Löe H, Anerud A, Boysen H, Morrison E (1986) Natural history of periodontal disease in man. Rapid, moderate and no loss of attachment in Sri Lankan labourers 14–46 years of age. *J Clin Periodontol* **13**: 431–40.

Loesche WJ, Bretz WA, Kerschensteiner D et al. (1990) Development of a diagnostic test for anaerobic periodontal infections based on plaque hydrolysis of benzoyl-DL-arginine-naphthylamide. *J Clin Microbiol* **28**: 1551–9.

López NJ, Mellado JC, Leighton GX (1996) Occurrence of *Actinobacillus actinomycetemcomitans*, *Porphyromonas gingivalis* and *Prevotella intermedia* in juvenile periodontitis. *J Clin Periodontol* **23**: 101–5.

Mandell RL, Ebersole JL, Socransky SS (1987) Clinical, immunologic and microbiologic features of active disease sites in juvenile periodontitis. *J Clin Periodontol* **14**: 534–40.

Matsson L (1978) Development of gingivitis in preschool children and young adults. A comparative experimental study. *J Clin Periodontol* **5**: 24–34.

Matsson L, Goldberg P (1985) Gingival inflammatory reaction in children at different ages. *J Clin Periodontol* **12**: 98–103.

Meskin LH, Farsht EM, Anderson DL (1968) Prevalence of *Bacteroides melaninogenicus* in the gingival crevice area of institutionalized trisomy 21 and cerebral palsy patients and normal children. *J Periodontol* **39**: 326–8.

Meyle J (1994) Leukocyte adhesion deficiency and prepubertal periodontitis. *Periodontol 2000* **6**: 26–36.

Michalowicz BS, Ronderos M, Camara-Silva R et al. (2000) Human herpesviruses and *Porphyromonas gingivalis* are associated with early-onset periodontitis. *J Periodontol* (in press).

Mishkin DJ, Grant NC, Bergeron RA, Young WL (1986) Prepubertal periodontitis: a recent defined clinical entity. *Pediatr Dent* **8**: 235–8.

Modeer T, Barr M, Dahllof G (1990) Periodontal disease in children with Down's syndrome. *Scand Dent Res* **98**: 228–34.

Mombelli A, Nyman S, Brägger U et al. (1995) Clinical and microbiological changes associated with an altered subgingival environment induced by periodontal pocket reduction. *J Clin Periodontol* **22**: 780–7.

Moore WE, Holdeman LV, Smibert RM et al. (1982) Bacteriology of experimental gingivitis in young adult humans. *Infect Immun* **38**: 651–667.

Moore LV, Moore WE, Riley C et al. (1993) Periodontal microflora of HIV positive subjects with gingivitis or adult periodontitis. *J Periodontol* **64**: 48–56.

Murayama Y, Kurihara H, Nagai A et al. (1994) Acute necrotizing ulcerative gingivitis: risk factors involving host defense mechanisms. *Periodontol 2000* **6**: 116–24.

Murray PA (1994) Periodontal diseases in patients infected by human immunodeficiency virus. *Periodontol 2000* **6**: 50–67.

Nakagawa S, Fujii H, Machida Y, Okuda K (1994) A longitudinal study from prepuberty to puberty of gingivitis. Correlation between the occurrence of *Prevotella intermedia* and sex hormones. *J Clin Periodontol* **21**: 658–65.

Nakou M, Kamma JJ, Andronikaki A, Mitsis F (1998) Subgingival microflora associated with nifedipine-induced gingival overgrowth. *J Periodontol* **69**: 664–9.

Newman MG, Socransky SS, Savitt ED et al. (1976) Studies of the microbiology of periodontosis. *J Periodontol* **47**: 373–9.

Petti S, Barbato E, Simonetti D'Arca A (1997) Effect of orthodontic therapy with fixed and removable appliances on oral microbiota: a six-month longitudinal study. *New Microbiol* **20**: 55–62.

Rams TE, Andriolo M, Feik D et al. (1991) Microbiological study of HIV-related periodontitis. *J Periodontol* **62**: 74–81.

Rosenberg ES, Torosian JP, Hammond BF, Cutler SA (1993) Routine anaerobic bacterial culture and systemic antibiotic usage in the treatment of adult periodontitis: a 6-year longitudinal study. *Int J Periodont Rest Dent* **13**: 213–43.

Saglie FR, Carrenza FA, Newman MG et al. (1982) Identification of tissue-invading bacteria in human periodontal disease. *J Periodont Res* **17**: 452–5.

Sasaki N, Nakagawa T, Seida K et al. (1989) Clinical, microbiological and immunological studies of post-juvenile periodontitis. *Bull Tokyo Dent Coll* **30**: 205–11.

Sastrowijoto SH, van der Velden U, van Steenbergen TJ et al. (1990) Improved metabolic control, clinical periodontal status and subgingival microbiology in insulin-dependent diabetes mellitus. A prospective study. *J Clin Periodontol* **17**: 233–42.

Savitt ED, Kent RL (1991) Distribution of *Actinobacillus actinomycetemcomitans* and *Porphyromonas gingivalis* by subject age. *J Periodontol* **62**: 490–4.

Scully C, Monteil R, Sposto MR (1998) Infectious and topical diseases affecting the human mouth. *Periodontol 2000* **18**: 47–79.

Shenker BJ, Kusher ME, Tsai CC (1982) Inhibition of fibroblast proliferation by *Actinobacillus actinomycetemcomitans*. *Infect Immun* **38**: 986–92.

Slots J (1976) The predominant cultivable organisms in juvenile periodontitis. *Scand J Dent Res* **84**: 1–10.

Slots J, Rams TE (1992) Microbiology of periodontal disease. In: Slots J, Taubman MA (eds). *Contemporary Oral Microbiology and Immunology*. St Louis: Mosby-Year Book, pp. 425–43.

Slots J, Rosling BG (1983) Suppression of the periodontopathic microflora in localized juvenile periodontitis by systemic tetracycline. *J Clin Periodontol* **10**: 465–86.

Slots J, Ting M (1999) *Actinobacillus actinomycetemcomitans* and *Porphyromonas gingivalis* in human periodontal disease: occurrence and treatment. *Periodontol 2000* **20**: 82–121.

Slots J, Reynolds H, Genco R (1980) *Actinobacillus actinomycetemcomitans* in human periodontal disease: a cross-sectional microbiological investigation. *Infect Immun* **29**: 1013–20.

Slots J, Zambon JJ, Rosling BG et al. (1982) *Actinobacillus actinomycetemcomitans* in human periodontal disease. Association, serology, leukotoxicity, and treatment. *J Periodont Res* **17**: 447–8.

Smith QT, Wilson MM, Germaine GR, Pihlstrom BL (1983) Microbial flora and clinical parameters in phenytoin associated gingival overgrowth. *J Periodont Res* **18**: 56–66.

Stevens RH, Gatewood C, Hammond BF (1983) Cytotoxicity of the bacterium *Actinobacillus actinomycetemcomitans* extracts in human gingival fibroblast. *Arch Oral Biol* **28**: 981–7.

Stevens RH, Lillard SE, Hammond BF (1987) Purification and biochemical properties of a bacteriocin from *Actinobacillus actinomycetemcomitans*. *Infect Immun* **55**: 692–7.

Sweeney EA, Alcoforado GAP, Nyman S, Slots J (1987) Prevalence and microbiology of localized prepubertal periodontitis. *Oral Microbiol Immunol* **2**: 65–70.

Taichman NS, Simpson DL, Sakurada S et al. (1987) Comparative studies on the biology of *Actinobacillus actinomycetemcomitans* leukotoxin in primates. *Oral Microbiol Immunol* **2**: 97–104.

Tanner A, Lai CH, Maiden M (1992) Characteristics of oral gram-negative species. In: Slots J, Taubman MA (eds) *Contemporary Oral Microbiology and Immunology*. St Louis: Mosby-Year Book, pp. 299–341.

Tanner A, Maiden MF, Macuch PJ et al. (1998) Microbiota of health, gingivitis, and initial periodontitis. *J Clin Periodontol* **25**: 85–98.

Ting M, Contreras A, Slots J (2000) Herpesviruses in localized juvenile periodontitis. *J Periodont Res* **35**: 17–25.

Tuan MC, Nowzari H, Slots J (2000) Clinical and microbiological study of apically positioned flaps, with and without osseous surgery. *Int J Periodont Rest Dent* (in press).

Umeda M, Chen C, Bakker I et al. (1998) Risk indicators for harboring periodontal pathogens. *J Periodontol* **69**: 1112–19.

van Winkelhoff AJ, Tijhof CJ, de Graaff J (1992) Microbiological and clinical results of metronidazole plus amoxicillin therapy in *Actinobacillus actinomycetemcomitans*-associated periodontitis. *J Periodontol* **63**: 52–7.

Velazco CH, Coelho C, Salazar F et al. (1999) Microbiological features of Papillon–Lefèvre syndrome periodontitis. *J Clin Periodontol* **26**: 622–7.

Wilson M, Holt R, Abdullah US (1992) Mycoplasmas in the plaque and saliva of children. *Microbios* **72**: 221–6.

Yalda B, Offenbacher S, Collins JG (1994) Diabetes as a modifier of periodontal disease expression. *Periodontol 2000* **6**: 37–49.

Zambon JJ, Reynolds HS, Genco RJ (1990) Studies of the subgingival microflora in patients with acquired immunodeficiency syndrome. *J Periodontol* **61**: 699–704.

9

Genetic aspects of periodontal diseases

Thomas C. Hart

Periodontal diseases are a heterogeneous group of diseases characterized by varying degrees of pathological changes in the periodontium. Periodontal diseases may be broadly grouped into two types, *gingivitis* and *periodontitis*. Gingivitis is inflammation of the gingiva in the absence of clinical attachment loss (see Figure 1.1a, b). Periodontitis is inflammation of the gingiva and the adjacent attachment apparatus (see Figure 1.2a–i). While gingivitis is reversible, periodontitis is characterized by loss of clinical attachment due to destruction of the periodontal ligament and loss of the adjacent supporting bone (AAP, 1996a). Each of these disease groups may be subclassified according to etiology, clinical presentation or associated findings (AAP, 1992, 1995). Despite the considerable amounts of time and effort expended in investigating the molecular pathogenesis of periodontal diseases (see Chapter 7), we still do not understand many specific components of the disease process (Offenbacher, 1996; Page and Kornman, 1997). However, several principles have emerged. Microbial infection and subsequent host inflammatory responses are believed to be primary etiologic factors (see Chapter 8). There are many different clinical presentations of periodontal diseases, and most can be viewed as occurring along a continuum of disease, loosely described as "mild" to "severe" (Caton, 1989). While the worldwide prevalence of periodontal diseases is high, all individuals do not appear to be at equal risk of these diseases, and small proportions of the population experience the most severe, destructive forms of disease (Johnson et al., 1988; Papapanou, 1996; Oliver et al., 1998).

In part because our understanding of periodontal diseases is incomplete, and the diseases themselves are variable in terms of etiologic factors, age of onset, clinical presentation, response to treatment, relation to systemic disease, relation to microbial factors, and clinical progression, existing classifications of periodontal diseases are unsatisfactory (Lang and Karring, 1994; Armitage, 1996). However, it is necessary to classify periodontal diseases within the framework of existing clinical and scientific knowledge. Simplified disease classifications suggested by several consensus workshops are shown in Table 9.1. These classifications are provided for practical purposes. Their creators are cognizant that there is an extensive overlap between

Table 9.1 Classification of periodontal diseases.

American Academy of Periodontology, 1989
I   Adult periodontitis
II Early onset periodontitis
    a.   Prepubertal periodontitis
    b.   Juvenile periodontitis
    c.   Rapidly progressive periodontitis
III Periodontitis associated with systemic disease
IV Necrotizing ulcerative periodontitis
V Refractory periodontitis

European Workshop, 1994
Gingivitis
Early onset periodontitis
Adult periodontitis
Necrotizing periodontitis

The age of 35 years has been suggested to delineate between the early onset periodontitis and adult periodontitis. The basis for this chronological distinction was epidemiological data that indicate periodontitis is relatively uncommon in individuals below the age of 35.

various disease forms in the proposed classification systems and that there is a need for development of evidence-based descriptors for the diseases at sites and in individuals in order to identify cause-and-effect relationships (Armitage, 1996). A review of previous classifications of periodontal disease and a new classification in children and adolescents are presented in Chapter 5.

Genetics and periodontal diseases

In spite of the probable etiologic diversity of periodontal diseases, there is consensus that oral microbes play a primary causative role (Ranney et al., 1981; Page, 1986; Socransky and Haffajee, 1991). The microbial challenge that initiates disease is modulated by other environmental, dietary, behavioral, and systemic factors (Offenbacher, 1996). While it is difficult to determine the relative importance of specific etiologic factors in periodontal disease, particularly on an individual basis, it is increasingly apparent that the genetic complement of the host is an important determinant of periodontal disease initiation, progression, and response to treatment (Baer and Lieberman, 1960; Michalowicz, 1993; Hart and Kornman, 1997). Host genetic factors controlling specific aspects of the growth and development of periodontal tissues such as cementum, collagen, epithelium, and root form may play a part in some forms of periodontitis (Page and Baab, 1985; Preus, 1988; Hartsfield and Kousseff, 1990; Hou and Tsai, 1993). However, because microbial infection is present in all periodontal disease, attention is currently focused on genetic regulation of the host immune responses that are likely to affect periodontal disease susceptibility and outcome (Offenbacher, 1996; Qureshi et al.,1999).

Emerging critical pathway models of several common diseases such as cardiovascular disease, arthritis, and asthma suggest that gene–environment interactions are etiologically important in disease pathogenesis. Additionally, studies suggest that disease risk and outcome may be influenced by the propensity of specific environmental agents to elicit host immune responses which are in large part genetically determined. Both human and animal studies demonstrate the importance of the host genetic background in modulating inflammation, tissue destruction, and restoration of tissue homeostasis (Skamene and Pietrangeli, 1991; Nadeau et al., 1995; Daser et al., 1996; Abel and Dessein, 1997; Qureshi et al., 1999). Given the primary role of oral microbes in periodontal diseases, it is logical to hypothesize that genetic regulation of inflammatory response will be a significant determinant of periodontal disease. Genetic regulation of inflammatory response involves many gene products interacting with each other and with environmental factors, and is incompletely understood—as yet fewer than 25% of human genes have been characterized. Identification of the specific genetic determinants of immune response will provide the foundation for new diagnostic tests and ultimately for treatments tailored to specific forms of disease (Hart et al., 2000a).

Considerations of gene action in periodontal disease

Many human diseases are influenced by heritable alterations in the structure or function of genes. It has been well established that humans and other mammals vary in the quality and quantity of their immune responses to infectious agents, and that a significant proportion of this variance is genetically determined (Skamene and Pietrangeli, 1991; Nadeau et al., 1995; Daser et al., 1996; Abel and Dessein, 1997). Recent advances in molecular genetics have enabled the genetic dissection of inflammatory responses for both acute and chronic inflammation. As a result the genetics of inflammation is central to studies seeking to identify susceptibility and resistance for a range of common human diseases including periodontal disease, diabetes, cardiovascular disease, and pulmonary disease (Nadeau et al., 1995; Hart and Kornman, 1997; Schmitz et al., 1998; Wiesch et al., 1999).

The interplay between humans and infective agents that has occurred for millennia is complex, and has undoubtedly influenced the evolution of both (Fischer et al., 1998). Host genetics, environmental factors, and the immune system do not function independently, but are characterized by the complex interactions that involve the interaction of thousands of gene products (Qureshi et al., 1999; Wiesch et al., 1999). The estimated number of human genes now exceeds 100 000, and of these, fewer than 25% are known and characterized. Future research will identify many genes that were not known to be involved in modulation of immune response in general and for periodontal diseases specifically. Currently, most of the gene candidates being investigated in relation to the genetics of inflammatory response were identified from pathophysiologic knowledge of specific diseases and subsequent epidemiological studies.

As our understanding of human genetics grows, genetic principles will be increasingly incorporated into the management of periodontal diseases. It is likely that identification of the genetic basis of periodontal disease will contribute to a new nosology, as well as to the development of new diagnostic and treatment strategies. Many of the genes important in development of periodontitis will probably also have a role in other systemic conditions such as diabetes and cardiovascular disease (Meyer and Fives-Taylor, 1998; Page, 1998; Valtonen, 1999). Understanding the etiologic relationship of systemic diseases will depend upon the identification of genes that influence susceptibility to periodontal disease as well as genes that regulate how the host responds to environmental and systemic factors.

Genetic disease models: simple versus multifactorial genetic traits

The search for genes important in genetic susceptibility to disease can be broadly divided into the search for genes of major effect, such as those responsible for genetic conditions that are transmitted as simple Mendelian traits, and genes of lesser effect that collectively are responsible for complex multifactorial genetic traits.

Traditional paradigms of genetic diseases are those of Mendelian genetics. In these cases, alterations of critical genes (mutations), significantly alter or even obliterate function of a gene or gene product, directly causing a disease phenotype. Often the presence of the gene mutation is itself sufficient to cause the disease. Diseases of this type include achondroplastic dwarfism (MIM100800), cystic fibrosis (MIM219700), and sickle cell anemia (MIM603903). These diseases are often serious but are also rare on a population level. They are usually inherited in a predictable pattern, and can often be correlated with a specific alteration (or alterations) of a common gene. They are therefore said to be inherited in a simple Mendelian fashion (Cummings, 1994). Although environmental, systemic, and other genetic factors may influence the expression of a Mendelian trait, the underlying major gene mutation is the key determinant of whether disease occurs, and also its severity. These forms of disease were the first to be identified as genetic in origin and—in many cases—understood at the molecular level. However, Mendelian diseases are not responsible for common diseases in most populations.

Common human diseases such as diabetes, cancer, and cardiovascular disease appear to be genetically complex. In contrast to simple Mendelian traits, which may result from a single gene mutation, complex diseases usually result from the interactive effect of multiple gene products and are usually significantly modulated by environmental agents. Traits or diseases that result from these gene–environment interactions are described as *multifactorial* (Cummings, 1994). The genes responsible are usually not altered (mutated) to produce very dysfunctional gene products; instead they are likely to exist in multiple different forms (alleles) which differ relatively little in terms of function. Groups of different genes functioning in a common biological pathway may themselves be molecular targets of environmental agents, e.g., carcinogens or infectious agents. Unlike Mendelian diseases, in which the mutant genes usually function very differently from the allelic normal gene and therefore tend to cause disease regardless of the environment, multifactorial diseases are caused by alleles that differ functionally very little from each other, but these functional differences can be enhanced by certain environments. While the effect of any one of these genetic variants is unlikely to produce a noticeable clinical phenotype, in combination such *functional* polymorphisms can significantly increase the risk of certain diseases when exposed to specific environmental challenges.

Multifactorial diseases differ from simple Mendelian diseases in other important ways. First, while mutations of a specific gene are typically rare (often less than 1% of the population), functional polymorphisms are much more common, and therefore, a much greater proportion of the population is likely to be a carrier of a given genetic allele. Second, while it is relatively easy to estimate the disease impact of a Mendelian mutation on a population, it is much more difficult to estimate the degree of interaction between a range of genotypes and the environment and predict phenotype. In the latter case, we must examine the total variation in phenotype exhibited by a population of individuals. The phenotypic variability is derived from two sources: the presence of different genotypes in members of the population; and the presence of different environments in which all the genotypes have been expressed (Cummings, 1994).

Many carcinogen-induced cancers are probably examples of multifactorial disease. For example, functional variation in the ability of phase I and phase II xenobiotic metabolizing enzymes may result in very different risks for genetically different individuals exposed to similar environmental challenges from carcinogens (Idle, 1991). While it is important to remember that multifactorial diseases involve multiple gene–gene and gene–environment interactions, it is necessary to identify and characterize each individual component to fully understand the disease and to apply genetic principles to treatment of individuals. In the case of periodontitis, for instance, microbial lipopolysaccharide (LPS) is known to induce a variety of cellular responses from different cells. In monocytes, microbial LPS can induce production of the proinflammatory cytokine interleukin-1 (IL-1) by the IL-1 gene on chromosome 2 (Duff, 1994). This gene is known to exist in several different forms: cells with different genetic forms produce different amounts of IL-1 when stimulated with microbial LPS (Duff, 1994; Cork et al., 1996). This is an example of a functional polymorphism. The presence of specific IL-1 alleles alone is not sufficient to cause disease, but combinations of this gene, with other genes and environmental factors, have been associated with a variety of inflammatory diseases including psoriasis, arthritis, cardiovascular disease, and periodontitis (Cox et al., 1999; Jouvenne et al., 1999; Kornman et al., 1999).

Implications

Collectively, multifactorial diseases such as diabetes, cancer, cardiovascular disease, arthritis, and asthma are responsible for a much greater disease burden than simple Mendelian diseases in most populations. While Mendelian diseases are in many ways easier to study and understand, disease management may be more feasible for many complex or multifactorial diseases. Because the relative effect of each gene is much smaller, and often dependent upon exposure to specific environmental agents, these conditions may be more amenable to effective management. The disease pathogenesis for these conditions are understood in terms of the functional genetic polymorphisms involved and the molecular targets of environmental agents. As this happens, it is likely they can be managed through a combination of presymptomatic identification of individuals at risk, behavior modification to avoid disease-associated environmental agents, and potential modulation of unfavorable genetic polymorphisms, for example with pharmacologic agents that ameliorate unfavorable biologic function. Such presymptomatic testing and intervention is likely to form the cornerstone of future preventive health care (Hart et al., 2000a).

Application of genetic principles to periodontal diseases

Gingivitis

Chronic gingivitis is common in children and is characterized by the presence of gingival inflammation without detectable loss of bone or clinical attachment (AAP, 1996a). Estimates of gingivitis in children range from less than 25% to over 70%, increase with age, and vary depending on measurement methods, behavioral and socioeconomic factors, and access to care (Bhowate et al., 1994; Arnlaugsson and

Magnusson, 1996; Bimstein and Matsson, 1999). Inflammation of the periodontium may result from varied causes, many of which have genetic components, but the growth and accumulation of microbial factors are believed to be the primary etiologic factor in gingivitis (Löe et al., 1965; Page and Schroeder, 1976; Ranney, 1993; Mariotti, Chapter 3). While differences in the microbial flora are likely to account for some of the variance in gingivitis between individuals, it is increasingly evident that the innate host response to microbial challenge plays a significant part in the development of disease, and that this response is genetically determined.

To date few formal studies have evaluated the relative role of host genetics on the observed variance of gingivitis, and the relative importance of genes versus environment for gingivitis is unclear. Population studies suggest that parental consanguinity and racial admixture may influence the propensity for gingivitis (Chung and Niswander, 1975; Chung et al., 1977). One method of evaluating the relative contribution of genetics to a phenotypic trait involves the study of twins. Because identical (monozygotic) twins have all their genes in common, and fraternal (dizygotic) twins have on average 50% of their genes in common, monozygotic twins are more concordant for genetic traits (Neale and Cardon, 1992). Although studies of concordance in twins do not provide information about the specific genes responsible for a trait, they can provide estimates of the effect of heredity versus environment. Twin studies suggest that the tendency for gingivitis has a significant heritable component (Michalowicz, 1993), however, few twin studies have been performed in children, and those have involved small numbers of twins (Ciancio et al., 1969; Hassell and Harris, 1995). While twin studies do suggest a genetic component for gingivitis risk, the relative contributions of environmental risk and genetic risk are not easily distinguished (Beaty et al., 1993).

Genes and environment do not act independently of each other, so that the appearance or magnitude of hereditability estimates may differ with various environments. Genetic studies are also complicated in gingivitis because so many contributing variables also change with age, (composition of the microbial flora, hormone levels, behavior), making it difficult to sort out dependent and independent variables. For instance, findings in twin studies that the tendency to form calculus may also have a genetic component adds complexity to distinguishing between environmental and genetic risks for periodontal disease (Reiser and Vogel, 1958). Microbial colonization as well as qualitative and quantitative aspects of the host inflammatory response are determined to a significant extent by the underlying host genotype (Malo and Skamene, 1994; Hill, 1996; Abel and Dessein, 1997; Pietrzak et al., 1998). It is also likely that differences exist in the inflammatory response to de novo plaque formation in young and old individuals (Fransson et al., 1996, 1999). While all these factors probably have etiological implications for gingivitis, specific genetic components have not been identified sufficiently to permit identification of polymorphisms contributing to gingivitis at the gene level. Additionally, while certain microbial profiles may be associated with periodontitis, microbial accumulations in gingivitis may be non-specific, and as a result microbial load may be a more significant factor in gingivitis (Zambon, 1996). To date there is no evidence of a major gene for gingivitis. The correlation of gingivitis and periodontitis is unclear. Gingivitis is a poor predictor of periodontitis in subjects less than 30 years of age, suggesting that the genetic susceptibilities for gingivitis and periodontitis may be distinct (Prayitno et al., 1993).

Periodontitis

Periodontitis is an inflammation-associated disease of the periodontium which results in destruction of the gingival and periodontal fibers, resorption of alveolar bone, and ultimately apical migration of the clinical attachment. While microbial factors have been consistently identified as primary etiologic agents in periodontitis, emerging evidence suggests that this microbial challenge together with other environmental and behavioral characteristics modulate the host response, which collectively determines the clinical presentation of periodontitis (Offenbacher, 1996; Zambon, 1996). A significant proportion of the host response to microbial infection is genetically determined and therefore unique to each individual (Nadeau et al., 1995; Offenbacher, 1996; Hart and Kornman, 1997; Kelso, 1998).

Depending on the genetic complement of each individual, similar microbial challenges may elicit different host responses which ultimately influence the risk for and the course of periodontitis. Although several different forms of periodontitis exist, we lack the molecular biomarkers to distinguish between them, making the identification of disease-associated genetic polymorphisms more difficult.

Periodontitis is generally reported to increase with age. Although most epidemiological studies have concentrated on adult populations, an increase in prevalence of the multifactorial forms of periodontitis is reported after age 35 years (Albandar et al., 1999; Streckfus et al., 1999). Although there is an increasing emphasis on identification of genetic risk factors in periodontitis, most studies attempting to relate specific genotypes for inflammatory-related genes (e.g. for 1-IL-1, tumor necrosis factor alpha) with multifactorial forms of periodontitis have studied adult populations (Offenbacher, 1996). As a result, little is known about the genetics of multifactorial types of periodontitis in children and adolescents. Most genetic studies of periodontitis in children have focused on forms of early onset periodontitis (EOP), which appears to be transmitted more as a simple Mendelian trait.

Periodontal diseases are estimated to affect hundreds of millions of adults worldwide, but periodontal diseases in general and the more destructive forms in particular are generally acknowledged to be less common in children and adolescents. Periodontitis may afflict both deciduous and permanent dentitions, although the former is much less common. Estimates of periodontitis in children and adolescents vary in different ethnic and geographic groups, ranging from 1% to 46% (Wei et al., 1986; Pilot et al., 1987; Wolfe and Carlos, 1987; Bimstein et al., 1988, 1994; Durward and Wright, 1989; Miyazaki et al., 1989; Perry and Newman, 1990; AAP, 1996b; Cortelli et al., 1996). Most estimates for significant periodontitis in children and adolescents range from below 1% to 3% (Papapanou, 1996).

Early onset periodontitis (aggressive periodontitis)

Epidemiologic studies of periodontitis suggest that although it may begin in adolescence, it is often not clinically evident until the patient's mid-30s (Löe et al., 1978; 1986; Listgarten, 1986). The prevalence of periodontitis increases sharply after age 35 years in most populations. As a result, periodontitis was formerly classified as "early onset periodontitis" when identified in individuals below age 35 years and as "adult periodontitis" in individuals over age 35 years. Today, we understand that the age cut-offs are arbitrary, and EOP has been reclassified as "aggressive periodontitis" (AP) (Chapter 5). However, for the purposes of the following review, the term EOP will be used as it represents the classification criteria current at the time of the research. Early onset periodontitis is estimated to affect 0.1–3% of children depending on the specific form of disease and the population studied (Löe and Brown, 1991; Papapanou, 1996). The condition is clinically heterogeneous, and includes forms of disease clinically indistinguishable from other types of periodontitis, as well as forms remarkable for causing significant destruction at a very early age. These latter forms of disease were subclassified as prepubertal periodontitis (presently childhood periodontitis), and juvenile periodontitis. Childhood and juvenile forms of periodontitis can appear clinically in localized or generalized forms (see Figure 1.2c–h) (Caton, 1989; Albandar et al., 1997). The distinction between clinically different forms is unclear, and various presentations of EOP have been reported to occur in the same nuclear family (Spektor et al., 1985; Long et al., 1987; Lopez, 1992; Novak and Novak, 1996; Bimstein et al., 1997). These severe forms of EOP, not associated with other systemic pathology (non-syndromic EOPs), are characterized by dramatic tissue destruction, often with significant alveolar bone loss, in otherwise healthy children and adolescents. These conditions also show a remarkable familial aggregation (reviewed by Schenkein and Van Dyke, 1994; Novak and Novak, 1996). The familial aggregation of certain EOPs and the consistent prevalence estimates for specific racial groups even in different geographic locations suggest genetic factors may be important determinants for susceptibility. However, a common environment can also account for familial aggregation of a trait, and formal genetic analyses are needed to evaluate support for genetic influence on a trait.

Initial reports of familial aggregation for EOP were interpreted as supportive of a major gene

Table 9.2 Genetic polymorphisms or mutations correlated with risk for early onset periodontitis (EOP) or clinical characteristics of EOP.

Gene locus	Polymorphism/mutation/clinical correlate	MIM catalogue number*	Reference
FMLP receptor (formyl peptide receptor 1)	Molecular alteration in the second intracellular loop of the FMLP receptor molecules may play a role in the decreased chemotactic activity reported for some LJP patients	136537	Gwinn et al. (1999)
IgG2 (immunoglobulin Gm 2)	Increased antibody titer levels of IgG2 correlated with limited/localized disease expression in EOP. Smoking reduces serum IgG2 in some subsets of EOP patients	147110	Lu et al. (1994) Marazita et al. (1996) Tangada et al. (1997)
FcγRIIa (Fc fragment of IgG, low affinity IIa)	Allelic variants (H131/R131) of Fc gamma receptor type IIa confer distinct phagocytic capabilities through differential ability to bind IgG2	146790	Salmon et al. (1996) Wilson and Kalmar (1996)
Vitamin D receptor	An exon 9 restriction fragment length polymorphism correlates with localized form of expression	601769	Hennig et al. (1999)
Il-1β (interleukin-1 beta)	Linkage disequilibrium suggests the IL-1β variant may be a risk factor for EOP	147720	Diehl et al. (1999)
TNF-α (tumor necrosis factor alpha)	LPS-stimulated TNF-α release significantly higher in EOP patients than in non-EOP controls. IL-1 genotype may modulate TNF-α production	191160	McFarlane et al. (1990) Kornman and di Giovine (1998)

*The MIM catalogue number refers to Online Mendelian Inheritance in Man, available through the Human Genome Data Base Project, Johns Hopkins University.
EOP, early onset periodontitis; FMLP, formyl peptide; Ig, immunoglobulin; IL, interleukin; LJP, localized juvenile periodontitis; LPS, lipopolysaccharide; TNF, tumor necrosis factor.

locus for EOP, with autosomal recessive and X-linked inheritance (Saxen and Nevanlinna, 1984; Long et al., 1987). While autosomal recessive forms of EOP appear in northern Europe, results of genetic studies (segregation analysis and linkage analysis) are most consistent with autosomal dominant inheritance for EOP in the USA, although other forms of inheritance cannot be excluded (Boughman et al., 1986; Hart et al., 1992; Marazita et al., 1994). Prepubertal periodontitis is a particularly rare form of childhood periodontitis, and both autosomal dominant and autosomal recessive inheritance have been reported (Shapira et al., 1997; Hart et al, 2000c). It is likely that there are several types of EOP, due to different gene defects. A gene for at least one form of EOP has been localized to chromosome 4 (Boughman et al., 1986); however, the existence of at least one other gene for non-syndromic EOP has also been demonstrated (Hart et al., 1993).

Genes of major effect responsible for most non-syndromic EOPs have not been identified, although a mutation in the lysosomal protease cathepsin C has been identified in two related families with prepubertal periodontitis (Hart et al., 2000c). Affected family members experienced severe periodontitis of their primary dentition, with no other systemic effects. Mutations of the cathepsin C gene have also been reported in individuals with Papillon–Lefèvre syndrome, a condition clinically characterized by severe EOP and palmoplantar keratoderma (Hart et al., 1999; Toomes et al., 1999).

Although there does appear to be support for the existence of genes of major effect for some forms of non-syndromic EOP, most have not yet been identified. The presence of a common cathepsin C gene mutation in individuals with clinical expression of prepubertal periodontitis and also in some individuals with the more extensive Papillon–Lefèvre syndrome phenotype suggest that other genes and/or environmental factors may modulate clinical manifestations of cathepsin C gene mutations. Variable clinical expression of a common gene mutation exists for other genetic conditions such as craniosynostosis due to mutations of the fibroblast growth factor 3 gene (MIM134934). The variable clinical expression arising from cathepsin C mutations highlights the interrelationship between oral and extraoral diseases. The apparent modulation of phenotype by other genetic and/or environmental factors is consistent with current interpretations of the genetics of AP.

Modifying genes for aggressive periodontitis

Studies of AP have identified a number of microbial, environmental, and genetic factors that appear—at least in some cases—to correlate with the clinical presentation of disease (Novak and Novak, 1996; Bueno et al., 1998; Schenkein, 1998). Non-microbial factors include cigarette smoking, mutations of the formylpeptide (FMLP) receptor, immunoglobulin G2 production, and FcγRIIa receptor heterogeneity (Wilson and Kalmar, 1996; Marazita et al., 1996; Tangada et al., 1997; Gwinn et al., 1999). Other mediators of inflammation that may be important determinants of periodontitis expression include prostaglandin E_2 production, interleukin-1 polymorphisms, tumor necrosis factor alpha polymorphisms and vitamin D receptor gene polymorphisms (reviewed by Offenbacher, 1996; Hennig et al., 1999). Table 9.2 summarizes genetic polymorphisms and mutations reported to correlate with clinical expression of some forms of periodontitis that manifest early expression. Studies to date suggest these factors may affect individual disease risk as well as outcome, but the interrelationship between many of these factors is unknown (Colombo et al., 1998). The potential relationship of microbial, environmental, systemic, and genetic factors to clinical expression of AP is presented in Figure 9.1.

Several forms of AP appear to segregate in families, and provide evidence that a single gene may be etiologically important in determining susceptibility. However, it is likely that most common forms of periodontitis are genetically

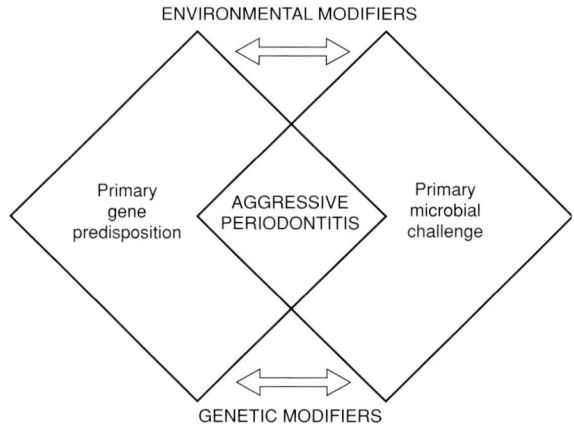

Figure 9.1

The clinical phenotype of aggressive periodontitis (AP) is determined by gene–environment interactions in the periodontium. For AP to occur, an individual must carry a primary genetic predisposition (gene of major effect) and experience a primary microbial challenge. The existence of either primary factor alone is not sufficient to cause disease: both must be present. Once an individual has developed AP, phenotypic characteristics such as extent, severity, rate of progression, and response to treatment may be influenced by environmental modifiers (e.g., smoking, diet, additional microbial challenge, and systemic disease) and also by genetic modifiers (e.g., IgG2 response, PGE_2 levels). Disease modifiers may act synergistically, for example in cases of systemic disease effects.

different from AP. Whereas some forms of AP may be thought of primarily as Mendelian diseases, modified by other genetic and environmental factors, the more common forms of disease may result from a combination of functional polymorphisms that influence quantitative and qualitative aspects of the individual's immune system, inflammatory response, and wound healing, that in specific combinations and in interaction with specific environmental challenges (e.g., microbial challenge, smoking), behavioral patterns (oral hygiene, stress), and systemic factors (diabetes, diet, lipids) act in concert to predispose an individual to periodontitis. The extent to which genetic factors responsible for periodontitis are important in periodontitis of children and adolescents is unknown (Hart and Kornman, 1997).

Table 9.3 Examples of syndromic diseases that often have early onset periodontitis as an associated clinical finding.

Condition	Inheritance	Chromosome	MIM	Gene defect
Chédiak–Higashi syndrome	AR	1q42.1–q42.2	214500	Lysosomal trafficking regulator gene
Papillon–Lefèvre syndrome	AR	11q14	245000	Cathepsin C
Haim–Munk syndrome	AR	11q14	245010	Cathepsin C
Cyclic neutropenia	AD	19p13.3	162800	Neutrophil elastase
Leukocyte adhesion deficiency type 1	AR	21q22.3	116920	Integrin beta chain, beta 2
Chronic neutropenia	AD, AR	?	162700	?
Ehlers–Danlos syndrome type 8	AD	?	130080	Collagen
Hypophosphatasia, childhood	AR, AD	1p36–p34	241510	Alkaline phosphatase, liver/bone/kidney type

AD, autosomal dominant inheritance; AR, autosomal recessive inheritance; MIM, Online Mendelian Inheritance in Man catalogue number for each condition.

Syndromic associations of periodontitis

In addition to isolated AP, which occurs in the absence of other systemic pathology, periodontitis is known to occur in association with a number of pathologic states. These conditions are typically rare, and inherited as Mendelian traits. For many of these conditions the underlying gene defect is known. Many of these syndromic forms of periodontitis have a pronounced predisposition to other, extraoral infections, reflecting significant defects in the immune response to microbial infections. Given that periodontitis is a disease of inflammation, this is not surprising. However, AP has also been associated with defects of structural components of the periodontium including collagen and cementum. Identification of the different genes involved with syndromic periodontitis extends our general understanding of genetic risk for periodontitis, and may ultimately help in clarifying disease pathogenesis pathways at the molecular level.

Syndromic forms of periodontitis

Periodontitis affecting young individuals has been associated with a number of genetic diseases (Table 9.3).

Chédiak–Higashi syndrome

The features of Chédiak–Higashi syndrome are decreased pigmentation of hair and eyes (partial albinism), photophobia, nystagmus, large eosinophilic, peroxidase-positive inclusion bodies in the myeloblasts and promyelocytes of the bone marrow, neutropenia, abnormal susceptibility to infection, and peculiar malignant lymphoma. Both childhood and adult onset forms of the condition are known, and mutations of the lysosomal trafficking regulator gene are responsible for the condition.

Papillon–Lefèvre syndrome

Papillon–Lefèvre syndrome (PLS) is characterized by palmoplantar keratosis and severe EOP (see Figures 1.7e–f) (Bimstein et al., 1990). Skin lesions can also be found on the knees and elbows. It has been classified as a type IV ectodermal dysplasia (Stevens et al., 1996). A variety of other clinical findings including cranial calcifications and an increased susceptibility to infections have been reported, but it is unclear if these are related to the primary gene defect or to the increased frequency of parental consanguinity in reported cases of PLS (Gorlin et al., 1964; Haneke, 1979). Mutations of the cathepsin C gene are responsible for PLS. This gene is a lysosomal trafficking protease, and may have important functions both in host response to microbial infection and in maintenance of epithelial integrity. Haim–Munk syndrome is an allelic variant of PLS, and is also due to mutations of the cathepsin C gene (Hart et al, 2000c).

Cyclic neutropenia

Cyclic neutropenia is characterized by 15- to 35-day cyclic fluctuations in formed elements of blood. As a result, individuals experience recurring fever and malaise, oral ulcerations and skin infections. Clinical manifestations usually begin in childhood and improve thereafter. However, the generalized increased susceptibility to infections can be life-threatening without treatment intervention. During intervals of neutropenia, affected individuals are at risk of opportunistic infection. Mutations have been found in a neutrophil elastase gene, a target for protease inhibition by alpha-1–antitrypsin, and its unopposed release destroys tissue at sites of inflammation, as occurs in gingivitis and periodontitis.

Leukocyte adhesion deficiency

One form of prepubertal onset periodontitis has been associated with the syndrome leukocyte adhesion deficiency (LAD) type 1. As a result of a defective surface adhesion glycoprotein, lymphocyte function-associated antigen 1 (LFA-1), affected individuals have delayed separation of the umbilical cord and defective neutrophil mobility. They suffer from widespread bacterial infections including recurrent skin infections, otitis media, septicemia, impaired pus formation and delayed wound healing. The glycoprotein complex LFA-1 is involved in T helper cell responses, natural killing, antibody-dependent cellular cytotoxicity, and lymphocyte aggregation. [Editors' note: in the new classification of periodontal diseases of children, prepubertal periodontitis (PPP) is not included as a form of aggressive periodontitis. Rather, prepubertal periodontitis associated with LAD is classified as "periodontitis associated with systemic disease". Non-syndromic forms of PPP are classified as idiopathic, but are not clinically or medically distinguishable from other forms of commonly occurring periodontitis, and are, therefore, classified simply as childhood periodontitis.]

Ehlers–Danlos syndrome

The underlying genetic defects in collagen synthesis, seen in Ehlers–Danlos syndrome (EDS) types IV, VIII, and IX (Stewart et al., 1977; Linch and Acton, 1979; Nelson and King, 1981; Hartsfield and Kousseff, 1990; Khosravi and Weaver, 1993), appear to increase susceptibility for rapidly progressive periodontal destruction in some individuals with these forms of EDS. Increased susceptibility to periodontitis associated with a structural defect in collagen in the periodontal supporting tissues suggests that genetic susceptibility to disease need not directly involve a primary defect of immune response mechanisms.

Hypophosphatasia

Defective cementum is a feature of childhood hypophosphatasia (Watanabe et al., 1993; Bimstein et al., 1998) due to defects in the alkaline phosphatase (liver/bone/kidney type) gene. Affected individuals typically prematurely exfoliate primary teeth (see Figure 1.7b). Inflammation of the gingiva is often a feature of this condition, but it is unclear whether infectious aspects of the process are primary or secondary factors in the premature tooth exfoliation. Histological studies suggest defective cementum and insertion of collagen fiber bundles into roots are the reasons for premature teeth loss. In addition to the cementogenesis defect, a number of other clinical findings may be present, including craniostenosis, microcephaly, rachitic skeletal changes, bone pain, osteogenesis defects, and neurological seizures.

Other chromosomal defects

In addition to genetic defects of Mendelian types, increased susceptibility to periodontitis has also been reported in chromosomal aberrations such as trisomy 21 (Cichon et al., 1998). The critical region present in triplicate in trisomy 21 spans a chromosomal region that includes the integrin beta chain, beta 2 gene. Mutations of this gene are believed to be responsible for causing LAD-1. Whether aberrant regulation of this gene secondary to altered gene dosage is important in the reported increased propensity for inflammatory-based periodontal disease associated with trisomy 21 is unknown.

Variations of clinical presentation of syndromic periodontitis

The recent identification of cathepsin C mutations in non-syndromic childhood periodontitis demonstrates that mutations of this gene are sufficient to cause periodontitis without other systemic pathology. Identification of the genetic basis of this form of periodontitis indicates that periodontitis might be the only manifestation of disease in a syndrome that usually presents with dermatologic manifestations. The variable clinical expression of cathepsin C mutations suggests that other genes and possibly environmental factors are also important determinants of the disease phenotype (Hart et al., 2000c). While the generality of this finding needs to be explored, this discovery raises the possibility that periodontitis, previously studied as a distinct pathologic entity, may in fact share a genetic etiologic basis with some extraoral dermatological pathologic infections. Establishment of this form of periodontitis as an allelic variant of the type IV palmoplantar ectodermal dysplasias suggests that at least a subset of the non-syndromic periodontitis conditions may be oral manifestations of dermatologic disease. This suggestion carries broad implications for the nosology of periodontitis disease states.

Gingival enlargement

In addition to inflammation-related diseases of the periodontium, several other pathologic states are known which have a significant genetic etiology. These include several conditions characterized by gingival enlargement.

Gingival enlargement may result from chronic gingival inflammation (Pihlstrom and Ammons, 1997). It may also occur as a drug-related side-effect in some individuals (see Figures 1.1f, 3.3a–e). Several classes of pharmacological agents (calcium channel blockers, phenytoin, cyclosporin) have been associated with this adverse effect (Hassell and Hefti, 1991), and the predisposition itself is likely to have a significant although currently unidentified genetic component (Pernu et al., 1994).

In addition to inflammation-associated and drug-induced gingival enlargement, pronounced gingival enlargement occurs in a genetic form called hereditary gingival overgrowth (HGF). In HGF gingival enlargement is characterized by a slowly progressive benign enlargement of the gingival tissues. As a result, teeth are partially or

totally engulfed by keratinized gingiva causing esthetic and functional problems. While gingival fibromatosis can occur as part of a syndromic presentation—e.g., gingival fibromatosis with progressive deafness (MIM135550); with hypertrichosis (MIM135400); with distinctive facies (MIM228560); with abnormal fingers, fingernails, nose and ears, and splenomegaly (MIM135500) —or in association with other diseases— e.g., aspartylglucosaminuria (MIM208400) and gangliosidosis (MIM230500)—the condition occurs most frequently as an isolated clinical finding. The most common forms of non-syndromic HGF (MIM135300) are inherited as autosomal dominant traits, although autosomal recessive inheritance has been reported. Several clinical reports describe variable clinical expression for HGF, which may be due to variable clinical expression of a common gene mutation or arise from different genetic forms of the disease (Jorgenson and Cocker, 1974; Raeste et al., 1978). Although a major gene locus for HGF has been localized to chromosome 2p21–22, at least one other genetic form of the condition is known to exist (Hart et al., 1998, 2000d).

Conclusions

The periodontal diseases gingivitis and periodontitis are a heterogeneous group of conditions that share common characteristics of inflammation and/or destruction of the periodontium. Oral microbes are primary etiologic agents in inflammatory periodontal diseases, but the consequence of microbial challenges is dependent upon the genetic background of the host. The propensity of the host to develop periodontal disease, particularly in its more severe form, periodontitis, is dependent on the complex interactions of microbial challenge, host immune response, host inflammatory response, and wound healing. This dynamic microbial–host interaction is modulated by other environmental and systemic factors. Data from epidemiological studies of periodontitis suggest that these host responses are variable, and a large part of this variance is determined at the genomic level. While considerable progress has been made in understanding the molecular pathogenesis of periodontal diseases, for most forms of these diseases the specific genetic basis of susceptibility is not sufficiently well known to affect diagnosis and treatment in individual patients. This is not surprising, given the diversity and complexity of periodontal diseases. Recent estimates of the number of human genes have increased to more than 100 000. Of this estimated total, less than 25% have been identified and characterized. A fully developed understanding of how these genes are regulated and how the gene products affect growth and development in health as well as in disease is far from complete. However, as the genetic basis for these conditions are elucidated, and the molecular targets of environmental agents important in disease pathogenesis are identified, we can expect to improve our understanding of the molecular pathogenesis of periodontal diseases and their genetic regulation. This understanding will ultimately lead to a more practical nosology for periodontal diseases, and development of appropriate etiology-based treatment intervention strategies.

References

[AAP] American Academy of Periodontology (1992) The etiology and pathogenesis of periodontal diseases [position paper]. Chicago: American Academy of Periodontology.

[AAP] American Academy of Periodontology (1995) Diagnosis of periodontal diseases [position paper]. Chicago: American Academy of Periodontology.

[AAP] American Academy of Periodontology (1996a) Parameters of care. Chicago: American Academy of Periodontology.

[AAP] American Academy of Periodontology (1996b) Periodontal diseases of children and adolescents. *J Periodontol* **67**: 57–62.

Abel L, Dessein AJ (1997) The impact of host genetics on susceptibility to human infectious diseases. *Curr Opin Immunol* **9**: 509–16.

Albandar JM, Brown LJ, Genco RJ, Löe H (1997) Clinical classification of periodontitis in adolescents and young adults. *J Periodontol* **68**: 545–55.

Albandar JM, Brunelle JA, Kingman A (1999) Destructive periodontal disease in adults 30 years of age and older in the United States, 1988–1994. *J Periodontol* **70**: 13–29 [published erratum appears in *J Periodontol* **70**: 351, 1999].

Armitage GC (1996) Periodontal diseases: diagnosis. *Ann Periodontol* **1**: 37–215.

Arnlaugsson S, Magnusson TE (1996) Prevalence of gingivitis in 6-year-olds in Reykjavik, Iceland. *Acta Odontol Scand* **54**: 247–50.

Baer P, Lieberman J (1960) Periodontal disease in six strains of inbred mice. *J Dent Res* **39**: 215.

Beaty TH, Colyer CR, Chang YC et al. (1993) Familial aggregation of periodontal indices. *J Dent Res* **72**: 544–51.

Bhowate RR, Borle SR, Chinchkhede DH, Gondhalekar RV (1994) Dental health amongst 11–15-year-old children in Sevagram, Maharashtra. *Indian J Dent Res* **5**: 65–8.

Bimstein E, Matsson L (1999) Growth and development considerations in the diagnosis of gingivitis and periodontitis in children. *Pediatr Dent* **21**: 186–91.

Bimstein E, Delaney JE, Sweeney EA (1988) Radiographic assessment of the alveolar bone loss in children and adolescents. *Pediatr Dent* **10**: 199–204.

Bimstein E, Lustman J, Sela MN et al. (1990) Periodontitis associated with Papillon–Lefèvre syndrome. *J Periodontol* **61**: 373–7.

Bimstein E, Treasure ET, Williams SM, Denver JG (1994) Alveolar bone loss in 5-year-old New Zealand children: its prevalence and relationship to caries prevalence. Socioeconomic status and ethnic origin. *J Clin Periodontol* **21**: 447–50.

Bimstein E, Sela MN, Shapira L (1997) Clinical and microbial considerations for the treatment of an extended kindred with seven cases of prepubertal periodontitis: a 2-year follow-up. *Pediatr Dent* **19**: 396–403.

Bimstein E, Wagner M, Nauman RK et al. (1998) Root surface characteristics of primary teeth from children with prepubertal periodontitis. *J Periodontol* **69**: 337–47.

Boughman JA, Halloran SL, Roulston D et al. (1986) An autosomal-dominant form of juvenile periodontitis: its localization to chromosome 4 and linkage to dentinogenesis imperfecta and Gc. *J Craniofac Genet Dev Biol* **6**: 341–50.

Bueno LC, Mayer MP, Di Rienzo JM (1998) Relationship between conversion of localized juvenile periodontitis-susceptible children from health to disease and *Actinobacillus actinomycetemcomitans* leukotoxin promoter structure. *J Periodontol* **69**: 998–1007.

Caton J (1989) Periodontal diagnosis and diagnostic aids. *World Workshop in Clinical Periodontics*. Chicago: American Academy of Periodontology.

Chung CS, Niswander JD (1975) Genetic and epidemiologic studies of oral characteristics in Hawaii's schoolchildren. V. Sibling correlations in occlusion traits. *J Dent Res* **54**: 324–9.

Chung CS, Kau MC, Chung SS, Schendel SA (1977) A genetic and epidemiologic study of periodontal disease in Hawaii. I. Racial and other epidemiologic factors. *J Periodont Res* **12**: 148–59.

Ciancio SG, Hazen SP, Cunat JJ (1969) Periodontal observations in twins. *J Periodont Res* **4**: 42–5.

Cichon P, Crawford L, Grimm WD (1998) Early-onset periodontitis associated with Down's syndrome–clinical interventional study. *Ann Periodontol* **3**: 370–80.

Colombo AP, Eftimiadi C, Haffajee AD et al. (1998) Serum IgG2 level, Gm(23) allotype and FcgammaRIIa and FcgammaRIIIb receptors in refractory periodontal disease. *J Clin Periodontol* **25**: 465–74.

Cork MJ, Crane AM, Duff GW (1996) Genetic control of cytokines. Cytokine gene polymorphisms in alopecia areata. *Dermatol Clin* **14**: 671–8.

Cortelli JR, Pallos D, Albuquerque CFM et al. (1996) Prevalence of periodontal disease in young individuals: a clinical and radiographic study. *Biociencias* **2**: 101–6.

Cox A, Camp NJ, Cannings C et al. (1999) Combined sib-TDT and TDT provide evidence for linkage of the interleukin-1 gene cluster to erosive rheumatoid arthritis. *Hum Mol Genet* **8**: 1707–13.

Cummings MR (1994) *Human Heredity: Principles and Issues*, 3rd edn. St Paul: West Publishing.

Daser A, Mitchison H, Mitchison A, Muller B (1996) Non-classical-MHC genetics of immunological disease in man and mouse. The key role of pro-inflammatory cytokine genes. *Cytokine* **8**: 593–7.

Diehl SR, Wang Y, Brooks CN et al. (1999) Linkage disequilibrium of interleukin-1 genetic polymorphisms with early-onset periodontitis. *J Periodontol* **70**: 418–30.

Duff GW (1994) Molecular genetics of cytokines: cytokines in chronic inflammatory disease. In: Thompson A (ed.) *The Cytokine Handbook*, 2nd edn. London: Academic Press, pp. 21–30.

Durward CS, Wright FA (1989) The dental health of Indo-Chinese and Australian-born adolescents. *Aust Dent J* **34**: 233–9.

Fischer C, Jock B, Vogel F (1998) Interplay between humans and infective agents: a population genetic study. *Hum Genet* **102**: 415–22.

Fransson C, Berglundh T, Lindhe J (1996) The effect of age on the development of gingivitis. Clinical, microbiological and histological findings. *J Clin Periodontol* **23**: 379–85.

Fransson C, Mooney J, Kinane DF, Berglundh T (1999) Differences in the inflammatory response in young and old human subjects during the course of experimental gingivitis. *J Clin Periodontol* **26**: 453–60.

Gorlin RJ, Sendano H, Anderson VE (1964) The syndrome of palmo-plantar hyperkeratosis and premature periodontal destructure of the teeth. *J Pediatr* **65**: 896–908.

Gwinn MR, Sharma A, De Nardin E (1999) Single nucleotide polymorphisms of the N-formyl peptide receptor in localized juvenile periodontitis. *J Periodontol* **70**: 1194–201.

Haneke E (1979) The Papillon–Lefèvre syndrome. Keratosis palmoplantaris with periodontopathy. Report of a case and review of the cases in the literature. *Hum Genet* **51**: 1–35.

Hart TC (1996) Genetic risk factors for early-onset periodontitis. *J Periodontol* **67**: 355–66.

Hart TC, Kornman KS (1997) Genetic factors in the pathogenesis of periodontitis. *Periodontol 2000* **14**: 202–15.

Hart TC, Marazita ML, Schenkein HA, Diehl SR (1992) Re-interpretation of the evidence for X-linked dominant inheritance of juvenile periodontitis. *J Periodontol* **63**: 169–73.

Hart TC, Marazita ML, McCanna KM et al. (1993) Reevaluation of the chromosome 4q candidate region for early onset periodontitis. *Hum Genet* **91**: 416–22.

Hart TC, Pallos D, Bowden DW et al. (1998) Genetic linkage of hereditary gingival fibromatosis to chromosome 2p21. *Am J Hum Genet* **62**: 876–83.

Hart TC, Hart PS, Bowden DW et al. (1999) Mutations of the cathepsin C gene are responsible for Papillon–Lefèvre syndrome. *J Med Genet* **36**: 881–7.

Hart TC, Marazita ML, Wright JT (2000a) The impact of molecular genetics on oral health paradigms. *Crit Rev Oral Biol Med* **11**: 26–56.

Hart TC, Pallos D, Bozzo L, Cortelli J (2000b) Genetic heterogeneity for hereditary gingival fibromatosis. *J Dent Res* (in press).

Hart TC, Hart PS, Michalec MD et al. (2000c) Localisation of a gene for prepubertal periodontitis to chromosome 11q14 and identification of a cathepsin C gene mutation. *J Med Genet* **37**: 95–101.

Hart TC, Hart PS, Michalec MD et al. (2000d) Haim–Munk syndrome and Papillon–Lefèvre syndrome are allelic mutations in cathepsin C. *J Med Genet* **37**: 88–94.

Hartsfield JK, Kousseff BG (1990) Phenotypic overlap of Ehlers–Danlos syndrome types IV and VIII. *Am J Med Genet* **37**: 465–70.

Hassell TM, Harris EL (1995) Genetic influences in caries and periodontal diseases. *Crit Rev Oral Biol Med* **6**: 319–42.

Hassell TM, Hefti AF (1991) Drug-induced gingival overgrowth: old problem. new problem. *Crit Rev Oral Biol Med* **2**: 103–37.

Hennig BJ, Parkhill JM, Chapple IL et al. (1999) Association of a vitamin D receptor gene polymorphism with localized early-onset periodontal diseases. *J Periodontol* **70**: 1032–8.

Hill AV (1996) Genetics of infectious disease resistance. *Curr Opin Genet Dev* **6**: 348–53.

Hou GL, Tsai CC (1993) Relationship between palatoradicular grooves and localized periodontitis. *J Clin Periodontol* **20**: 678–82.

Idle JR (1991) Is environmental carcinogenesis modulated by host polymorphism? *Mutat Res* **247**: 259–66.

Johnson NW, Griffiths GS, Wilton JM et al. (1988) Detection of high-risk groups and individuals for periodontal diseases. Evidence for the existence of high-risk groups and individuals and approaches to their detection. *J Clin Periodontol* **15**: 276–82.

Jorgenson RJ, Cocker ME (1974) Variation in the inheritence and expression of gingival fibromatosis. *J Periodontol* **45**: 472–7.

Jouvenne P, Chaudhary A, Buchs N et al. (1999) Possible genetic association between interleukin-1alpha gene polymorphism and the severity of chronic polyarthritis. *Eur Cytokine Netw* **10**: 33–6.

Kelso A (1998) Cytokines: principles and prospects. *Immunol Cell Biol* **76**: 300–17.

Khosravi M, Weaver DD (1993) Ehlers–Danlos syndrome type IX (occipital horn syndrome): report of an additional case. *American Journal of Human Genetics* **53**: suppl. Program and Abstracts of the Annual Meeting of the American Society of Human Genetics, Abstr. 1548.

Kornman KS, di Giovine FS (1998) Genetic variations in cytokine expression: a risk factor for severity of adult periodontitis. *Ann Periodontol* **3**: 327–38.

Kornman KS, Pankow J, Offenbacher S et al. (1999) Interleukin-1 genotypes and the association between periodontitis and cardiovascular disease [in process citation]. *J Periodont Res* **34**: 353–7.

Lang NP, Karring T (1994) *Proceedings of the First European Workshop on Periodontology*. London: Quintessence.

Linch DC, Acton CH (1979) Ehlers–Danlos syndrome presenting with juvenile destructive periodontitis. *Br Dent J* **147**: 95–6.

Listgarten MA (1986) Pathogenesis of periodontitis. *J Clin Periodontol* **13**: 418–30.

Löe H, Brown LJ (1991) Early onset periodontitis in the United States of America. *J Periodontol* **62**: 608–16.

Löe H, Theilade E, Jensen SB (1965) Experimental gingivitis in man. *J Periodontol* **36**: 177–87.

Löe H, Anerud A, Boysen H, Smith M (1978) The natural history of periodontal disease in man. The rate of periodontal destruction before 40 years of age. *J Periodontol* **49**: 607–20.

Löe H, Anerud A, Boysen H, Morrison E (1986) Natural history of periodontal disease in man. Rapid, moderate and no loss of attachment in Sri Lankan laborers 14 to 46 years of age. *J Clin Periodontol* **13**: 431–45.

Long JC, Nance WE, Waring P et al. (1987) Early onset periodontitis: a comparison and evaluation of two proposed modes of inheritance. *Genet Epidemiol* **4**: 13–24.

Lopez NJ (1992) Clinical, laboratory, and immunological studies of a family with a high prevalence of generalized prepubertal and juvenile periodontitis. *J Periodontol* **63**: 457–68.

Lu H, Wang M, Gunsolley JC et al. (1994) Serum immunoglobulin G subclass concentrations in periodontally healthy and diseased individuals. *Infect Immun* **62**: 1677–82.

Malo D, Skamene E (1994) Genetic control of host resistance to infection. *Trend Genet* **10**: 365–71.

Marazita ML, Burmeister JA, Gunsolley JC et al. (1994) Evidence for autosomal dominant inheritance and race-specific heterogeneity in early-onset periodontitis *J Periodontol* **65**: 623–30.

Marazita ML, Lu H, Cooper ME et al. (1996) Genetic segregation analyses of serum IgG2 levels. *Am J Hum Genet* **58**: 1042–9.

McFarlane CG, Reynolds JJ, Meile MC (1990) The release of interleukin-1 beta, tumor necrosis factor-alpha and interferon-gamma by cultured peripheral blood mononuclear cells from patients with periodontitis. *J Periodont Res* **25**: 207–14.

Meyer DH, Fives-Taylor PM (1998) Oral pathogens: from dental plaque to cardiac disease. *Curr Opin Microbiol* **1**: 88–95.

Michalowicz BS (1993) Genetic and inheritance considerations in periodontal disease. *Curr Opin Periodontol* **2**: 11–17.

Miyazaki H, Hanada N, Andoh MI et al. (1989) Periodontal disease prevalence in different age groups in Japan as assessed according to the CPITN. *Commun Dent Oral Epidemiol* **17**: 71–4.

Nadeau JH, Arbuckle LD, Skamene E (1995) Genetic dissection of inflammatory responses. *J Inflamm* **45**: 27–48.

Neale M, Cardon L (1992) *Methodologies for Genetic Studies of Twins and Families*. Boston: Kluwer.

Nelson DL, King RA (1981) Ehlers-Danlos syndrome type VIII. *J Am Acad Dermatol* **5**: 297–303.

Nevins M, Becker W, Kornman K (1989) *Proceedings of the World Workshop in Clinical Periodontics*. Chicago: American Academy of Periodontology, I-1–I-31.

Novak MJ, Novak KF (1996) Early-onset periodontitis. *Curr Opin Periodontol* **3**: 45–58.

Offenbacher S (1996) Periodontal diseases: pathogenesis. *Ann Periodontol* **1**: 821–78.

Oliver RC, Brown LJ, Löe H (1998) Periodontal diseases in the United States population. *J Periodontol* **69**: 269–78.

Page RC (1986) Gingivitis. *J Clin Periodontol* **13**: 345–59.

Page RC (1998) The pathobiology of periodontal diseases may affect systemic diseases: inversion of a paradigm. *Ann Periodontol* **3**: 108–20.

Page RC, Baab DA (1985) A new look at the etiology and pathogenesis of early-onset periodontitis. Cementopathia revisited. *J Periodontol* **56**: 748–51.

Page RC, Kornman KS (1997) The pathogenesis of human periodontitis: an introduction. *Periodontol 2000* **14**: 9–11.

Page RC, Schroeder HE (1976) Pathogenesis of inflammatory periodontal disease. A summary of current work. *Lab Invest* **34**: 235–49.

Papapanou PN (1996) Periodontal diseases: epidemiology. *Ann Periodontol* **1**: 1–36.

Pernu HE, Knuuttila ML, Huttunen KR, Tiilikainen AS (1994) Drug-induced gingival overgrowth and class II major histocompatibility antigens. *Transplantation* **57**: 1811–3.

Perry DA, Newman MG (1990) Occurrence of periodontitis in an urban adolescent population. *J Periodontol* **61**: 185–8.

Pietrzak ER, Polak B, Walsh LJ et al. (1998) Characterization of serum antibodies to *Porphyromonas gingivalis* in individuals with and without periodontitis. *Oral Microbiol Immunol* **13**: 65–72.

Pihlstrom BL, Ammons WF (1997) Treatment of gingivitis and periodontitis. Research, Science and Therapy Committee of the American Academy of Periodontology. *J Periodontol* **68**: 1246–53.

Pilot T, Barmes DE, Leclercq MH et al. (1987) Periodontal conditions in adolescents, 15–19 years of age: an overview of CPITN data in the WHO Global Oral Data Bank. *Commun Dent Oral Epidemiol* **15**: 336–8.

Prayitno SW, Addy M, Wade WG (1993) Does gingivitis lead to periodontitis in young adults? [see comments]. *Lancet* **342**: 471–2.

Preus HR (1988) Treatment of rapidly destructive periodontitis in Papillon–Lefèvre syndrome. Laboratory and clinical observations. *J Clin Periodontol* **15**: 639–43.

Qureshi ST, Skamene E, Malo D (1999) Comparative genomics and host resistance against infectious diseases. *Emerg Infect Dis* **5**: 36–47.

Raeste AM, Collan Y, Kilpinen E (1978) Hereditary fibrous hyperplasia of the gingiva with varying penetrance and expressivity. *Scand J Dent Res* **86**: 357–65.

Ranney RR (1993) Classification of periodontal diseases. *Periodontol 2000* **2**: 13–25.

Ranney RR, Debski BF, Tew JG (1981) Pathogenesis of gingivitis and periodontal disease in children and young adults. *Pediatr Dent* **3**: 89–100.

Reiser H, Vogel F (1958) Ueber die erblichkeit der zahnsteinbildung beim menschen. *Dtsch Zahnarztl Zschr* **13**: 1355–8.

Salmon JE, Millard S, Schachter LA et al. (1996) Fc gamma RIIA alleles are heritable risk factors for lupus nephritis in African Americans. *J Clin Invest* **97**: 1348–54.

Saxen L, Nevanlinna HR (1984) Autosomal recessive inheritance of juvenile periodontitis: test of a hypothesis. *Clin Genet* **25**: 332–5.

Schenkein HA (1998) Etiology of localized juvenile periodontitis. *J Periodontol* **69**: 1068–9.

Schenkein HA, Van Dyke TE (1994) Early-onset periodontitis: systemic aspects of etiology and pathogenesis. *Periodontol 2000* **6**: 7–25.

Schmitz G, Aslanidis C, Lackner KJ (1998) Recent advances in molecular genetics of cardiovascular disorders. Implications for atherosclerosis and diseases of cellular lipid metabolism. *Pathol Oncol Res* **4**: 152–60.

Shapira L, Schlesinger M, Bimstein E (1997) Possible autosomal-dominant inheritance of prepubertal periodontitis in an extended kindred. *J Clin Periodontol* **24**: 388–93.

Skamene E, Pietrangeli CE (1991) Genetics of the immune response to infectious pathogens. *Curr Opin Immunol* **3**: 511–17.

Socransky SS, Haffajee AD (1991) Microbial mechanisms in the pathogenesis of destructive periodontal diseases: a critical assessment. *J Periodont Res* **26**: 195–212.

Spektor MD, Vandesteen GE, Page RC (1985) Clinical studies of one family manifesting rapidly progressive, juvenile and prepubertal periodontitis. *J Periodontol* **56**: 93–101.

Stevens HP, Kelsell DP, Bryant SP et al. (1996) Linkage of an American pedigree with palmoplantar keratoderma and malignancy (palmoplantar ectodermal dysplasia type III) to 17q24. Literature survey and proposed updated classification of the keratodermas. *Arch Dermatol* **132**: 640–51.

Stewart RE, Hollister DW, Rimoin DL (1977) A new variant of Ehlers–Danlos syndrome: an autosomal dominant disorder of fragile skin, abnormal scarring, and generalized periodontitis. *Birth Def Orig Artic Ser* **13**: 85–93.

Streckfus CF, Parsell DE, Streckfus JE et al. (1999) Relationship between oral alveolar bone loss and aging among African-American and Caucasian individuals. *Gerontology* **45**: 110–14.

Tangada SD, Califano JV, Nakashima K et al. (1997) The effect of smoking on serum IgG2 reactive with *Actinobacillus actinomycetemcomitans* in early-onset periodontitis patients. *J Periodontol* **68**: 842–50.

Toomes C, James J, Wood AJ et al. (1999) Loss-of-function mutations in the cathepsin C gene result in periodontal disease and palmoplantar keratosis [see comments]. *Nat Genet* **23**: 421–4.

Valtonen VV (1999) Role of infections in atherosclerosis. *Am Heart J* **138**: S431–S433.

Watanabe H, Umeda M, Seki T, Ishikawa I (1993) Clinical and laboratory studies of severe periodontal disease in an adolescent associated with hypophosphatasia. A case report. *J Periodontol* **64**: 174–80.

Wei SHY, Yang S, Barmes DE (1986) Needs and implementation of preventive dentistry in China. *Commun Dent Oral Epidemiol* **14**: 19–23.

Wiesch DG, Meyers DA, Bleecker ER (1999) Genetics of asthma. *J Allerg Clin Immunol* **104**: 895–901.

Wilson ME Kalmar JR (1996) Fc-gamma-RIIA (DC32)—a potential marker defining susceptibility to localized juvenile periodontitis. *J Periodontol* **67**: 323–31.

Wolfe MD, Carlos JP (1987) Epidemiological findings in Navajo Indians. *Comm Dent Oral Epidemiol* **15**: 33–40.

Zambon JJ (1996) Periodontal diseases: microbial factors. *Ann Periodontol* **1**: 879–925.

PART V

Treatment

10
Promotion of gingival and periodontal health from childhood

Harold D. Sgan-Cohen and Rina Adut

Oral hygiene—its rise, fall, and rise again

Historically, preventive dentistry placed primary emphasis on oral hygiene. In fact, the single most continuous theme of preventive dentistry and dental public health appears to have been the cleaning of teeth. The first toothbrushes can be traced as far back as 1000 CE in China, but the more common bristle brush dates from the late eighteenth and early nineteenth centuries (Fischman, 1997).

By 1890, W. D. Miller had performed extensive research on dental problems. His work culminated in establishing the cause of dental caries: oral bacteria, feeding on food particles, produce acids that give rise to tooth decay. Armed with this knowledge, the era of prevention had begun. Empowered with a new slogan, "A clean tooth never decays," dentists initiated periodic dental prophylaxis. From an early age children were urged to brush twice a day and the public was encouraged to improve their oral hygiene habits (Fischman, 1997).

A trend to minimize the role of oral hygiene and the importance of gingivitis became evident in the 1970s and 1980s, although attitudes differed widely between parts of the world such as the USA, Britain, and Scandinavia. A marked skepticism could already be noted in 1958, as expressed in the book *Dentistry for Children* (Brauer et al., 1958), where Massler questioned the feasibility of oral hygiene in young children. He wrote, "Toothbrushing performed at the beginning or the end of the day serves a real cosmetic function but bears little relation to the prevention of dental caries. Children in general do not use the toothbrush frequently or effectively." No reference to the importance of oral hygiene in preventing gingival disease was made, and the author stated that "gingivitis is common in the adult but rare in the healthy child."

Dental public health literature placed increasing emphasis on caries as the primary concern and on fluoride in general, and fluoridated dentifrice in particular, as the almost universal panacea. Scientific articles describing preventive dentistry and health education among children were dominated by emphasis on the role of fluoride (Frazier, 1980; Horowitz, 1980; Klein et al., 1985; Horowitz and Frazier, 1986). This decreased emphasis on the role of oral hygiene education and promotion among children was particularly evident in the USA; authors did not completely ignore the role of oral hygiene and gingivitis, but mention of these topics was marginal. The pervading message of the time was: "Promote children's oral health with fluoride and sealants." An American Dental Association slogan read: "Fluoride + Sealants = Healthy Teeth."

The British school seems to have presented an intermediate stand between that of the USA and Scandinavia. The British Health Education Authority has regularly stressed the role of oral hygiene, and in 1997 reported that "Reduction in plaque levels almost always, but not invariably, leads to reductions in inflammation and bleeding of the gingivae." The Authority recommended that, "Caries preventive efforts should be focused on children as the benefits are cumulative." This last sentence could have rationally and scientifically included gingivitis, but did not (British Health Education Authority, 1997).

This fall in the importance associated with oral hygiene stemmed from a scientific and logical source and could be traced to the following factors:

- an acknowledgment that fluoride is the central most effective contributor to the decline in dental caries
- a recognition that dental caries is the primary dental public health concern relating to children
- an inadequate basis of sound scientific reports (apart from the Scandinavian school) associating oral hygiene with dental caries
- a lack of recognition that periodontal health promotion among children is an important concern for dental public health
- a belief that optimal oral hygiene, among children, is unrealistic
- inadequate data on the cost-effectiveness of oral hygiene attempts in the prevention of caries and gingivitis (Burt, 1978).

The Scandinavian literature, over the same period, presented an almost completely different school of thought. By 1972, Löe and his colleagues had demonstrated that caries could be inhibited by plaque control (Löe et al., 1972). Other Scandinavian studies reported a significant association between oral hygiene and caries, especially on smooth dental surfaces (Kleemola-Kujala, 1978; Bellini et al., 1980; Hamp and Johanssen, 1982; Kleemola-Kujala and Räsänen, 1982). Scandinavian trials, recognizing that the skill and perseverance needed to maintain an adequate level of oral hygiene may exceed the average ability of children, initiated supervised tooth-cleaning programs. These efforts were documented and demonstrated a significant reduction of gingivitis and caries in children and adults (Ramfjord et al., 1973; Axelsson and Lindhe, 1974, 1978; Axelsson et al., 1991; Mattila et al., 1998). Few of these efforts to prevent both caries and gingivitis were duplicated in other Western countries. School-based supervised plaque removal programs in the USA have, however, been demonstrated as effective in the reduction of gingivitis (Horowitz et al., 1977).

Gingival and periodontal health is important among children, and improved oral hygiene is the dominant—if not the only—method of achieving this goal. Oral health is concerned with teeth, periodontal tissue, and the other soft and hard oral tissues. The health of these components are often associated with the same, or similar, predisposing environmental and microbial variables (Babaahmady et al., 1998).

Although not all gingivitis will inevitably lead to destructive periodontal disease, it is now clear that most periodontal diseases are preceded by gingivitis. The prevention of periodontal disease is therefore dependent on the prevention of gingivitis (Löe, 1999). Moreover, gingivitis itself can significantly impair wellbeing.

Oral health has to be viewed and promoted in its entirety. With the decline in caries prevalence (Anderson et al., 1982; Brunelle and Carlos, 1982; Downer, 1984), the dental profession and public health leaders need to shift their emphases to previously neglected areas. Periodontal disease and dental caries have always been recognized as the paramount dental pathologies and in fact are the most prevalent human diseases. The time, therefore, is ripe for dental public health to redirect its focus towards promoting periodontal health in children. Even if periodontal disease is less prevalent in children than adults, it should be recognized that the disease is progressive and that appropriate prevention has to start at an early age. The reluctance of the public to adopt optimal oral hygiene suggests that the profession should strive to encourage it at the earliest possible age (Sheiham, 1990).

The European Workshop on Mechanical Plaque Control adopted the following policy statement in 1998: "Forty years of experimental research, clinical trials and demonstration projects in different geographical and social settings have confirmed that effective removal of dental plaque is essential to dental and periodontal health throughout life. Therefore, we recommend that this be reflected in the development of explicit oral health promotion policies at the national and community levels" (Lang et al., 1998). This is an important new challenge for comprehensive dental public health policy.

The epidemiology and etiology of gingival and periodontal health in children

Epidemiology

Whereas dental caries has been present as a widespread epidemic for less than five hundred years, since the development of the flour and sugar industries, periodontal disease has been prevalent since the beginning of humankind. Symptoms of periodontal bone loss have been found in Neanderthal human skulls dating from 60 000 years ago. The World Health Organization (WHO) Global Oral Data Bank reports that adults "with a healthy periodontium are virtually absent in most surveys" (Pilot, 1998).

As early as 1933, it was reported that gingivitis was very common among children (McCall, 1933). Both gingivitis and periodontitis are still reported to be prevalent, but less extensively and less severe than previously (Löe, 1999). An improvement in periodontal health has been especially noted among children and adults in industrialized countries (Anderson, 1981; Douglass et al., 1983; Cutress, 1986; Hugoson et al., 1986; Sheiham et al., 1986; Brown et al., 1989; Frode Hansen et al., 1990). This improvement has been explained by a concurrent increase in oral hygiene. In industrialized countries 80–90% of the population brush their teeth once or twice a day (Saxer and Yankell, 1997).

According to the WHO Global Oral Data Bank, there are currently 190 sets of community periodontal index (CPI) data from 100 countries for subjects aged 15–19 years. According to these data, gingival inflammation, accompanied by bleeding, plaque and calculus, is more severe and more prevalent in developing countries than in industrialized countries. Periodontal pocketing accompanied by attachment loss among adolescents was rare but was found in most populations of developing or industrialized countries (Pilot, 1998).

Etiology

The etiological basis of gingivitis at the beginning of the twentieth century was attributed to a wide range of factors, including dental caries and dental trauma (McCall, 1933), mouth breathing, and vitamin C deficiency (Brucker, 1943). Oral hygiene levels were associated with course, soft or sticky foods (Wallace, 1935; Klatsky, 1937). Brucker in 1943 wrote, "The merit of the toothbrush as an aid in preventing dental ills, including gingivitis, appears to be debatable." He also added, "No one denies that gingival diseases may develop despite meticulous observances of good oral hygiene" (Brucker, 1943).

It was not until 1965 that Löe and colleagues firmly established a positive association between gingivitis and dental plaque. Since then the undisputed method of choice for preventing gingival and periodontal disease has been optimal oral hygiene. The microbial composition of plaque is similar in children and in adults (Löe et al., 1965; Mackler and Crawford, 1973), although it has been suggested that young children may be more resistant to gingival inflammation (Matsson, 1978).

Mechanical methods of oral hygiene

There is no "natural cleansing" of teeth. Especially in cervical and proximal areas, plaque will always accumulate. No foods—not even apples or carrots, as has sometimes been suggested—can clean these areas (Löe, 1999). Plaque can only be successfully removed by mechanical methods. The most common and effective system of tooth cleansing is the toothbrush. The only problem with this method is the difficulty in removing interdental plaque (Löe, 1999).

Toothbrush design

The European Workshop on Mechanical Plaque Control (Lang et al., 1998), cited the following attributes of an acceptable toothbrush:

- a handle size appropriate to user age and dexterity
- a head size appropriate to the size of the patient's mouth
- end-rounded nylon or polyester filaments no larger than 0.009 inch (0.225 mm) in diameter
- soft bristle configuration as defined by the acceptable international industry standards
- bristle patterns that enhance plaque removal in the approximal spaces and along the gum line.

As far as infants, children, and adolescents are concerned, the above directives should be interpreted to provide the size and design of brush

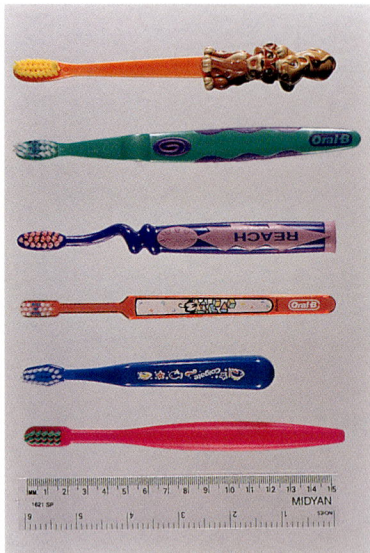

a

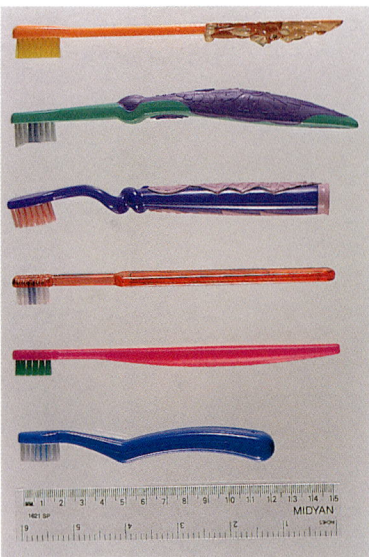

b

Figure 10.1

Brushes for children aged 0–5 years. The heads are approximately 1.5 cm long; the handles are large, easy to grip, and attractive to young children.

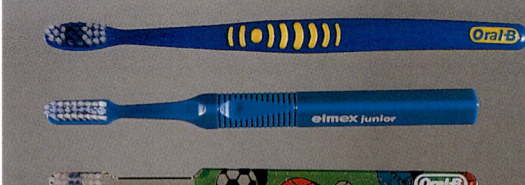

a

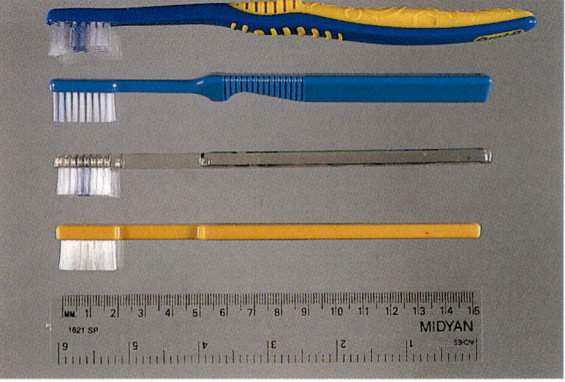

b

Figure 10.2

Brushes for children aged 6–11 years. The heads are approximately 2 cm long.

(usually the smaller the better) that suits the individual child. Modern brushes, which often are endorsed, accepted, or recommended by local dental health agencies, are usually of a high standard of quality. The smallest heads should be recommended for infants (Figure 10.1), medium for young children (Figure 10.2), and regular for adolescents (Figure 10.3). It is often correctly recommended that infants' brushes have large handles which facilitate manual dexterity. Brushes should be replaced once the bristles are splayed.

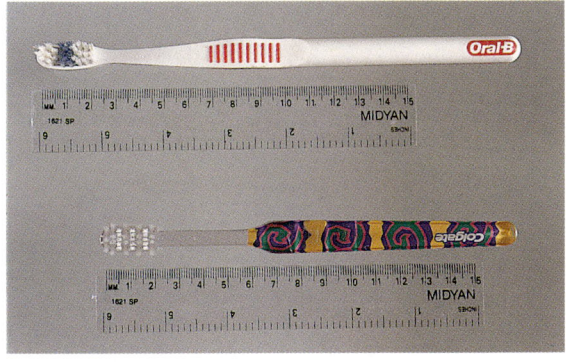
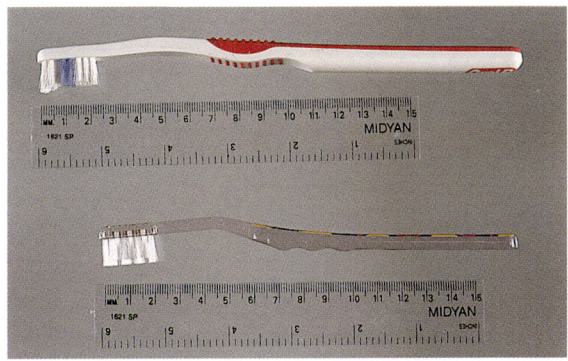

a   b

Figure 10.3

Brushes for children aged 12–18 years. The heads are approximately 2.5 cm long. Most regular small adult brushes can be used in this age group.

Electric toothbrushes are not necessary for well-motivated and properly instructed individuals. For the less motivated and those lacking the necessary dexterity, electrical brushes may be more efficient in maintaining oral hygiene. A review by Wejden et al. (1998) has shown that powered toothbrushes can remove more plaque, especially from the dental proximal areas, and can be particularly beneficial for children, especially those undergoing orthodontic treatment. Other studies of powered toothbrushes have demonstrated similar efficacy, especially in the interproximal areas (Sahota et al., 1998; Heasman and McCracken, 1999; Barnes et al., 1999). Electrical tooth brushing has been shown to be of significant value in reducing gingivitis in orthodontic patients (Clerehugh et al., 1998). In general, electric toothbrushes are recommended for children with suboptimal plaque control and for those who are at high risk of caries and periodontal disease.

Countless toothbrush designs have been suggested and marketed, ranging from multi-headed brushes (Zimmer et al., 1999), differing bristle feathering and outside row dimensions (Yankell et al., 1998), to "manually rotating" brushes (Sgan-Cohen et al., 1995). Most of these designs have been similarly effective. Concern has been voiced regarding the potential abrasion of dental and gingival tissue by tooth brushing,

but research has demonstrated that with rounded filament brushes, regardless of brushing force or speed, there should be no basis for this concern (Danser et al., 1998).

Brushing techniques

The most commonly recommended methods of tooth brushing include the following.

- The Bass technique: introduced in the early 1950s, this method is aimed at cleaning the buccal and lingual cervical areas, with emphasis on the gingival sulcus. The bristles are placed at an angle of 45° towards the apical direction of the tooth and vibrated horizontally, with the bristles lodged gently within the gingival sulcus (Robinson, 1976).
- The horizontal scrubbing method: the most common technique used by people who have never received professional instruction. The brush is held at a 90° angle to the tooth axis and moved back and forth on the buccal, lingual, and occlusal surfaces (Anaise, 1975; Robinson, 1976).
- The Charters method: aimed at reaching the interdental proximal areas (Charters, 1932).

The bristles are placed at approximately 45° towards the occlusal plane. Pressure is applied as the brush is vibrated between the teeth.

Other methods exist which cannot all be described here; few have been demonstrated to be scientifically superior. In the "toothpick" method, the bristles are placed on the gingival margin at an angle of 30° towards the crown (similar to the Charters method). The bristles are then pressed into the interdental spaces and pulled out like a toothpick. This has been reported to be more effective than the Bass technique in removing plaque from proximal surfaces (Morita et al., 1998).

A study conducted *in vitro* has shown that toothbrush design has more effect on interproximal plaque than the brushing technique (Bruun et al., 1998). Most studies demonstrate little significant difference in the effectiveness of the different techniques whether used by children or adults (McClure, 1966; Anaise, 1975; Sangnes, 1974; Robinson, 1976; Gibson and Wade, 1977).

The horizontal scrub technique is the easiest and is therefore recommended as the first method to teach parents who are brushing infants' teeth. Studies have demonstrated that this method was more effective in young children (McClure, 1966; Sangnes, 1974; Anaise, 1975). When the child reaches school age the Bass technique can be adopted. Sheiham has recommended modifying and improving the scrub method by using a 'finger pen' instead of fist grip while holding the brush (Sheiham, 1983, 1990).

Löe, at the FDI Second World Conference on Oral Health Promotion in 1999, stated that the Charters method of 1932, "may be more demanding than other techniques; it may require more detailed instructions, and is more time consuming, but it does what the more common brushing methods fail to do, i.e. address the problem of plaque removal on interdental surfaces".

Interdental cleaning

Even optimal tooth brushing cleans only the buccal, lingual, and occlusal surfaces. Occlusal pits and fissures, proximal and interdental surfaces cannot be reached by the bristles, and these are the most common areas for caries and periodontal disease initiation. Pits and fissures can be sealed against caries, and proximal and interdental surfaces can be cleaned using dental floss, tape, interdental sticks, and other devices. No one method suits all people.

A survey of oral hygiene habits among children in 22 European countries and Canada (Kuusela et al., 1997) revealed that flossing was rare; the highest level, only 25%, was found among Canadian adolescents. In general girls flossed more frequently than boys. Similar results have been reported in other epidemiological studies (Honkala et al., 1990; Stevens et al., 1992). Despite these data, it is encouraging to note that training children to floss has been shown to be effective (Rodrigues et al., 1996). Flossing, like tooth brushing, has been shown to be related to social group among adolescents (Macgregor et al., 1997). The problem is therefore clearly cultural and the solution needs to be found at the community level. Löe (1999) suggested that "children and young adults with reasonably normal mesial-distal contact between their teeth, and with gingival papillae filling the interdental area, may be advised to use dental floss or tape."

It should be noted that in less Westernized countries alternative methods are preferred to toothbrushes. These include chewing sticks and chewing sponges (Clerehugh et al., 1995; Fischman, 1997). When these methods are effective they should not be discouraged.

The only way a dentist or hygienist can definitively endorse a specific brush, brushing technique or interdental cleaning method for a specific patient is by actually monitoring its use. The behavior needs to be tailored to each individual child. Whichever technique achieves optimal oral hygiene is the best and should be recommended. The dentist or hygienist can only ascertain this by direct continued observation.

Tooth-brushing initiation and frequency

Regular tooth brushing has been strongly encouraged since the inception of the modern dental profession. However, as late as the 1950s, this has been advocated only from the age of about 2–3 years, after eruption of the second deciduous molars.

Today it is usually recommended that oral cleaning should commence even before and definitely immediately after tooth eruption. The British Dental Association (1997) has recommended that "toothbrushing needs to be introduced as soon as the first teeth appear. If a baby resists brushing, use a clean piece of moist gauze with a tiny spot of fluoride tooth paste, to wipe the teeth. By the age of 2 years, though, an infant toothbrush ought to be used, with twice daily brushing." The American Academy of Pediatric Dentistry (1999) recommends providing oral hygiene counseling to parents, guardians, and caregivers from birth to 24 months. From 24 months to 12 years, it is recommended to include the child in this counseling, and from age 12 years, only the child.

Early reports on the required frequency of tooth brushing were not always uniform in their recommendations, ranging from once to five times a day (Stanymeyer, 1957; Dale, 1969). Gingivitis is related more to plaque age than to amount (Löe et al., 1965; Theilade et al., 1966). The first subclinical tissue changes appear after 2 days of plaque accumulation (Löe and Holm Pedersen, 1965, 1967; Brecx et al., 1980), and it has therefore been suggested that it could be enough to remove plaque only once a day or even once every 2 days. Longer intervals are insufficient (Lang et al., 1973; Kelner et al., 1974; Bosman and Powell, 1977). There is no evidence-based directive as to the exact optimal frequency demanded to prevent caries and gingivitis. However, on a didactic and practical level it still is recommended that people continue the tradition of twice-daily brushing (Lang et al., 1998). There appears to be no scientific evidence basis on whether it is better to brush before or after meals; nevertheless, most people appreciate the feeling of cleanliness when brushing after meals. This subjective factor is important and should be acknowledged.

Dental cleaning guidelines, by age

Guidelines on oral hygiene maintenance have been drawn up according to age (Nowak and Crall, 1994). The following modified recommendations are suggested for both the individual and the community levels.

Birth to age 3 years

Plaque removal in children under 3 years old is often neglected and misunderstood. It is the responsibility of the parents to maintain optimal oral hygiene. Early initiation of an oral hygiene habit will enhance the potential of continued maintenance throughout life. Parents should be strongly encouraged by dental health professionals to clean and examine their infants' teeth. Any difficulties should be referred to dentists or hygienists.

The best location within the home for tooth cleaning is not necessarily the bathroom, which may be small and cramped. The regular diaper changing table can be practical. Laying the infant down on a table or bed may afford a better view of the mouth and teeth.

Before tooth eruption, the oral cavity should be cleaned with a gauze cloth wrapped around a finger. After eruption, teeth should be cleaned by parents, using the smallest available toothbrush (see Figure 10.1). These brushes should have small heads, soft bristles, and preferably large handles. Brushes should be moistened and a small drop of fluoridated toothpaste applied. The amount of paste has been recommended to be pea-sized or the size of the child's smallest fingernail. At this age infants are unable to expectorate efficiently, and excessive fluoride ingestion can and does cause fluorosis (Jackson et al., 1999).

Infants may object to tooth cleaning. Parents need to be persistent and to persevere, despite possible opposition. It is the responsibility of the dental team to invite all parents of newly born infants for instruction in oral hygiene methods, including methods of head stabilization, propping of the mouth, and reflection of the lips and cheeks. Parents are encouraged to aim for optimal oral hygiene, including all surfaces of the maxillary and mandibular teeth; nevertheless, it should be recognized that at this age this may not be practical. The three primary objectives therefore are:

• topical application of a small amount of fluoride
• removal of most dental plaque
• introduction of future life-time oral hygiene habits.

The optimal time for tooth brushing is before bedtime, often before or after a bath. It is

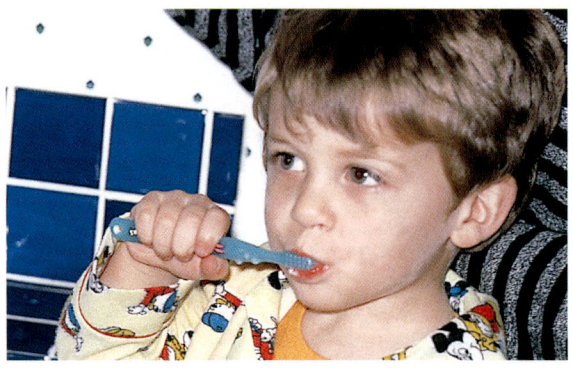

a

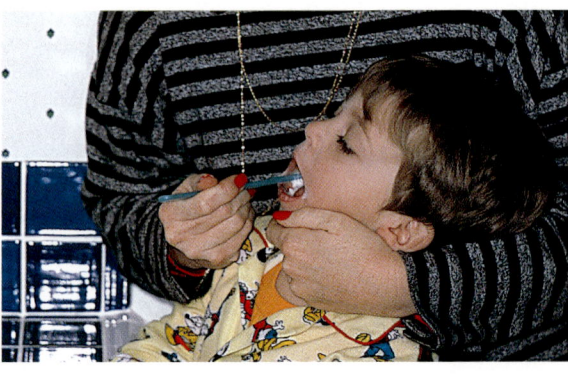

b

Figure 10.4

Adequate tooth brushing is achieved by combining independence with supervision: (a) the child brushes independently; (b) the parents clean thoroughly at bedtime. Courtesy of Dr Martin Sinai Rayman.

recommended that oral and general hygiene procedures are given in the same context.

Towards age 2–3 years, toddlers may want to start brushing their own teeth. This should be strongly encouraged. When brushing by themselves, toothpaste should not be freely supplied—only a wet toothbrush. Parents may dispense the correct amount of fluoridated toothpaste before handing the brush to the child. Another good idea at this age is for parents and toddlers to brush their teeth together. After toddlers have brushed their own teeth, parents should check their mouths, giving positive feedback, and rebrushing any surfaces that have not been reached. Flossing is not practical and not necessary at this age, as interdental spacing is usually present.

These recommendations are aimed at individuals, but optimal promotion of these objectives can only be achieved if they are incorporated within the culture of the community. Therefore these components should be included in all community health programs, which at this age are traditionally conducted from mother and child health and daycare centers. The best community health agents are public health nurses.

Ages 3–6 years

The independence of children in this age group is variable. Some children have adequate motor coordination, others do not; some need help from their parents, others do not. It is suggested that independence is combined with supervision, for example, the child brushes independently after meals, the parents clean more thoroughly at bedtime (Figure 10.4). Individual families can formulate their own systems.

Now is the optimal time to adopt the habit of cleaning teeth after meals and before bedtime. When the child finds it difficult or impractical to clean after meals, mouth rinsing with water, at least, should be encouraged. The dental team should become more involved in monitoring the family's oral hygiene efforts. As always, positive feedback is of utmost value. When needed, the dentist or hygienist should point out which oral areas have not been optimally cleaned, and give practical advice on improvement.

At this stage all primary teeth are present and interdental spaces are closing, making it more important to clean the gingival margins and the interproximal dental areas. This requires fine brushing and flossing skills, dedication, and a keen oral health awareness. It is recommended that expectations of the dental team, the parents, and the child, should not be too high in these matters. This can only lead to unneeded frustration. The primary objective is to introduce these subjects and convey the knowledge that careful brushing and flossing are important. If this step is achieved, it can be hoped that awareness and optimal behavior will follow at a later age. When parents are able and willing to floss their children's teeth, this should be encouraged. In these cases a floss holder can be helpful. Care must be taken by the parents not to injure the gingiva. Fluoride recommendations are similar to those for the previous age group.

At the end of this age period, deciduous teeth start exfoliating and swollen gingival tissue is common and physiologically normal. This needs to be explained to parents, together with encouragement that optimal cleansing will decrease the inflammation and discomfort.

In this age group the community level effort is of especial relevance. The dental health team needs to be familiar with the complete community profile, including socioeconomic, cultural, ethnic, and other factors. Methods such as flossing may be inappropriate and even wrong in some communities. Inappropriate health education strategies not only can be unsuccessful, but may alienate the health providers from their clients. The best community health agents are preschool (kindergarten) teachers.

Ages 6–12 years

At this age children become busier with school and other activities. These have to be considered when recommending oral hygiene practices. As before, the most important time to concentrate on oral hygiene efforts is at bedtime. At other times, when possible, children should be encouraged to brush; when not possible, at least to rinse.

Children should now be independently capable of optimal hygiene. As in other areas of parenting, this does not mean that monitoring and discipline are no longer required. This is the final stage when life-time habits are formed.

Slightly larger brushes are now indicated (see Figure 10.2). Bristles should still be soft. Many children will have attained the motor skills required for flossing, which should be learned and practiced. Floss holders may be used. Regarding toothpaste, children can now be taught to expectorate properly and independently use fluoridated dentifrice. When indicated, they are also capable of using mouth rinses.

Children should visit a dentist and hygienist annually. The dental team should supply general oral hygiene instruction and explain the potential cleaning problems involved with the gradual change from the deciduous to the full permanent dentition. The best community health agents are school teachers. It is the responsibility of the local dental health teams and officers to supply correct oral health education to teachers.

Ages 12 years to adolescence

The subject of oral hygiene cannot be disassociated from the general context of adolescence. Adolescents have the potential of independently achieving optimal hygiene, but they may lack motivation owing to other problems, or because oral hygiene habits were not initiated at an earlier age.

At this age full dental information can and should be supplied. Dental health education should be incorporated in the regular school curriculum. Teenagers should be told about gingivitis, its symptoms, and the fact that oral hygiene is the best method of prevention. The possibility of malodor due to poor oral hygiene should be stressed.

For adolescents brushes in the regular adult range should be chosen (see Figure 10.3). As for adults, smaller brushes are always recommended, as they can more conveniently reach all dental surfaces. When gingivitis is present, mouth rinses may be used in addition to improved oral hygiene techniques.

The best community health agents are now primary and high-school teachers. As before, it is the responsibility of the local dental health teams and officers to supply correct oral health education. In communities where not all children regularly attend high school, attempts should be made by the community dental team to identify alternative peer groups and opinion leaders.

Chemical agents for oral hygiene in children, adolescents, and young adults

Chlorhexidine is the primary evidence-based method of chemical plaque control. The potential of 0.2% chlorhexidine gluconate mouth rinse to prevent plaque, gingivitis, and caries development has been clearly confirmed (Rölla and Melsen, 1975; Bonesvoll and Gjermo, 1978; Zickert et al., 1982). For decades in Europe, and more recently in the USA, chlorhexidine has been the treatment of choice and the "gold standard" in clinical trials.

The main problems with the use of chlorhexidine are its taste, and stain formation on the teeth and tongue. These are of no serious health concern. The stain is removable by pumice polishing, and the taste can be masked by flavor agents. Apprehension about biological shifts in the oral microflora and changes in keratinization of the oral mucosa has not been substantiated in a 2-year daily rinsing study (McKenzie et al., 1976; Nuki et al., 1976). Dental professionals traditionally do not prescribe chlorhexidine for more than 2–3 weeks and then only to special cases or groups.

Because of these concerns, few studies have been conducted in children. Chlorhexidine has, however, been demonstrated to be effective in removing oral bacteria from both the permanent and the deciduous dentitions of children aged 4–12 years (Achong et al., 1999), to be more effective in removing interdental plaque than flossing in adolescents aged 15–16 years (Emilson et al., 1999), and to be significantly effective in improving gingival health in children aged 11–15 years (Valente et al., 1996).

The use of chlorhexidine rinses, gels, sprays, and varnishes has been encouraged and evaluated in populations who are incapable of achieving optimal oral hygiene through regular mechanical methods. These include children with physical or mental disabilities (Shapira et al., 1994; Laher and Cleaton-Jones, 1996; Steelman et al., 1996), children undergoing oncological chemotherapy (Levy-Polack et al., 1998), and children receiving orthodontic treatment (Anderson et al., 1997; Ögaard et al., 1997). In most of these cases chlorhexidine—in the form of rinses, sprays, or varnishes—is used as an adjunct to manual hygiene methods. Once an optimal level of plaque control and gingival health has been reached, a return to regular mechanical oral hygiene practices is usually recommended. All mouth rinses should be given to young children under supervision, to avoid the risk of swallowing.

Other chemical agents reported to be effective in reducing plaque and gingivitis include rinses and pastes containing triclosan with copolymer (Deasy et al., 1992; Worthington et al., 1993), cetylpyridinium chloride (Lobene et al., 1979), sanguinaria (Lobene et al., 1986), Listerine antiseptic (Mankodi et al., 1987), and others. Dentifrices containing triclosan have also been reported to prevent calculus formation (Svatun et al., 1993; Volpe et al., 1996) and the incidence of periodontal attachment loss in adolescents (Ellwood et al., 1998).

Fluoride, the almost omnipotent anticarious agent, also holds promise for controlling gingivitis, by reducing the surface energy of enamel, its tendency to adsorb protein, and its effect on bacterial metabolism and on dental plaque (Glantz, 1969; Ericsson and Ericsson, 1967). Sodium fluoride has been found to possess an altering effect on microbial metabolism of plaque (Genco and Picozzi, 1986), amine fluoride has a plaque-reducing effect (Shern et al., 1970), and the stannous ion in stannous fluoride was found to have a preventive effect on both plaque and gingivitis (Tinanoff et al., 1980; Sgan-Cohen et al., 1996).

Chemical agents in toothpastes

Tooth brushing is the easiest and most common procedure in the promotion of oral hygiene, so it is pertinent to investigate the role of chemical agents in different dentifrices.

The few studies on chlorhexidine fully formulated (not included with other therapeutic agents) in toothpastes have demonstrated effects ranging from moderate (Kornman, 1986) to significant (Sanz et al., 1994) on plaque and gingivitis. The recurrent problem with toothpastes containing chlorhexidine has been the significant increase in tooth staining.

Triclosan has recently been studied as a potential antiplaque and antigingivitis agent in toothpastes. An additive and potentially synergistic activity has been observed when it has been combined with zinc citrate (Cummins, 1991; Gjermo and Saxton, 1991; Svatun et al., 1993). In clinical studies, 0.3% triclosan has been successfully combined with 2% polyvinylmethyl ether–maleic acid copolymer (PVM/MA) to give a decrease of 15–20% in plaque and 30–50% in gingivitis (Cubells et al., 1991; Denepitiya et al.,

1992; Lindhe et al., 1993). The evidence so far suggests that this agent has a promising potential for plaque and calculus prevention, and gingival and periodontal health promotion.

The potential of the zinc ion as a plaque inhibitor has been demonstrated: zinc citrate in toothpastes had a moderate inhibitory effect on plaque formation (Addy et al., 1983; Saxton et al., 1987).

Stannous fluoride has a significant plaque and gingivitis inhibitory effect, probably due to the stannous ion (Bay and Rölla, 1980; Boyd and Chun, 1994; Tinanoff, 1995). Toothpastes containing amine fluoride combined with stannous fluoride significantly reduced gingivitis, specifically gingival bleeding (Banoczy et al., 1989; Sgan-Cohen et al., 1996). Like chlorhexidine, but to a lesser and more manageable extent, the problem with stannous fluoride is mild tooth staining.

Studies of other potential antigingivitis toothpaste components such as sanguinarine, peroxides, enzymes, and herbal extracts, have revealed preliminary, inadequate, or conflicting results.

Plaque indices

Plaque indices were primarily designed for epidemiological surveys. However, they are useful in individual oral hygiene instruction as a numerical method of plaque assessment. The child or adolescent patient can be given a plaque "score" at each visit with the dentist or hygienist, thus achieving a measurable goal for future improvement. Many indices exist. Some involve the use of a disclosing agent (e.g., erythrosine), and some examine "index" teeth, usually six: one premolar, one incisor and one molar in the mandible and in the maxilla respectively (Ramfjord, 1959).

Indices should be chosen according to the purposes of the examination. One of the simplest methods, the oral hygiene index of Greene and Vermillion (1960), divides the facial areas of teeth into thirds, which are scored as follows: 0, no plaque; 1, one-third covered with plaque; 2, more than one-third but less than two-thirds; 3, more than two-thirds of the tooth covered with plaque. Using a disclosing solution makes this index easy to demonstrate to the child patient.

Another common method is the plaque index of Löe (1967), where detected plaque (using a periodontal probe) is scored as follows: 0, no plaque in gingival area; 1, a film of plaque adhering to the free gingival margin and adjacent area, may only be recognized using probe; 2, moderate accumulation of soft deposits at gingival margin, seen by naked eye; 3, abundance of soft matter at gingival margin. The method demands training, but is simple, takes little time and supplies information about the gross amount of plaque.

When more information is called for alternative indices can be used. The Turesky modification of the Quigley–Hein plaque index (Turesky et al., 1970) emphasizes the gingival margin: 0, no plaque; 1, specks of plaque on the gingival margin; 2, a continuous line of plaque on the margin; 3, one-third of the tooth covered with plaque; 4, two-thirds of the tooth covered with plaque; 5, the whole tooth covered with plaque. A disclosing solution is normally used.

The patient hygiene performance (PHP) index of Podshadley and Haley (1968) emphasizes the proximal surfaces: 0 is no plaque; a separate score is added for each of the following surfaces: mesial, distal, gingival, middle, occlusal, giving a total of 5 for a tooth completely covered with plaque. The PHP index is usually assessed with the aid of a disclosing solution.

In epidemiological surveys these indices are applied to index teeth (Ramfjord, 1959). In individual use the goal of a numerical score can be obtained by measuring index teeth alone, but dentists and hygienists are obligated to demonstrate to their patients the location of dental plaque on all surfaces of all teeth. When used, indices should be appropriate to the patient's age group and needs. In small children the simple plaque index of Löe (1967) may be quick and effective in revealing gross plaque bulk, whereas in teenagers the practitioner may want to pinpoint areas pertinent to gingival and periodontal diseases, employing more sensitive indices such as those of Podshadley and Haley (1968), Turesky et al. (1970) or others.

Individual and community programs for the promotion of periodontal health in children

Significant improvements in oral hygiene and oral hygiene awareness have been noted in many (mainly industrialized) countries. The majority of people recognize the benefit of oral health and the contributory role of oral hygiene. Clean teeth have become an integral part of Westernized urban society, alongside weight control, jogging, cessation of smoking, healthy diet practices, and generally increased health awareness (Löe, 1999). It is the belief of this chapter's authors that the improvement in oral health, with reductions in both dental caries and periodontal disease, in many countries (including the USA), is due not only to fluoride use but also to improved oral hygiene.

This chapter has focused on the role of oral hygiene improvement in gingival and periodontal health promotion among children. Research in recent years has demonstrated an inescapable association between smoking and periodontal disease (Goultschin et al., 1990; Akef et al., 1992; Thomson MR et al., 1993; Machuca et al., 2000; Bergstrom et al., 2000). Smoking is an addictive habit, initiated in adolescence and even childhood, with strong psychological and sociological contributing factors. Once started the addiction is extremely difficult to end. Avoidance of smoking, therefore, needs to be included as an integral component of dental and periodontal health education efforts from an early age.

The problems

The problems of initiating and implementing community programs of oral hygiene promotion for children are numerous. As in all of medicine, diagnosis of the problems is a major step in identifying the solutions:

- Most people in Westernized countries possess toothbrushes and most people exercise some degree of oral hygiene, but wide variations exist in the levels of dental cleanliness attained (Löe, 1999).
- Considerable differences exist between and within countries as to the emphasis placed on oral hygiene, owing to different traditions, cultures, and social atmosphere (Gift, 1993; Ronis et al., 1998).
- The basic premise of public health is the "herd" concept. Individuals living in a community not conducive to oral hygiene

promotion will find it difficult to modify their own behavior.
- Children at a young age possess inadequate manual dexterity for optimal tooth brushing. This, however, improves with age (Unkel et al., 1995).
- Establishment of optimal oral care home habits involves modifications in lifestyle, priorities, and other factors associated with an already full daily schedule (Renvert and Glavind, 1998).
- Parents need to set aside time and effort, not only for their own oral hygiene, but also for that of their young children.
- Many parents are not aware that children's teeth should be cleaned at an early age. Brushing teeth before the age of 1 year appeared, at first, to be an unrealistic objective for public health nurses participating in a Jerusalem oral health promotion program for infants (Sgan-Cohen, 1997).
- Most children predominantly brush the occlusal and buccal surfaces of the anterior teeth. Posterior and lingual surfaces are often neglected (Simmons et al., 1983; Honkala et al., 1986).
- Many children brush quickly and not for the time required for optimal hygiene (Honkala et al., 1986).
- For many children, and even some adults, brushing the palatinal dental areas causes a gag reflex.
- Very few individuals, especially young children, pay any attention to interdental cleaning (Löe, 1999).
- There have been many organized community efforts at oral hygiene improvement, but few of them have been successful (Feldman et al., 1988; Russell et al., 1989; Rayner, 1992; van Palenstein et al., 1997; Bartold et al., 1998).
- When community efforts have been successful, there has been a marked regression to former inferior oral hygiene, in the absence of reinforcement efforts, after the program's termination (Anaise and Zilkah, 1976).
- Patients in general and children in particular often fail to be able to see dental plaque and the accompanying symptoms of gingivitis.
- Plaque disclosing solutions are often messy (especially if used in the classroom) and are not practical in a daily, lifelong regimen. They often dye most of the mouth (especially erythrosine),

making it no easier for an unprofessional eye to detect where the real plaque is present. Moreover, the large extent of the staining can discourage the patient as to the feasibility of successfully cleaning all the plaque.

- The more effective tooth-brushing methods and use of interdental cleaning devices are difficult for most young children to master (Löe, 1999).
- Electric toothbrushes are not affordable for everyone.
- In the presence of optimal daily fluoride exposure, many members of the dental profession are unconvinced of the importance of oral hygiene promotion among children.
- Oral hygiene instruction by dentists or dental hygienists is not inexpensive.

Summary of recommendations

Individual efforts

- Oral hygiene, from the earliest age, should be an integral part of total body hygiene.
- Parents should initiate brushing with the eruption of the child's first tooth. From about the age of 2–3 years, children should be encouraged to clean their own teeth, at the same age that they start bathing themselves.
- Begin cleaning with the smallest toothbrush, employing the simplest horizontal scrub method.
- Children should be encouraged to brush teeth together with their parents.
- Good oral routines have to be established early in life.
- Oral hygiene instructions should be simple and easy to adopt.
- Cleaning instructions should emphasize the brushing duration—at least 2 minutes (Honkala et al., 1986).
- Easier systems for self-inspection and identification of plaque need to be devised and evaluated (Baab and Weinstein, 1983).
- Dentists and hygienists should demonstrate plaque to children without using disclosing solutions. The gingival margins and proximal areas should be emphasized. The child should be shown how to detect plaque by employing a simple toothpick. There seems no reason why dentists and hygienists can see plaque and patients cannot. The same can be said for the first symptoms of gingivitis.

- The detection of plaque by the patient and duration of brushing are more important than elaborate brushing techniques.
- Dental educators should stress to children the importance of the posterior and lingual dental surfaces. This is best demonstrated in the patient's own mouth; an artificial mouth model, as the next best system, should only be used when a personal oral demonstration cannot be performed.
- Mouth rinses, as adjuncts to tooth brushing, should only be recommended when regular brushing does not succeed in achieving optimal hygiene. Rinsing should only be recommended to older children, under supervision, avoiding swallowing.
- Tooth cleaning needs to be emphasized as an integral component of general personal hygiene and grooming. This is especially important for adolescents.
- Avoidance of smoking has to be identified by the dental team as an important contributing factor to dental and periodontal disease. This message needs to be stressed to child, adolescent and young adult patients.

Community efforts

- Early clinical detection of periodontal pocketing is of paramount importance in detecting high-risk groups. Community screening programs should be considered.
- Once detected, high-risk groups require intense and continuing therapy. This includes optimal mechanical oral hygiene efforts, together with the use of chemical agents, antibiotic therapy, and clinical treatment (calculus removal, root planing, etc.) when needed.
- For the general population, a "whole population strategy" is strongly advised (Rose, 1993). A population strategy aims to "reduce the plaque level of the whole population; moving the distribution curve to the left" (Sheiham, 1990). This strategy will, in general, promote health, because there are more low-risk people than high-risk people. It has to be remembered that the concept of "low risk" is relative. People at low risk are by definition still "at risk". Moreover, many are in reality at high risk but have not been diagnosed as

such. The procedures for high-risk periodontal disease diagnosis are complicated, often expensive and not always of high sensitivity and specificity (Johnson, 1991).

- In order to reach as much of the population as possible, public health programs should be developed within a coherent, comprehensive, and explicit national and community-based health policy (Schou, 1998). Educational approaches must be adapted to the different needs and stages of behavior change among different sub-groups of the population (Sheiham, 1990).
- Concepts of oral health and care awareness in each community are important and need to be improved. The oral hygiene of individuals is closely integrated with that of the larger group within which they live. Therefore community and national programs, policies, and a generally positive oral health "atmosphere" are of paramount importance.
- In the education of dental professionals, the importance of oral hygiene in preventing both caries and periodontal disease must be emphasized.
- Non-dental education and health professionals (kindergarten and school teachers, nurses, health educators, etc.) should be supplied with the materials and knowledge to provide basic information and guidance on oral hygiene promotion. One does not need a dentist or hygienist to explain the importance of cleaning the proximal, posterior, and lingual surfaces of teeth.
- It is advised to supply free toothbrushes to children. These "gifts" have been shown to be an effective incentive for increased oral hygiene behavior (Torpaz et al., 1984; Sgan-Cohen, 1997).
- Oral hygiene education should be included within the regular health education curricula of the general education system.
- The mass media should be involved. Televised toothpaste commercials have probably contributed more to caries prevention than much of the dental profession, and this avenue should also be explored in oral hygiene promotion. National governmental health agencies should provide appropriate incentives to commercial organizations.
- The earlier the intervention, the more effective is the result (Sheiham, 1990). It is advised to start oral hygiene education in mother and child health centers and programs (Sgan-Cohen, 1997).
- Community, public, and health staff should all participate in the planning, formulation, implementation, and evaluation of a community program.
- A community atmosphere of positive reinforcement for improved oral hygiene should be fostered. This is a more difficult goal, but it cannot be ignored.
- Smoking is an addiction with strong social undertones. All community efforts, aimed at promoting dental and periodontal health, need to stress the importance of avoiding this harmful habit.

References

Achong RA, Briskie DM, Hildebrandt GH et al. (1999) Effect of chlorhexidine varnish mouthguards on the levels of selected oral microorganisms in pediatric patients. *Pediatr Dent* **21**: 169–75.

Addy M, Willis L, Moran J (1983) Effect of toothpaste rinses compared with chlorhexidine on plaque formation during a 4–day period. *J Clin Periodontol* **10**: 89–99.

Akef J, Weine FS, Weissman DP (1992) The role of smoking in the progression of periodontal disease: A literature review. *Compend Contin Educ Dent* **13**: 526–30.

American Academy of Pediatric Dentistry (1999) Periodicity of examination, preventive dental services, and oral treatment for children. *Pediatr Dent* (special issue: Reference Manual) **21**: 79.

Anaise JZ (1975) The toothbrush in plaque removal. ASDC *J Dent Child* **42**: 186–9.

Anaise JZ, Zilkah E (1976) Effectiveness of a dental education program on oral cleanliness of school children in Israel. *Commun Dent Oral Epidemiol* **4**: 186–9.

Anderson RJ (1981) The changes in dental health of 12-year-old school children in two Somerset schools. A review after an interval of 15 years. *Br Dent J* **150**: 218–21.

Anderson RJ, Bradnock G, Beal JF, James PMC (1982) The reduction of dental caries prevalence in English schoolchildren. *J Dent Res* **61**: 1311–16.

Anderson GB, Bowden J, Morrison EC, Caffesse RG (1997) Clinical effects of chlorhexidine mouthwashes on patients undergoing orthodontic treatment. *Am J Orthod Dentofac Orthop* **111**: 606–12.

Axelsson P, Lindhe J (1974) The effect of a preventive program on dental plaque, gingivitis and caries in school children. Results after one and two years. *J Clin Periodontol* **1**: 126–38.

Axelsson P, Lindhe J (1978) Effect of controlled oral hygiene procedures on caries and periodontal disease in adults. *J Clin Periodontol* **5**: 133–51.

Axelsson P, Lindhe J, Nyström B (1991) On the prevention of caries and periodontal disease. Results of a 15-year-longitudinal study in adults. *J Clin Periodontol* **13**: 182–9.

Baab DA, Weinstein P (1983) Oral hygiene instruction using a self inspection plaque index. *Commun Dent Oral Epidemiol* **11**: 174–9.

Babaahmady KG, Challacombe SJ, Marsh PD, Newman HN (1998) Ecological study of Streptococcus mutans, Streptococcus sobrinus and Lactobacillus spp. At subsites from approximal dental plaque from children. *Caries Res* **32**: 51–8.

Banoczy J, Szoke J, Kertesz P et al. (1989) Effect of amine fluoride/stannous fluoride containing toothpaste and mouthrinsings on dental plaque, gingivitis, plaque and enamel F-accumulation. *Caries Res* **23**: 284–8.

Barnes CM, Russel CM, Weatherford TW (1999) A comparison of the efficacy of 2 powered toothbrushes in affecting plaque accumulation, gingivitis, and gingival bleeding. *J Periodontol* **70**: 840–7.

Bartold PM, Seymour GJ, Cullinan MP, Westerman B (1998) Effect of increased community and professional awareness of plaque control on the management of inflammatory periodontal diseases. *Int Dent J* **48**: 282–9.

Bay LM, Rölla G (1980) Plaque inhibition and improved gingival condition by use of a stannous fluoride toothpaste. *Scand J Dent Res* **88**: 313–15.

Bellini HT, Arneberg P, von der Fehr FR (1980) Oral hygiene and caries. *Acta Odontol Scand* **39**: 257–65.

Bergstrom J, Eliasson S, Dock J (2000) Exposure to tobacco smoking and periodontal health. *J Periodontol* **27**: 61–8.

Bonesvoll P, Gjermo P (1978) A comparison between chlorhexidine and some quaternary ammonium compounds with regard to retention, salivary concentration and plaque inhibiting effect in the human mouth after mouthrinses. *Arch Oral Biol* **27**: 861–8.

Bosman CW, Powell RN (1977) The reversal of localized experimental gingivitis. *J Clin Periodontol* **4**: 161–72.

Boyd RL, Chun YS (1994) Eighteen-month evaluation of the effects of a 0.4% stannous fluoride gel on gingivitis in orthodontic patients. *Am J Orthodont Dentofac Orthoped* **105**: 35–41.

Brauer JC, Demeritt WM, Higley LB et al. (1958) *Dentistry for Children*. New York: McGraw-Hill.

Brecx M, Theilade J, Attström R (1980) Influence of optimal and excluded oral hygiene on early formation of dental plaque on plastic films. *J Clin Periodontol* **7**: 361–73.

British Dental Association (1997) Fact files: Toothbrushes and toothbrushing. *Fact Files*, September. London: BDA.

British Health Education Authority (1997) *Effectiveness of Oral Health Promotion*. Health Promotion Effectiveness reviews, Summary Bulletin 7. London: Health Education Authority.

Brown LJ, Oliver RC, Löe H (1989) Periodontal diseases in the U.S. in 1981: prevalence, severity, extent, and role in tooth mortality. *J Periodontol* **60**: 363–70.

Brucker M (1943) Studies on the incidence and cause of dental defects in children. III. Gingivitis. *J Dent Res* **22**: 309–14.

Brunelle JA, Carlos JP (1982) Changes in the prevalence of dental caries in US schoolchildren 1961–1982. *J Dent Res* **61**: 1346–51.

Bruun C, Ekstrand KR, Andreasen KB (1998) A new in vitro method for testing the interproximal cleaning potential of toothbrushing. *J Clin Dent* **9**: 11–15.

Burt BA (1978) *The relative efficiency of methods of caries prevention in dental public health*. Proceedings of a workshop at the University of Michigan. Ann Arbor: University of Michigan.

Charters WJ (1932) Eliminating mouth infections with the toothbrush and other stimulating instruments. *Dent Dig* **38**: 130–6.

Clerehugh V, Laryea U, Worthington HV (1995) Periodontal condition and comparison of toothcleaning using chewing sticks and toothbrushes in 14-year-old schoolchildren in Ghana. *Commun Dent Oral Epidemiol* **23**: 319–20.

Clerehugh V, Williams P, Shaw WC et al. (1998) A practice-based randomised controlled trial of the efficacy of an electric and a manual toothbrush on gingival health in patients with fixed orthodontic appliances. *J Dent* **26**: 633–9.

Cubells AB, Dalmau LB, Petrone ME et al. (1991) The effect of a triclosan/polymer/fluoride dentifrice on plaque formation and gingivitis: a six month clinical study. *J Clin Dent* **2**: 63–9.

Cummins D (1991) Zinc citrate/triclosan: a new anti-plaque system for the control of plaque and the prevention of gingivitis: short-term clinical and mode of action studies. *J Clin Periodontol* **18**: 455–61.

Cutress TW (1986) Periodontal health and disease in young people: global epidemiology. *Int Dent J* **36**: 146–51.

Dale JW (1969) Toothbrushing frequency and its relationship to dental caries and periodontal disease. *Austr Dent J* **14**: 120–3.

Danser MM, Timmerman MF, Ijzerman Y et al. (1998) Evaluation of the incidence of gingival abrasion as a result of toothbrushing. *J Clin Periodontol* **25**: 701–6.

Deasy MJ, Battisda G, Rustogi KN, Volpe AR (1992) Antiplaque efficacy of a triclosan/copolymer pre-brush rinse: a plaque prevention clinical trial. *Am J Dent* **5**: 91–4.

Denepitiya JL, Fine D, Singh SM et al. (1992) Effect upon plaque formation and gingivitis of a triclosan/copolymer/fluoride dentifrice. A 6-month clinical study. *Am J Dent* **5**: 307–11.

Douglass CW, Gillings D, Sollecito W, Gammon M (1983) National trends in the prevalence and severity of the periodontal diseases. *J Am Dent Assoc* **107**: 403–12.

Downer MC (1984) Changing patterns in the western world. In: Guggenheim B (ed.) *Cariology Today*. Basel: Karger.

Ellwood RP, Worthington HV, Blinkhorn ASB et al. (1998) Effect of a triclosan/copolymer dentifrice on the incidence of periodontal attachment loss in adolescents. *J Clin Periodontol* **25**: 363–7.

Emilson CG, Gisselsson H, Birkhed D (1999) Recolonisation pattern of mutans streptococci after suppression by three modes of chlorhexidine gel application. *Eur J Oral Sci* **107**: 170–5.

Ericsson T, Ericsson Y (1967) The effect of partial fluoride substitution of the phosphate change and protein adsorption of hydroxylapatite. *Acta Ondontol Helv* **11**: 10–4.

Feldman CA, Bentley JM, Oler J (1988) The rural dental health program: long-term impact of two dental delivery systems on children's oral health. *J Publ Health Dent* **48**: 201–7.

Fischman SL (1997) The history of oral hygiene products: how far have we come in 6000 years? *Periodontology* **15**: 7–14.

Frazier PJ (1980) School-based instruction for improving oral health: closing the knowledge gap. *Int Dent J* **30**: 257–68.

Frode Hansen B, Bjertness E, Gjermo P (1990) Changes in periodontal disease indicators in 35-year-old Oslo citizens from 1973 to 1984. *J Clin Periodontol* **17**: 249–54.

Genco R, Picozzi A (1986) Workshop reports and recommendations–antimicrobials. In: Löe H, Kleinman DV (eds) *Dental Plaque Control Measures and Oral Hygiene Practices*. Oxford: IRL Press, pp. 256–61.

Gibson MT, Wade AB (1977) Plaque removal by Bass and roll brushing techniques. *J Periodontol* **48**: 456–9.

Gift HC (1993) Social factors in oral health promotion, In: Schou L, Blinkhorn AS (eds) *Oral Health Promotion*. Oxford: Oxford Medical.

Gjermo P, Saxton CA (1991) Antibacterial dentifrices. Clinical data and relevance with emphasis on zinc/triclosan. *J Clin Periodontol* **18**: 468–73.

Glantz PO (1969) On wetability and adhesiveness. A study of enamel, dentine, some restorative materials and dental plaque. *Odontol Rev* **20** (suppl 17): 1–32.

Goultschin J, Sgan-Cohen HD, Donchin M et al. (1990) Association of smoking with periodontal treatment needs. *J Periodontol* **61**: 364–7.

Greene JC, Vermillion JR (1960) The oral hygiene index; a method for classifying oral hygiene status. *J Am Dent Assoc* **61**: 172–9.

Hamp SE, Johanssen LA (1982) Dental prophylaxis for youths in their late teens. *J Clin Periodontol* **9**: 22–34.

Heasman PA, McCracken GI (1999) Powered toothbrushes: a review of clinical trials. *J Clin Periodontol* **26**: 407–20.

Honkala E, Nyyssönen V, Knuuttila M, Markkanen H (1986) Effectiveness of children's habitual toothbrushing. *J Clin Periodontol* **13**: 81–5.

Honkala E, Kannas L, Rise J (1990) Oral health habits of schoolchildren in 11 European countries. *Int Dent J* **40**: 211–17.

Horowitz HS (1980) Established methods of prevention. *Br Dent J* **149**: 311–18.

Horowitz AM, Frazier PJ (1986) Effective oral health programs in school settings. In: Clark JW (ed.) *Clinical Dentistry*, vol. 2. Philadelphia: Harper & Row, pp. 1–15.

Horowitz AM, Suomi JD, Peterson JK, Lyman BA (1977) Effects of supervised daily dental plaque removal by children: II. 24 months' results. *J Publ Health Dent* **3**: 180–8.

Hugoson A, Koch G, Bergendal T et al. (1986) Oral health of individuals aged 3–80 years in Jonkoping, Sweden, in 1973 and 1983. II. A review of clinical and radiographic findings. *Swed Dent J* **10**: 175–94.

Jackson RD, Kelly SA, Katz B et al. (1999) Dental fluorosis in children residing in communities with different water fluoride levels: 33-month follow-up. *Pediatr Dent* **21**: 248–54.

Johnson NW (1991) *Risk markers for oral diseases. Vol. 3. Periodontal diseases. Part 2. Methods for the characterization of high risk groups and individuals*. Cambridge University Press.

Kelner RM, Wohl BR, Deasy MJ, Formicola AJ (1974) Gingival inflammation as related to frequency of plaque removal. *J Periodontol* **45**: 302–7.

Klatsky M (1937) A comparative analysis of masticatory function and its relation to dental disease in ancient and in modern man. *J Am Dent Assoc* **24**: 932–42.

Kleemola-Kujala E (1978) Oral hygiene and its relationship to caries prevalence in Finnish rural children. *Proc Finn Dent Soc* **74**: 76–85.

Kleemola-Kujala E, Räsänen L (1982) Relationship of oral hygiene and sugar consumption to risk of caries in children. *Commun Dent Oral Epidemiol* **10**: 224–33.

Klein SP, Bohannan HM, Bell RM et al. (1985) The cost effectiveness of school-based preventive dental care. *Am J Publ Health* **75**: 382–94.

Kornman KS (1986) Antimicrobial agents. In: Löe H, Kleinman DV (eds) *Dental Plaque Control Measures and Oral Hygiene Practices*. Washington: IRL Press, pp. 121–42.

Kuusela S, Honkala E, Kannas L et al. (1997) Oral hygiene habits of 11-year-old schoolchildren in 22 European countries and Canada in 1993/1994. *J Dent Res* **76**: 1602–9.

Laher A, Cleaton-Jones PE (1996) Chlorhexidine rinsing in physically handicapped pupils in Katlehong. *J Dent Assoc S Afr* **51**: 343–6.

Lang NP, Cumming BR, Löe H (1973) Toothbrushing frequency as it relates to plaque development and gingival health. *J Periodontol* **44**: 396–405.

Lang NP, Attström R, Löe H (1998) *Proceedings of the European Workshop on Mechanical Plaque Control*. Berlin: Quintessence.

Levy-Polack MP, Sebelli P, Polack NL (1998) Incidence of oral complications and application of a preventive protocol in children with acute leukemia. *Spec Care Dent* **18**: 189–93.

Lindhe J, Rosling B, Socransky SS, Volpe AR (1993) The effect of triclosan-containing dentifrice on established plaque and gingivitis. *J Clin Periodontol* **20**: 327–34.

Lobene RR, Kashket S, Soparkar PM et al. (1979) The effect of cetylpyridinium chloride on human plaque bacteria and gingivitis. *Pharmacol Therapeut Dent* **4**: 33–47.

Lobene RR, Pramod MS, Soparkar M, Newman MB (1986) The effects of a sanguinaria dentifrice on plaque and gingivitis. *Compend Contin Educ Dent* **7** (suppl): 185–8.

Löe H (1967) The gingival index, the plaque index and the retention index systems. *J Periodontol* **38**: 610–16.

Löe H (1999) Oral hygiene in the prevention of caries and periodontal disease. In: *The FDI's Second World Conference on Oral Health Promotion: Core Messages in Oral Health Education*. London: FDI.

Löe H, Holm Pedersen P (1965) Absence and presence of fluid from normal and inflamed gingiva. *Periodontology* **3**: 171–7.

Löe H, Theilade E, Jensen SB (1965) Experimental gingivitis in man. *J Periodontol* **36**: 177–87.

Löe H, Theilade E, Jensen SB (1967) Experimental gingivitis in man. III. The influence of antibiotics on gingival plaque development. *J Periodontol Res* **2**: 282–9.

Löe H, von der Fehr FR, Schiött CR (1972) Inhibition of experimental caries by plaque prevention. *Scand J Dent Res* **80**: 1–9.

Macgregor ID, Regis D, Balding J (1997) Self-concept and dental health behaviours in adolescents. *J Clin Periodontol* **24**: 335–9.

Machuca G, Rosales I, Lacalle JR et al. (2000) Effect of cigarette smoking on periodontal status of healthy young adults. *J Periodontol* **71**: 73–8.

Mackler SB, Crawford JJ (1973) Plaque development and gingivitis in the primary dentition. *J Periodontol* **44**: 18–24.

Mankodi S, Ross NM, Mostler K (1987) Clinical efficacy of listerine in inhibiting and reducing plaque and experimental gingivitis. *J Clin Periodontol* **14**: 285–8.

Mattila ML, Paunio P, Rautava P et al. (1998) Changes in dental health and dental health habits from 3 to 5 years of age. *J Publ Health Dent* **58**: 270–4.

Mattson L (1978) Development of gingivitis in preschool children and young adults. A comparative experimental study. *J Clin Periodontol* **5**: 24–34.

McCall JP (1933) The periodontist looks at children's dentistry. *J Am Dent Assoc* **20**: 1518–21.

McClure DB (1966) Comparison of toothbrushing technics for the preschool child. *ASDC J Dent Child* **33**: 205–10.

McKenzie IC, Nuki K, Löe H, Schiött CR (1976) Two years of oral use of chlorhexidine in man. V. Effects on stratum corneum of oral mucosa. *J Periodontol Res* **11**: 165–71.

Morita M, Nishi K, Watanabe T (1998) Comparison of 2 toothbrush methods for efficacy in supragingival plaque removal. The Toothpick method and the Bass method. *J Clin Periodontol* **25**: 829–31.

Nowak A, Crall J (1994) Prevention of dental disease. In: Pinkham JR (ed.) *Pediatric Dentistry: Infancy Through Adolescence*, 2nd edn. Philadelphia: WB Saunders, pp. 192–208, 278–86, 445–50, 576–80.

Nuki K, Schlenker R, Löe H, Schiött CR (1976) Two years oral use of chlorhexidine in man. VI. Effect on oxidative enzymes in oral epithelia. *J Periodontol Res* **11**: 172–5.

Ögaard B, Larsson E, Glans R et al. (1997) Antimicrobial effect of a chlorhexidine-thymol varnish (Cervitec) in orthodontic patients. A prospective, randomized clinical trial. *J Orofac Orthop* **58**: 206–13.

Pilot T (1998) The periodontal disease problem. A comparison between industrialised and developing countries. *Int Dent J* **48** (suppl 1): 221–32.

Podshadley AG, Haley JV (1968) A method for evaluating oral hygiene performance. *Publ Health Rep* **83**: 259–64.

Ramfjord SP (1959) Indices for prevalence and incidence of periodontal disease. *J Periodontol* **30**: 51–9.

Ramfjord SP, Knowles JW, Nissle RR (1973) Longitudinal study of periodontal therapy. *J Periodontol* **44**: 66–77.

Rayner JA (1992) A dental health education programme, including home visits, for nursery school children. *Br Dent J* **172**: 57–62.

Renvert S, Glavind L (1998) Individualized instruction and compliance in oral hygiene practices. Recommendations and means of delivery. In: Lang NP, Attström R, Löe H (eds) *Proceedings of the European Workshop on Mechanical Plaque Removal*. Berlin: Quintessence. 300–9.

Robinson E (1976) A comparative evaluation of the scrub and Bass methods of toothbrushing with flossing as an adjunct (in fifth and sixth graders). *Am J Publ Health* **66**: 1078–81.

Rodrigues CR, Ando T, Singer JM, Issao M (1996) The effect of training on the ability of children to use dental floss. *ASDC J Dent Child* **63**: 39–41.

Rölla G, Melsen B (1975) On the mechanism of the plaque inhibition by chlorhexidine. *J Dent Res* **54**: 57–62.

Ronis DL, Lang WP, Antonakos CL, Borgnakke WS (1998) Preventive oral health behaviors among African-Americans. *J Publ Health Dent* **58**: 234–40.

Rose G (1993) The population strategy of prevention. In: *The Strategy of Preventive Medicine*. Oxford University Press.

Russell BA, Horowitz AM, Frazier PJ (1989) School-based preventive regimens and oral health knowledge and practices of sixth graders. *J Publ Health Dent* **49**: 192–200.

Sahota H, Landini G, Walmsley AD (1998) A testing system for electric toothbrushes. *Am J Dent* **11**: 271–5.

Sangnes G (1974) Effectiveness of vertical and horizontal toothbrushing in the removal of plaque. II. Comparison of brushing by six-year-old children and their parents. *ASDC J Dent Child* **41**: 119–23.

Sanz M, Vallcorba N, Fabregues S et al. (1994) The effect of a dentifrice containing chlorhexidine and zinc on plaque, gingivitis, calculus and tooth staining. *J Clin Periodontol* **21**: 431–7.

Saxer UP, Yankell SL (1997) Impact of improved toothbrushes on dental disease. *Quintess Int* **28**: 573–93.

Saxton CA, Lane RM, van der Ouderaa F (1987) The effects of a dentifrice containing a zinc salt and a non-cationic antimicrobial agent on plaque and gingivitis. *J Clin Periodontol* **14**: 144–48.

Schou L (1998) Behavioral aspects of dental plaque control measures. An oral health promotion perspective. In: Lang NP, Attström R, Löe H (eds) *Proceedings of the European Workshop on Mechanical Plaque Removal*. Berlin: Quintessence. 287–99.

Sgan-Cohen HD (1997) Healthy teeth for infants—a mother and child community oral health program in Jerusalem. *Sixth World Congress on Preventive Dentistry*, Cape Town, South Africa.

Sgan-Cohen HD, Babayof I, Zadik D, Mann J (1995) One month evaluation of the manually rotating "Bio-Bright" toothbrush for clinical safety and efficacy. *J Clin Dent* **6**: 120–3.

Sgan-Cohen HD, Gat E, Schwartz Z (1996) The effectiveness of an amine fluoride/stannous fluoride dentifrice on the gingival health of teenagers: results after six months. *Int Dent J* **46**: 340–5.

Shapira J, Sgan-Cohen HD, Stabholz A et al. (1994) Clinical and microbiological effects of chlorhexidine and arginine sustained-release varnishes in the mentally retarded. *Spec Care Dent* **14**: 158–63.

Sheiham A (1990) *Public Health Approaches to the Promotion of Periodontal Health*. Monograph Series no. 3. London: University College.

Sheiman A (1983) Promoting periodontal health–effective programmes of education and promotion. *Int Dent J* **33**: 182–7.

Sheiham A, Smales FC, Cushing AM, Cowell CR (1986) Changes in periodontal health in a cohort of British workers over a 14-year period. *Br Dent J* **160**: 125–7.

Shern RJ, Swing KW, Crawford JJ (1970) Prevention of plaque formation by organic fluorides. *J Oral Med* **25**: 93–7.

Simmons S, Smith R, Gelbier S (1983) Effect of oral hygiene instruction on brushing skills in preschoolchildren. *Commun Dent Oral Epidemiol* **11**: 193–9.

Stanymeyer WR (1957) A measure of tissue response to frequency of toothbrushing. *J Periodontol* **28**: 17–22.

Steelman R, Holmes D, Hamilton M (1996) Chlorhexidine spray effects on plaque accumulation in developmentally disabled patients. *J Clin Pediatr Dent* **20**: 333–6.

Stevens AM, Maes L, Peeters R (1992) Dental hygiene in 10-to-18-year-old youths in Flanders. *Rev Belg Med Dent* **47**: 51–6.

Svatun B, Saxton CA, Huntington E, Cummins D (1993) The effects of three silica dentifrices containing triclosan on supragingival plaque and calculus and on gingivitis. *Int Dent J* **43**: 441–52.

Theilade E, Wright WH, Jensen SB, Löe H (1966) Experimental gingivitis in man. II. A longitudinal clinical and bacteriological investigation. *J Periodontol Res* **1**: 1–13.

Thomson MR, Garito ML, Brown FH (1993) The role of smoking in periodontal diseases: A review of the literature. *Periodontal Abstracts* **41**: 5–9.

Tinanoff N (1995) Progress regarding the use of stannous fluoride in dentistry. *J Clin Dent* (special issue) **6**: 37–40.

Tinanoff N, Hock J, Camosci D, Hellden L (1980) Effect of stannous fluoride mouthrinse on dental plaque formation. *J Clin Periodontol* **7**: 232–41.

Torpaz E, Noam Y, Anaise JZ, Sgan-Cohen HD (1984) Effectiveness of dental health educational programs on oral cleanliness of school children in Israel. *Dent Hyg* April: 169–73.

Tureskey S, Gilmore ND, Glickman J (1970) Reduced plaque formation by chloromethyl analogue of Vitamin C. *J Periodontol* **41**: 41–3.

Unkel JH, Fenton SJ, Hobbs G, Frere CL (1995) Toothbrushing ability is related to age in children. *ASDC J Dent Child* **62**: 346–8.

Valente MI, Seabra G, Chiesa C et al. (1996) Effects of a chlorhexidine varnish on the gingival status of adolescents. *J Can Dent Assoc* **62**: 46–8.

Van Palenstein Helderman WH, Munck L, Mushendwa S et al. (1997) Effect evaluation of an oral health education programme in primary schools in Tanzania. *Commun Dent Oral Epidemiol* **25**: 296–300.

Volpe AR, Petrone ME, DeVizio W et al. (1996) A review of plaque, gingivitis, calculus and caries clinical efficacy studies with a fluoride dentifrice containing triclosan and PVM/MA copolymer. *J Clin Dent* **7** (suppl): S1–14.

Wallace JS (1935) Deficiency diseases, protective foods and dental caries. *J Am Dent Assoc* **22**: 1334–43.

Wejden GV, van der Timmerman MF, Danser MM, van der Velden U (1998) The role of electrical toothbrushes: advantages and limitations. In: Lang NP, Attström R, Löe H (eds) *Proceedings of the European Workshop on Mechanical Plaque Removal*. Berlin: Quintessence. 138–55.

Worthington HV, Davies RM, Blinkhorn AS et al. (1993) A six-month clinical study of the effect of a pre-brush rinse on plaque removal and gingivitis. *Br Dent J* **175**: 322–6.

Yankell SL, Shi X, Emling RC, Harris M (1998) Laboratory evaluation of the Reach tooth and gum toothbrush and three additional manual toothbrushes for subgingival access. *J Clin Dent* **9**: 1–4.

Zickert I, Emilson CG, Krasse B (1982) Effects of caries preventive measures in children highly infected with the bacterium streptococcus mutans. *Arch Oral Biol* **27**: 861–8.

Zimmer S, Didner B, Roulet JF (1999) Clinical study on the plaque-removing ability of a new triple-headed toothbrush. *J Clin Periodontol* **26**: 281–5.

11

Treatment of gingival and periodontal diseases

Gary C. Armitage

Importance of early diagnosis

Routine periodontal examination

Epidemiologic studies have established that children, adolescents, and young adults can develop many forms of plaque-induced periodontal infections (Bhat, 1991; Noar and Portnoy, 1991; Aass et al., 1994; Bimstein et al., 1994; Clerehugh et al., 1995; Armitage and Van Dyke, 1996; Papapanou, 1996). Since effective treatment of these infections often depends on early detection and diagnosis, it is important that young people routinely receive periodontal examinations.

In adults, a periodontal examination includes visual inspection of the gingival tissues for signs of inflammation, abnormal contours, and mucogingival deformities. A complete periodontal examination requires measurement and recording of probing depths, clinical attachment loss, presence of furcation involvements, mobility, and other information that may be useful in making a diagnosis and formulating a treatment plan. In addition, intraoral radiographs can provide important information about the periodontium that cannot otherwise be easily obtained, such as root length, root form, presence of periapical lesions, and estimates of the amount of alveolar bone loss (Armitage, 1996). During the examination the presence and location of probable etiologic factors such as plaque, calculus, and defective restorations should also be noted.

In small children with only primary teeth and some adolescents with mixed dentition, modifications in periodontal examination procedures may be required. Although periodontal probing is the most reliable way of assessing periodontal

damage (Armitage, 1995), some children may not tolerate the slight discomfort involved. In such cases, it may be necessary to limit inspection of the gingiva to visual and radiographic findings. When this compromise is made, it is important to realize that important diagnostic information may be missed; it is therefore recommended that periodontal probing should be attempted in all children. If it is done gently, most children will tolerate the procedure. Nevertheless, if periodontal probing cannot be done, bite-wing radiographs can provide a good assessment of the presence or absence of early alveolar bone loss in children (Bimstein et al., 1988; Cogen et al., 1992; Sjödin et al., 1993; Sjödin and Matsson, 1994).

For children with primary teeth only it is usually not necessary to record in the child's dental chart probing depths at six sites per tooth (mesiobuccal, buccal, distobuccal, mesiolingual, lingual, distolingual) as is routine for adult patients. It is usually sufficient to write in the chart, "No probing depths greater than 2 mm" or a similar summary statement.

In children who have a mixed dentition with several erupting teeth, probing depths greater than 3 mm may indicate "pseudopocketing" rather than true loss of attachment. Probing depths of 4–5 mm around erupting permanent teeth are frequently found and are not necessarily a sign of periodontal damage. In such cases, radiographs are useful in determining if there is associated bone loss. It is important that sites with excessive probing depths be carefully inspected at subsequent visits to determine if there is periodontal damage. Adolescents and young adults who are well past the mixed dentition stage should receive the same type of periodontal examination as adults.

Types of gingival and periodontal infections

Plaque-induced periodontal infections in young people can be placed into five general categories:

- chronic gingivitis
- necrotizing ulcerative gingivitis
- aggressive periodontitis
- chronic periodontitis
- periodontitis associated with systemic disease.

Chronic gingivitis, or the presence of gingival inflammation without the loss of alveolar bone or clinical attachment, is a common finding in children and adolescents (Ismail et al., 1987; Guile et al., 1990; Ng'ang'a and Valderhaug, 1991; Koloway and Kailis, 1992; Cappelli et al., 1994). Its prevalence varies greatly depending on the method of assessment and the population surveyed (Mann et al., 1981). The importance of gingivitis is that it is a necessary precursor to periodontitis. It is generally believed that although not all cases of gingivitis progress to periodontitis, all cases of periodontitis are preceded by gingivitis (Attström and van der Velden, 1994). Therefore, theoretically it should be possible to prevent periodontitis by effectively treating gingivitis.

Necrotizing ulcerative gingivitis (NUG) is an acute periodontal infection which is now rarely seen in North American and European children under 10 years of age. In these populations, the disease primarily affects young adults and adolescents (Skach et al., 1970; Stevens et al., 1984; Claffey et al., 1986; MacCarthy and Claffey, 1991). In sharp contrast to the prevalence of NUG in North America and Europe, over 50% of cases of the disease in less developed areas of Africa (Sheiham, 1966; Enwonwu, 1972), Asia (Pindborg et al., 1966), and South America (Jiménez and Baer, 1975) occur in children under the age of 10 years. The reason why children in these countries have a higher prevalence of NUG is unknown. However, almost without exception, children who develop the disease have systemic problems such as malnutrition or serious infections (viral or parasitic) that can lead to immunosuppression. The two most significant clinical findings used in the diagnosis of NUG are the presence of interproximal necrosis and

ulceration and the rapid onset of gingival pain (Johnson and Engel, 1986; Armitage and Van Dyke, 1996).

Aggressive periodontitis is a complicated group of periodontal infections that affect children, adolescents, and young adults. Based on clinical characteristics, there are at least two general subgroups of aggressive periodontitis (AP): 1) localized AP and 2) generalized AP (Armitage, 1999). These infections result in the loss of clinical attachment and alveolar bone, but are otherwise clinically distinct. It is likely that each of the subgroups of AP comprises various periodontal infections with different microbiological and pathogenic mechanisms (Albandar et al., 1997).

Based on the conclusions from an international workshop on the classification of periodontal diseases, the term "prepubertal periodontitis" has been discarded since patients previously placed in this category did not have a single disease entity (Armitage, 1999). Indeed, it is now recognized that patients previously given the diagnosis of "prepubertal periodontitis" would more appropriately be categorized as having either chronic periodontitis, AP, or periodontitis associated with systemic disease. Most reported cases of so-called prepubertal periodontitis are probably due to increased susceptibility to infections secondary to certain systemic diseases, particularly those that interfere with neutrophil function (Meyle, 1994). Localized aggressive periodontitis (LAP) primarily affects permanent first molars and incisors of adolescents who have no clinical evidence of systemic disease (Baer, 1971). Some retrospective radiographic data suggest that LAP may start around primary teeth (Sjödin et al., 1993). Genetic analyses indicate that LAP may be a group of diseases with shared clinical characteristics (Boughman et al., 1986; Hart et al., 1993). Many patients with LAP do not form heavy deposits of plaque or calculus and exhibit minimal signs of gingival inflammation (Baer, 1971). Generalized aggressive periodontitis (GAP) affects most teeth and, unlike LAP, individuals with the disease have marked gingival inflammation and heavy deposits of plaque and calculus (Page et al., 1983). Although generally regarded as a disease of young adults, it can begin at or around puberty (Page et al., 1983; Spektor et al., 1985). Longitudinal data suggest that certain forms of untreated LAP may progress to GAP (Brown et al., 1996).

Many forms of AP tend to be more common in certain families and may have a significant genetic component (Van der Velden et al., 1993; Marazita et al., 1994; Hart, 1996; Diehl et al., 1999). Therefore, when individuals with AP are identified, other family members should routinely be examined for the disease. This practice frequently detects individuals with early periodontal damage and facilitates prompt and effective treatment.

Chronic periodontitis is the most common form of periodontitis affecting adults (Papapanou, 1996). Epidemiologic data and clinical experience suggest that this form of periodontitis can also be found in prepubertal children and adolescents (Papapanou, 1996). In children and adolescents, one of the main clinical differences between chronic and aggressive forms of periodontitis is that patients with chronic periodontitis have much less periodontal damage than their age-matched counterparts with AP.

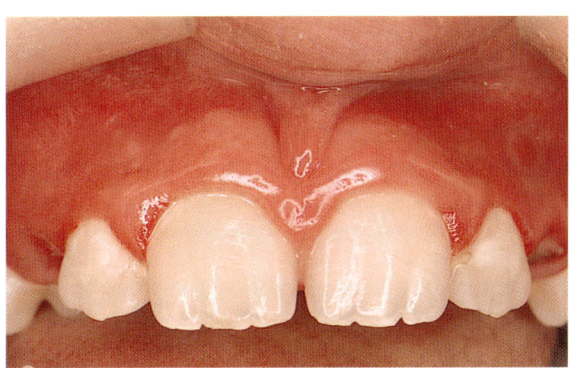

Figure 11.1

Mild chronic gingivitis in an 11-year-old boy. The interproximal gingival tissues exhibit redness and swelling. Management of the gingival disease in this patient required plaque control instructions, cleaning of the teeth, and periodic follow-up. Reprinted with permission from Armitage GC (1986) Periodontal diseases of children and adolescents. *J Calif Dent Assoc* **14** (Dec): 57–61.

Treatment planning

As with all plaque-induced periodontal diseases, treatment is easier and more effective if the diagnosis is made before extensive damage has occurred. The nature and timing of treatment depend on the diagnosis and severity of the disease as well as the overall medical and dental status of the patient. Even in chronic gingivitis, treatment may vary depending on the entire clinical picture. For example, Figure 11.1 shows an uncomplicated case of mild chronic gingivitis in an 11-year-old boy. Effective treatment of this patient required nothing more than plaque control instructions, cleaning of the teeth, and periodic follow-up. This contrasts with the case of the 10-year-old girl shown in Figure 11.2, who also had chronic gingivitis. This patient had a congenital heart defect that required surgical repair. Because the child was chronically ill, her parents and grandparents indulged her with an abundant supply of candy and other sucrose-containing foods. As a result, she developed severe gingivitis with marked inflammatory enlargement of the gingiva and generalized severe dental caries of both primary and permanent teeth. Treatment began with emergency extraction of primary teeth

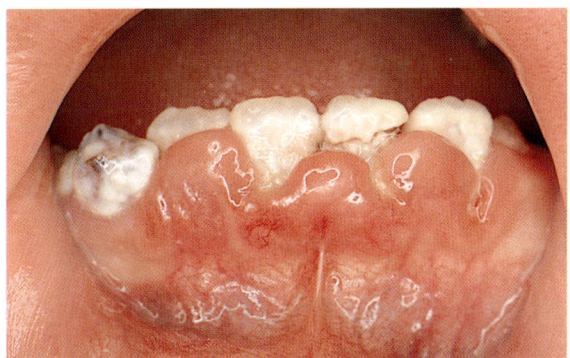

Figure 11.2

Severe chronic gingivitis with inflammatory gingival enlargement in a 10-year-old girl with a congenital heart defect. The patient had a high-sucrose diet and massive caries of her primary and permanent teeth. Initial management of the dental disease in this patient required emergency care, cleaning of the teeth, and provisional restorative care. After recovery from her heart surgery, the patient required a complex series of dental procedures of which periodontal care was a part, but not the highest priority treatment need. Reprinted with permission of Harcourt Health Sciences from Armitage GC, Miller SR (1980) Management of gingival lesions in children and adolescents. In: Braham RL, Morris ME (eds) *Textbook of Pediatric Dentistry*. Baltimore: Williams & Wilkins, pp. 362–372.

with massive carious lesions, initial cleaning of the teeth, and provisional caries control procedures. After recovery from heart surgery, the patient required additional cleaning of her teeth, extensive restorative care, space maintenance procedures, professional help with her plaque control, family dietary counseling, and careful follow-up periodontal and dental maintenance care. The point of this example is that periodontal care is not always the first item on the treatment plan, even for patients with chronic gingivitis. Other urgent treatment needs may have a higher priority.

In children and adolescents with periodontitis, the treatment again depends on the overall diagnosis. Since moderate to severe periodontitis is uncommon at this age it is important to determine if the young patient has an underlying systemic problem that may be contributing to the periodontal disease. After the periodontal examination and prior to treatment, practitioners must make some important diagnostic and treatment planning decisions. Questions that need to be answered are:

- Is a medical consultation needed to rule out the presence of significant systemic or medical contributory factors?
- Is concurrent medical treatment needed to enhance the effectiveness of periodontal treatment?
- Will conventional mechanical therapy suffice to control the disease?
- Are systemic or locally applied antimicrobial agents necessary or advisable?
- When is the strategic extraction of periodontitis-affected primary teeth indicated?

When is a medical consultation needed?

Patients with classical forms of LAP do not generally require a medical consultation since effective methods of treatment are well documented without concurrent management of underlying systemic conditions (Slots and Rosling ,1983; Christersson et al.,1985; Kornman and Robertson, 1985; Mandell et al., 1986b; Mandell and Socransky, 1988; Novak et al., 1988, 1991; Asikainen et al., 1990; Christersson and Zambon, 1993; Saxén and Asikainen, 1993). Similarly, patients with GAP usually do not require medical consultations. However, some patients who are given a preliminary diagnosis of GAP have covert underlying systemic problems, such as diabetes (Cianciola et al., 1982; Novaes et al., 1997) or neutropenia (Kirstilä et al., 1993), which greatly increase their susceptibility to periodontal infections. In young patients with severe periodontitis that is not easily explained by local factors, it may be advisable to seek a medical consultation. Patients with a presumptive diagnosis of "prepubertal periodontitis" frequently have contributory systemic problems; indeed, many published reports of patients who had been assigned the diagnosis of "generalized prepubertal periodontitis" indicate that they had systemic conditions such as leukocyte adhesion deficiency (Waldrop et al., 1987; Meyle, 1994), hypophosphatasia (Plagmann et al., 1994), congenital primary immunodeficiency (Batista et al., 1999), cyclic neutropenia (Prichard et al., 1984), or chronic neutrophil defects (Dougherty and Gataletto, 1995; Kamma et al., 1998). In such cases, information gained from a medical consultation may alter the periodontal treatment plan. It should be emphasized, however, that not all individuals with "prepubertal periodontitis" have a readily detectable underlying systemic disease (Bimstein et al., 1997).

Is concurrent medical treatment needed to enhance the effectiveness of periodontal treatment?

If a patient's systemic condition is an important contributor to periodontal disease susceptibility, it is reasonable to assume that controlling the systemic disease will make it easier to treat the periodontal disease. The validity of this assumption is supported by case reports where medical management of a patient's systemic disease was found to improve the response to conventional periodontal treatment such as scaling and root planing. For example, neutropenic patients treated with recombinant granulocyte colony-stimulating factor often respond well to anti-infective periodontal therapy (Kirstilä et al., 1993; Pernu et al., 1996; Seow et al., 1998).

In some instances, the host response defect in a child's underlying systemic disease is so extensive that local periodontal treatment is ineffective (Roberts and Atkinson, 1990). An example of such a systemic disease is leukocyte adhesion deficiency (LAD) in which certain cell surface integrins are poorly expressed or missing (Meyle, 1994). Individuals with LAD are highly susceptible to a variety of infections, some of them life-threatening. Medical management of LAD is difficult, although some success has been achieved in restoring near-normal neutrophil function using high-risk procedures such as bone marrow transplantation (Fischer et al., 1983; Le Deist et al., 1989; Fischer et al., 1994).

Will conventional mechanical therapy suffice to control the disease?

Before periodontal treatment is started, practitioners must decide if conventional mechanical therapy alone is likely to control the patient's periodontal disease, or whether antimicrobial agents are also required. This decision is often difficult. Clinical studies suggest that LAP does not respond well to scaling and root planing alone (Slots and Rosling, 1983; Kornman and Robertson, 1985), possibly because *Actinobacillus actinomycetemcomitans*, one of the putative pathogens of LAP, invades the gingival tissues, providing a reservoir for recolonization (Slots and Ting, 1999). This hypothesis is supported by several observations: (a) periodontal surgery improves the clinical status of children with LAP (Kim et al., 1992); (b) resective surgery is more effective in reducing recolonization by *A. actinomycetemcomitans* than non-resective surgery in patients with chronic periodontitis (Tuan et al., 1999); and (c) surgery plus antibiotics that suppress *A. actinomycetemcomitans* are an effective treatment for LAP (Saxén et al., 1990; Christersson and Zambon, 1993; Saxén and Asikainen 1993).

Are systemic or locally applied antimicrobial agents necessary or advisable?

The decision to use antimicrobial agents as part of the therapeutic regimen can be made at any time during the course of treatment. However, it is usually wise to refrain from using antimicrobial agents until treatment with plaque control instructions and professionally administered mechanical debridement has proved ineffective. There are exceptions to this general approach. If the patient has LAP it is generally agreed that antibiotics should be given in conjunction with mechanical debridement (Genco, 1981). In addition, if young patients have particularly severe cases of periodontitis, clinicians may use their clinical judgment to prescribe local (e.g., chlorhexidine mouthrinses) or systemic (e.g., antibiotics) antimicrobial agents.

When is the strategic extraction of periodontitis-affected primary teeth indicated?

In a child with severe periodontitis of the primary teeth, it is possible that the succedaneous permanent teeth are at an increased risk of colonization by a periodontitis-producing flora from the overlying primary teeth. Some authors have reported the eradication of *A. actinomycetemcomitans* (Ngan et al., 1985; Mandell et al., 1986a; Ram and Bimstein, 1994) and *Porphyromonas gingivalis* (Ram and Bimstein, 1994) after extraction of affected primary teeth. However, in other cases antibiotics plus extraction of affected primary teeth failed to eliminate these putative pathogens (Bimstein et al., 1997). Therefore, extraction of affected primary teeth by no means guarantees prevention of colonization of permanent teeth by periodontal pathogens, and may not eliminate other intraoral reservoirs or extraoral sources of pathogens. Nevertheless, strategic extraction of primary teeth should be considered if there is a strong clinical impression that their presence places the permanent teeth at an increased risk.

General treatment approaches

Plaque control instructions

Daily plaque removal by the patient is essential to successful periodontal therapy in children (Axelsson, 1994) and adults (Axelsson et al., 1991). Longitudinal studies of Swedish schoolchildren have shown that meticulous plaque control and a rigorous, professionally administered maintenance program can almost totally prevent dental caries and gingivitis (Axelsson and Lindhe, 1973, 1974, 1977; Axelsson et al., 1976). It is worth noting that children who participated in these school-based studies developed excellent oral hygiene habits and became less dependent on professionally administered maintenance care (Axelsson and Lindhe, 1977). An important message from these studies is that children can be taught plaque control procedures that effectively reduce the occurrence of caries and gingivitis. There are, however, data indicating that self-performed supragingival oral hygiene alone is not sufficient to prevent the progression of periodontitis in adolescents (Albandar et al., 1995). This is not surprising, since complete supragingival plaque removal is difficult for patients to achieve, especially at interproximal sites where most cases of periodontitis begin. In addition, supragingival oral hygiene alone is unlikely to effectively disrupt the subgingival flora and thus will have a minimal impact on the development of periodontitis. Professional intervention, in the form of scaling and root planing, is needed for effective subgingival debridement.

Scaling and root planing

Local debridement (scaling and root planing) is a powerful therapeutic procedure. Most authorities agree that carefully performed root planing is one of the most effective parts of periodontal therapy (Greenstein, 1992; Cobb, 1996). Alone or in combination with other therapeutic procedures it is universally employed in the treatment of periodontitis. The primary objectives of scaling and root planing are (a) to remove supra- and subgingival plaque and calculus, and (b) to reduce gingival inflammation and promote healing. Although scaling and root planing do not completely eliminate putative pathogens from the subgingival flora, they significantly reduce the overall bacterial load, including spirochetes (Mousquès et al., 1980; Hinrichs et al., 1985; Lavanchy et al., 1987; Loos et al., 1988) and *Porphyromonas gingivalis* (Van Winkelhoff et al., 1987; Renvert et al., 1990; Sbordone et al., 1990). After scaling and root planing, the time it takes for subgingival recolonization by putative pathogens is highly variable. In adults with periodontitis who do not practice optimal plaque control, recolonization to pretreatment levels can be expected within 2–4 months (Greenstein, 1992). Meticulous supragingival plaque control can, however, affect the composition of the subgingival flora (Lavanchy et al., 1987; Dahlén et al., 1992; Katsanoulas et al., 1992; McNabb et al., 1992; Hellström et al., 1996) and probably slows down the rate of subgingival recolonization by pathogenic species.

Within weeks after the completion of scaling and root planing, there is usually a substantial reduction in the extent and severity of clinically detectable inflammation. Subgingival instrumentation routinely results in sustained reductions in probing depths and in the percentage of sites that exhibit bleeding on probing (Van Winkelhoff et al., 1987; Loos et al., 1988, Pedrazzoli et al., 1991; Greenstein, 1992). Figure 11.3 shows the results of scaling and root planing 1 month after initial treatment in an 11-year-old boy with severe gingival inflammation and recession on a mal-positioned lower incisor. The initial anti-infective therapy resulted in a reduction in gingival inflammation and a remodeling of the gingival tissues.

Evaluation of response to initial treatment

One of the most important steps in the treatment of periodontal disease is the careful evaluation of the effectiveness of the initial anti-infective therapy (i.e., the patient's oral hygiene plus scaling and root planing). This evaluation should occur approximately 1 month after scaling and root planing. Its primary purpose is to determine if further therapy is needed or if the patient is

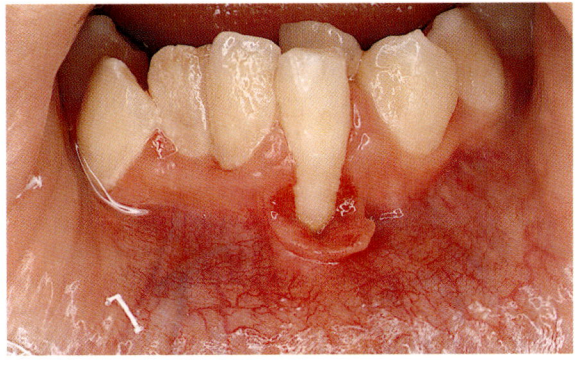
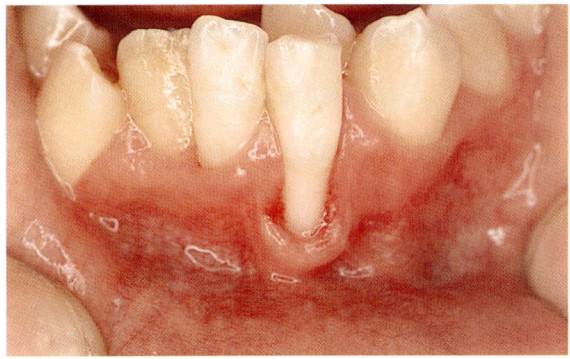

a
b

Figure 11.3

(a) Localized gingival recession and severe gingival inflammation on a malposed lower incisor in an 11-year-old boy. (b) Effects of a single session of scaling and root planing 1 month after instrumentation. Although the inflammation has not been completely resolved by this initial treatment, there has been a substantial reduction in its intensity. The treatment has also resulted in a substantial remodeling of the facial gingival tissues on the malposed tooth.

ready for maintenance care. Questions that need to be answered at this visit are:

- Has the patient's plaque control improved enough to minimize recurrence of disease?
- Is the scaling and root planing complete or is further instrumentation required?
- Has the disease been sufficiently controlled to permit placement of the patient on a periodontal maintenance care program?
- If so, what should the recall interval be?

At the first evaluation of the patient's plaque control following initial treatment, the therapist determines if there has been an improvement in the patient's oral hygiene. It is the therapist's hope that some improvement in oral hygiene will have occurred and the patient will have learned to remove supragingival plaque effectively. As a basis for comparison, it is advisable to record the patient's level of plaque control at the initial visit. A simple and reproducible system such as the plaque index (Silness and Löe, 1964) is usually sufficient. Patients who show no improvement in oral hygiene must receive additional instruction. When treating children it is advisable to involve parents in the oral hygiene program so they can help teach good plaque control habits (Rayner, 1992). It usually takes several visits to teach oral hygiene procedures effectively. Indeed, at each

visit it is important to evaluate or reinforce this critical component of self-care.

If scaling and root planing procedures have been effective, decreased gingival inflammation and a reduction in probing depths are usually observed within a month. If gingival inflammation persists, with bleeding on probing and no change in probing depths, it is likely that further treatment is needed; this may include further plaque control instructions, additional subgingival instrumentation, subgingival delivery of antimicrobial agents, or surgical intervention.

If the clinical response to plaque control instructions and subgingival instrumentation has been good, then the patient should be placed on a periodontal maintenance or recall program that minimizes the chances of disease recurrence. The optimal recall interval is not the same for all children who have been treated for periodontitis: those at higher risk (i.e., those with the most advanced disease) should be seen more frequently. In most cases, extension of the recall interval for low-risk patients does not increase their risk of disease progression (Wang and Holst, 1995). Young patients who have successfully been treated for periodontitis can be recalled at 3–month intervals. At any time during the maintenance program, the interval can be changed according to how well the patient's disease is being controlled.

Adjunctive use of antimicrobial agents

Antimicrobial mouthrinses are frequently used as local adjuncts to mechanical periodontal therapy (Drisko, 1996). No randomized, controlled clinical trial has evaluated the effectiveness of such mouthrinses in the treatment of periodontitis in children and adolescents. Nevertheless, reports on the treatment of periodontitis in young patients frequently include the use of chlorhexidine mouthrinses as part of the overall anti-infective therapy (Lindhe and Liljenberg, 1984; Wennström et al., 1986; Pedrazzoli et al., 1991; Pernu et al., 1996; Bimstein et al., 1997; Tinoco et al., 1998). Since it is well documented that chlorhexidine is an excellent antiplaque agent (Addy and Moran, 1997; Jones, 1997), it is reasonable to use it empirically in the treatment of periodontitis in young patients. It should be emphasized, however, that chlorhexidine and other ethanol-containing mouthrinses should be used under parental supervision because of the danger of acute ethanol toxicity. Indeed, in the period 1989–94 there were 2937 calls to poison control centers in the USA related to ethanol exposure due to overingestion of mouthrinses (Shulman and Wells, 1997).

In young patients with severe periodontitis, systemically administered antibiotics are frequently considered as important adjuncts to mechanical anti-infective therapy. In the case of LAP, several studies have reported some success in combining scaling and root planing (with or without surgical access) with systemically administered antibiotics. The antibiotics most often used include tetracycline (Lindhe, 1982; Slots and Rosling, 1983; Lindhe and Liljenberg, 1984; Kornman and Robertson, 1985; Christersson and Zambon, 1993; Saxén and Asikainen, 1993), doxycycline (Mandell et al., 1986b; Mandell and Socransky, 1988; Asikainen et al., 1990; Saxén et al., 1990), metronidazole alone (Saxén and Asikainen, 1993), or metronidazole plus amoxicillin (Van Winkelhoff et al., 1989, 1992; Pavicic et al., 1994; Bimstein et al., 1997; Tinoco et al., 1998). The therapeutic benefit of systemic antibiotics in the treatment of LAP is often attributed to their antibacterial effect on microorganisms believed to play a causative role in the disease, such as *P. gingivalis* and *A. actinomycetemcomitans*. Indeed, some success in resolving early lesions of LAP has been reported by using systemically administered tetracyclines without any scaling and root planing (Novak et al., 1988, 1991). However, since dental plaques are structured biofilms in which bacteria beneath the surface are somewhat protected from the effects of antibiotics (Socransky et al., 1999), it is likely that antibiotics are most effective when they are used in conjunction with mechanical therapy which disrupts the protective structure of biofilms. In addition, reliance on antibiotics alone to treat LAP should be viewed with caution since strains of *A. actinomycetemcomitans* resistant to tetracyclines are on the rise (Roe et al., 1995; Madinier et al., 1999).

Although there is convincing evidence that *A. actinomycetemcomitans* is a periodontal pathogen in susceptible hosts (Fives-Taylor et al., 1999, Slots and Ting, 1999), there is also good evidence that not all strains of this organism are strongly associated with periodontal disease (Asikainen et al., 1991, 1995; DiRienzo et al., 1994). Indeed, the organism can frequently be isolated from dental plaques of patients with healthy periodontal tissues (Gmür and Guggenheim, 1994; Hölttä et al., 1994; Müller et al., 1996; Bimstein et al., 1997). The existence of clonal variants of *A. actinomycetemcomitans* with vastly different virulence properties may partially explain why the organism can be found at healthy sites in some individuals (Haubek et al 1995, 1996; Bueno et al., 1998). The mere presence of *A. actinomycetemcomitans* in a plaque sample does not mean that the site is diseased. Furthermore, sites that harbor less virulent strains of the organism may not even be at risk of developing disease (DiRienzo et al., 1994). It has been suggested that LAP may be at least two different infections associated with either virulent or avirulent strains of *A. actinomycetemcomitans* (Haubek et al., 1995, 1996). These authors have speculated that the adjunctive use of antibiotics may be warranted only when the disease involves the virulent strains (Haubek et al., 1996).

In clinical practice, the decision to use systemic antibiotics is based primarily on clinical judgment, since there are few randomized, controlled clinical trials to guide the therapist. However, if the use of systemic antibiotics is contemplated, it is recommended that samples of subgingival plaque from affected sites be sent to a microbiology laboratory for cultural analysis and antibiotic

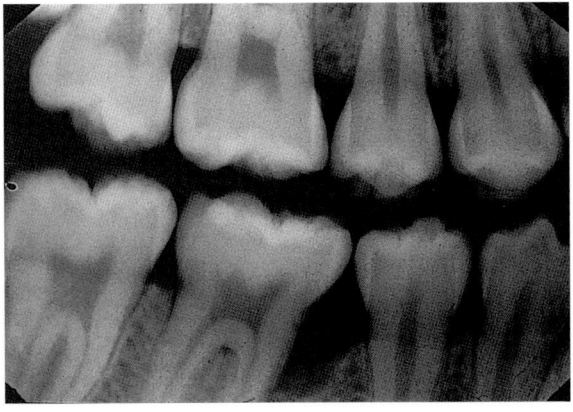

a

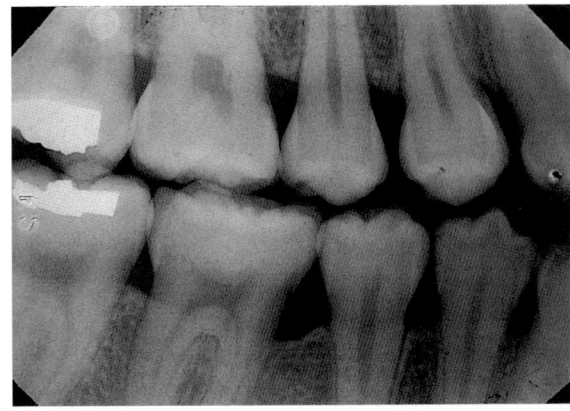

b

Figure 11.4

(a) Extensive bone loss on the mesial surface of a lower first permanent molar and slight bone loss on the mesial of an upper first permanent molar in a 16-year-old girl with LAP. (b) The result 18 months after surgery, with extensive fill of the osseous defects. Treatment involved surgical debridement of the sites and root planing (i.e., flap for access). No antibiotics were used.

sensitivity testing. Laboratory results can provide the therapist with valuable information regarding the types of putative pathogens at infected sites and the sensitivity of the bacteria to antibiotics. However, even with microbiological testing, clinicians cannot be absolutely certain that the bacteria cultured from a given periodontal pocket are the pathogens responsible for the patient's periodontal disease or that the antibiotic regimen recommended by the laboratory report will have a beneficial therapeutic effect (Armitage, 1996).

Periodontal surgery

One of the goals of periodontal therapy is to convert deep pockets—the principal habitat of periodontitis-producing bacteria—into shallow gingival crevices which are easier to maintain. Periodontal surgery is one way to reduce the depth of pockets. Other important reasons for performing periodontal surgery are to provide improved access for root planing; to remove inflamed tissue in osseous defects to promote healing; to modify or reshape the gingiva to facilitate easier plaque control; and to promote regeneration of lost periodontal tissues. Since most periodontal diseases are infections, surgical intervention only makes sense if it facilitates the overall anti-infective effort or is designed to

promote regeneration. Often it does both. Figure 11.4 shows the result of treatment of a patient with LAP 18 months after surgery, which provided access for scaling and root planing and facilitated removal of potentially infected tissues. The intervention resulted in an extensive fill of the osseous defect and clinical attachment gain. Although good results may be obtained by surgical intervention, the decision to operate in children and young patients should not be taken lightly, since adverse experiences in the dental office increase the chances of developing a fear of other dental procedures.

Evaluation following treatment

In general, this is similar to the evaluation of the response to initial treatment. However, there are some important differences. Prior to this visit, all forms of treatment that can be done to arrest the patient's disease have been completed, and the patient is ready for a program of long-term maintenance care. First, however, clinical attachment loss measurements should be taken. These measurements of the distance from the cementoenamel junction to the base of the probeable crevice serve as the baseline for determining disease progression during the maintenance program.

Long-term periodontal maintenance therapy

Young patients with a history of periodontitis are highly susceptible to disease recurrence. The two most important factors contributing to this susceptibility are the genetic predisposition of the patient (Marazita et al., 1994; Diehl et al., 1999), and the tendency of the original pathogenic flora to recover after treatment (Von Troil-Lindén et al., 1996; Saarela et al., 1999). Maintenance therapy can be effective, even in the most difficult-to-manage forms of periodontitis such as the Papillon–Lefèvre syndrome (Kim et al., 1997). The long-term prevention of recurrence of periodontitis is a labor-intensive endeavor that tests the diagnostic and therapeutic limits of the practitioner. A diligent and well-executed maintenance program, however, is the key to successful periodontal therapy.

References

Aass AM, Tollefsen T, Gjermo P (1994) A cohort study of radiographic bone loss during adolescence. *J Clin Periodontol* **21**: 133–8.

Addy M, Moran JM (1997) Clinical indications for the use of chemical adjuncts to plaque control: chlorhexidine formulations. *Periodontol 2000* **15**: 52–4.

Albandar JM, Buischi YAP, Oliveira LB, Axelsson P (1995) Lack of effect of oral hygiene training on periodontal disease progression over 3 years in adolescents. *J Periodontol* **66**: 255–60.

Albandar JM, Brown LJ, Genco RJ, Löe H (1997) Clinical classification of periodontitis in adolescents and young adults. *J Periodontol* **68**: 545–55.

Armitage GC (1995) Clinical evaluation of periodontal diseases. *Periodontol 2000* **7**: 39–53.

Armitage GC (1996) Periodontal diseases: diagnosis. *Ann Periodontol* **1**: 37–215.

Armitage GC (1999) Development of a classification system for periodontal diseases and conditions. *Ann Periodontol* **4**: 1–6.

Armitage GC, Van Dyke TE (1996) Position paper. Periodontal diseases of children and adolescents. *J Periodontol* **67**: 57–62.

Asikainen S, Jousimies-Somer H, Kanervo A, Saxén L (1990) The immediate efficacy of adjunctive doxycycline in treatment of localized juvenile periodontitis. *Arch Oral Biol* **35**: 231S–234S.

Asikainen S, Lai C-H, Alaluusua S, Slots J (1991) Distribution of *Actinobacillus actinomycetemcomitans* serotypes in periodontal health and disease. *Oral Microbiol Immunol* **6**: 115–18.

Asikainen S, Chen C, Slots J (1995) *Actinobacillus actinomycetemcomitans* genotypes in relation to serotypes and periodontal status. *Oral Microbiol Immunol* **10**: 65–8.

Attström R, van der Velden U (1994) Consensus report of session I. In: Lang NP, Karring T (eds) *Proceedings of the 1st European Workshop on Periodontology*. London: Quintessence, pp. 120–6.

Axelsson P (1994) Mechanical plaque control. In: Lang NP, Karring T (eds) *Proceedings of the 1st European Workshop on Periodontology*. London: Quintessence, pp. 219–43.

Axelsson P, Lindhe J (1973) The effect of controlled oral hygiene and topical fluoride application on caries and gingivitis in Swedish school children. *Commun Dent Oral Epidemiol* **1**: 9–16.

Axelsson P, Lindhe J (1974) The effect of a preventive programme on dental plaque, gingivitis and caries in schoolchildren. Results after one and two years. *J Clin Periodontol* **1**: 126–38.

Axelsson P, Lindhe J (1977) The effect of a plaque control program on gingivitis and dental caries in schoolchildren. *J Dent Res* **56** (special issue): C142–C148.

Axelsson P, Lindhe J, Wäseby J (1976) The effect of various plaque control measures on gingivitis and caries in school-children. *Commun Dent Oral Epidemiol* **4**: 232–9.

Axelsson P, Lindhe J, Nyström B (1991) On the prevention of caries and periodontal disease. Results of a 15-year longitudinal study in adults. *J Clin Periodontol* **18**: 182–9.

Baer PN (1971) The case for periodontosis as a clinical entity. *J Periodontol* **42**: 516–20.

Batista EL, Novaes AB, Calvano LM et al. (1999) Necrotizing ulcerative periodontitis associated with severe congenital immunodeficiency in a prepubescent subject: clinical findings and response to intravenous immunoglobulin treatment. *J Clin Periodontol* **26**: 499–504.

Bhat M (1991) Periodontal health of 14–17-year-old US schoolchildren. *J Publ Health Dent* **51**: 5–11.

Bimstein E, Delaney JE, Sweeney EA (1988) Radiographic assessment of the alveolar bone in children and adolescents. *Pediatr Dent* **10**: 199–204.

Bimstein E, Treasure ET, Williams SM, Dever JG (1994) Alveolar bone loss in 5-year-old New Zealand children: its prevalence and relationship to caries prevalence, socio-economic status and ethnic origin. *J Clin Periodontol* **21**: 447–50.

Bimstein E, Sela MN, Shapira L (1997) Clinical and microbial considerations for the treatment of an extended kindred with seven cases of prepubertal periodontitis: a 2-year follow-up. *Pediatr Dent* **19**: 396–403.

Boughman JA, Halloran SL, Roulston D et al. (1986) An autosomal-dominant form of juvenile periodontitis: its localization to chromosome 4 and linkage to dentinogenesis imperfecta and Gc. *J Craniofac Genet Dev Biol* **6**: 341–50.

Brown LJ, Albandar JM, Brunelle JA, Löe H (1996) Early-onset periodontitis: progression of attachment loss during 6 years. *J Periodontol* **67**: 968–75.

Bueno LC, Mayer MPA, DiRienzo JM (1998) Relationship between conversion of localized juvenile periodontitis-susceptible children from health to disease and *Actinobacillus actinomycetemcomitans* leukotoxin promoter structure. *J Periodontol* **69**: 998–1007.

Cappelli DP, Ebersole JL, Kornman KS (1994) Early-onset periodontitis in Hispanic-American adolescents associated with *A. actinomycetemcomitans*. *Commun Dent Oral Epidemiol* **22**: 116–21.

Christersson LA, Zambon JJ (1993) Suppression of subgingival *Actinobacillus actinomycetemcomitans* in localized juvenile periodontitis by systemic tetracycline. *J Clin Periodontol* **20**: 395–401.

Christersson LA, Slots J, Rosling BG, Genco RJ (1985) Microbiological and clinical effects of surgical treatment of juvenile periodontitis. *J Clin Periodontol* **12**: 465–76.

Cianciola LJ, Park BH, Bruck E et al. (1982) Prevalence of periodontal disease in insulin-dependent diabetes mellitus (juvenile diabetes). *J Am Dent Assoc* **104**: 653–60.

Claffey N, Russell R, Shanley D (1986) Peripheral blood phagocyte function in acute necrotizing ulcerative gingivitis. *J Periodont Res* **21**: 288–97.

Clerehugh V, Worthington HV, Lennon MA, Chandler R (1995) Site progression of loss of attachment over 5 years in 14- to 19-year-old adolescents. *J Clin Periodontol* **22**: 15–21.

Cobb CM (1996) Non-surgical pocket therapy: mechanical. *Ann Periodontol* **1**: 443–90.

Cogen RB, Wright JT, Tate AL (1992) Destructive periodontal disease in healthy children. *J Periodontol* **63**: 761–5.

Dahlén G, Lindhe J, Sato K et al. (1992) The effect of supragingival plaque control on the subgingival microbiota in subjects with periodontal disease. *J Clin Periodontol* **19**: 802–9.

Diehl SR, Wang YF, Brooks CN et al. (1999) Linkage disequilibrium of interleukin-1 genetic polymorphisms with early-onset periodontitis. *J Periodontol* **70**: 418–30.

DiRienzo JM, Slots J, Sixou M et al. (1994) Specific genetic variants of *Actinobacillus actinomycetemcomitans* correlate with disease and health in a regional population of families with localized juvenile periodontitis. *Infect Immun* **62**: 3058–65.

Dougherty N, Gataletto MA (1995) Oral sequelae of chronic neutrophil defects: case report of a child with glycogen storage disease type 1b. *Pediatr Dent* **17**: 224–9.

Drisko CH (1996) Non-surgical pocket therapy: pharmacotherapeutics. *Ann Periodontol* **1**: 491–566.

Enwonwu CO (1972) Epidemiological and biochemical studies of necrotizing ulcerative gingivitis and noma (cancrum oris) in Nigerian children. *Arch Oral Biol* **17**: 1357–71.

Fischer A, Pham HT, Descamps-Latscha B et al. (1983) Bone-marrow transplantation for inborn error of phagocytic cells associated with defective adherence, chemotaxis, and oxidative response during opsonised particle phagocytosis. *Lancet* **2**: 473–6.

Fischer A, Landais P, Friederich W et al. (1994) Bone marrow transplantation (BMT) in Europe for primary immunodeficiencies other than severe combined immunodeficiency: a report from the European Group for BMT and the European Group for Immunodeficiency. *Blood* **83**: 1149–54.

Fives-Taylor PM, Meyer DH, Mintz KP, Brissette C (1999) Virulence factors of *Actinobacillus actinomycetemcomitans*. *Periodontol 2000* **20**: 136–67.

Genco RJ (1981) Antibiotics in the treatment of human periodontal diseases. *J Periodontol* **52**: 545–58.

Gmür R, Guggenheim B (1994) Interdental supragingival plaque – a natural habitat of *Actinobacillus actinomycetemcomitans*, *Bacteroides forsythus*, *Campylobacter rectus*, and *Prevotella nigrescens*. *J Dent Res* **73**: 1421–28.

Greenstein G (1992) Periodontal response to mechanical non-surgical therapy. A review. *J Periodontol* **63**: 118–30.

Guile EE, Al-Shammary A, El-Backly M (1990) Prevalence and severity of periodontal diseases in Saudi Arabian schoolchildren aged 6, 9 and 12 years. *Commun Dent Health* **7**: 429–32.

Hart TC (1996) Genetic risk factors for early-onset periodontitis. *J Periodontol* **67**: 355–66.

Hart TC, Marazita ML, McCanna KM et al. (1993) Reevaluation of the chromosome 4q candidate region for early onset periodontitis. *Hum Genet* **91**: 416–22.

Haubek D, Poulsen K, Asikainen S, Kilian M (1995) Evidence for absence in northern Europe of especially virulent clonal types of *Actinobacillus actinomycetemcomitans*. *J Clin Microbiol* **33**: 395–401.

Haubek D, Poulsen K, Westergaard J et al. (1996) Highly toxic clone of *Actinobacillus actinomycetemcomitans* in geographically widespread cases of juvenile periodontitis in adolescents of African origin. *J Clin Microbiol* **34**: 1576–8.

Hellström M-K, Ramberg P, Krok L, Lindhe J (1996) The effect of supragingival plaque control on the subgingival microflora in human periodontitis. *J Clin Periodontol* **23**: 934–40.

Hinrichs JE, Wolff LF, Pihlstrom BL et al. (1985) Effects of scaling and root planing on subgingival microbial proportions standardized in terms of their naturally occurring distribution. *J Periodontol* **56**: 187–94.

Hölttä P, Alaluusua S, Saarela M, Asikainen S (1994) Isolation frequency and serotype distribution of mutans streptococci and *Actinobacillus actinomycetemcomitans*, and clinical periodontal status in Finnish and Vietnamese children. *Scand J Dent Res* **102**: 113–19.

Ismail AL, Burt BA, Brunelle JA (1987) Prevalence of dental caries and periodontal disease in Mexican American children aged 5 to 17 years: results from Southwestern HHANES, 1982–83. *Am J Publ Health* **77**: 967–70.

Jiménez LM, Baer PN (1975) Necrotizing ulcerative gingivitis in children: a 9 year clinical study. *J Periodontol* **46**: 715–20.

Johnson BD, Engel D (1986) Acute necrotizing ulcerative gingivitis. A review of diagnosis, etiology and treatment. *J Periodontol* **47**: 141–50.

Jones CG (1997) Chlorhexidine: is it still the gold standard? *Periodontol 2000* **15**: 55–62.

Kamma JJ, Lygidakis NA, Nakou M (1998) Subgingival microflora and treatment in prepubertal periodontitis associated with chronic idiopathic neutropenia. *J Clin Periodontol* **25**: 759–65.

Katsanoulas T, Reneè I, Attström R (1992) The effect of supragingival plaque control on the composition of the subgingival flora in periodontal pockets. *J Clin Periodontol* **19**: 760–5.

Kim KJ, Kim DK, Chung CP, Son S (1992) Longitudinal monitoring for disease progression of localized juvenile periodontitis. *J Periodontol* **63**: 806–11.

Kim J-B, Morita M, Kusumoto M et al. (1997) Preservation of permanent teeth in a patient with Papillon–Lefèvre syndrome by professional tooth-cleaning. *J Dent Child* **64**: 222–6.

Kirstilä V, Sewón L, Laine J (1993) Periodontal disease in three siblings with familial neutropenia. *J Periodontol* **64**: 566–70.

Koloway B, Kailis DG (1992) Caries, gingivitis and oral hygiene in urban and rural pre-school children in Indonesia. *Commun Dent Oral Epidemiol* **20**: 157–8.

Kornman KS, Robertson PB (1985) Clinical and microbiological evaluation of therapy for juvenile periodontitis. *J Periodontol* **56**: 443–6.

Lavanchy DL, Bickel M, Baehni PC (1987) The effect of plaque control after scaling and root planing on the subgingival microflora in human periodontitis. *J Clin Periodontol* **14**: 295–9.

Le Deist F, Blanche F, Keable H et al. (1989) Successful HLA nonidentical bone marrow transplantation in three patients with the leukocyte adhesion deficiency. *Blood* **74**: 512–16.

Lindhe J (1982) Treatment of localized juvenile periodontitis. In: Genco RJ, Mergenhagen SE (eds) *Host-Parasite Interactions in Periodontal Diseases*. Washington: American Society for Microbiology, pp. 382–94.

Lindhe J, Liljenberg B (1984) Treatment of localized juvenile periodontitis. Results after 5 years. *J Clin Periodontol* **11**: 399–410.

Loos B, Claffey N, Egelberg J (1988) Clinical and microbiological effects of root debridement in periodontal furcation pockets. *J Clin Periodontol* **15**: 453–63.

MacCarthy D, Claffey N (1991) Acute necrotizing ulcerative gingivitis is associated with attachment loss. *J Clin Periodontol* **18**: 776–9.

Madinier IM, Fosse TB, Hitzig C et al. (1999) Resistance profile survey of 50 periodontal strains of *Actinobacillus actinomycetemcomitans*. *J Periodontol* **70**: 888–92.

Mandell RL, Socransky SS (1988) Microbiological and clinical effects of surgery plus doxycycline on juvenile periodontitis. *J Periodontol* **59**: 373–9.

Mandell RL, Siegal MD, Umland E (1986a) Localized juvenile periodontitis of the primary dentition. *J Dent Child* **53**: 193–6.

Mandell RL, Tripodi LS, Savitt E et al. (1986b) The effect of treatment on *Actinobacillus actinomycetemcomitans* in localized juvenile periodontitis. *J Periodontol* **57**: 94–9.

Mann J, Cormier PP, Green P et al. (1981) Loss of periodontal attachment in adolescents. *Commun Dent Oral Epidemiol* **9**: 135–41.

Marazita ML, Burmeister JA, Gunsolley JC et al. (1994) Evidence for autosomal dominant inheritance and race-specific heterogeneity in early-onset periodontitis. *J Periodontol* **65**: 623–30.

McNabb H, Mombelli A, Lang NP (1992) Supragingival cleaning 3 times a week. The microbiological effects in moderately deep pockets. *J Clin Periodontol* **19**: 348–56.

Meyle J (1994) Leukocyte adhesion deficiency and prepubertal periodontitis. *Periodontol 2000* **6**: 26–36.

Mousquès T, Listgarten MA, Phillips RW (1980) Effect of scaling and root planing on the composition of the human subgingival microbial flora. *J Periodont Res* **15**: 144–51.

Müller H-P, Zöller L, Eger T et al. (1996) Natural distribution of oral *Actinobacillus actinomycetemcomitans* in young men with minimal periodontal disease. *J Periodont Res* **31**: 373–80.

Ngan PWH, Tsai C-C, Sweeney E (1985) Advanced periodontitis in the primary dentition; case report. *Pediatr Dent* **7**: 255–8.

Ng'ang'a PM, Valderhaug J (1991) Oral hygiene practices and periodontal health in primary school children in Nairobi, Kenya. *Acta Odontol Scand* **49**: 303–9.

Noar J, Portnoy S (1991) Dental status of children in a primary and secondary school in rural Zambia. *Int Dent J* **41**: 142–8.

Novaes AB, Silva MAP, Batista EL et al. (1997) Manifestations of insulin-dependent diabetes mellitus in the periodontium of young Brazilian patients. A 10-year follow-up study. *J Periodontol* **68**: 328–34.

Novak MJ, Polson AM, Adair SM (1988) Tetracycline therapy in patients with early juvenile periodontitis. *J Periodontol* **59**: 366–72.

Novak MJ, Stamatelakys C, Adair SM (1991) Resolution of early lesions of juvenile periodontitis with tetracycline therapy alone: long-term observations of 4 cases. *J Periodontol* **62**: 628–33.

Page RC, Altman LC, Ebersole JL et al. (1983) Rapidly progressive periodontitis. A distinct clinical condition. *J Periodontol* **54**: 197–209.

Papapanou PN (1996) Periodontal diseases: epidemiology. *Ann Periodontol* **1**: 1–36.

Pavicic MJAMP, van Winkelhoff AJ, Douqué NH et al. (1994) Microbiological and clinical effects of metronidazole and amoxicillin in *Actinobacillus actinomycetemcomitans*-associated periodontitis. A 2-year evaluation. *J Clin Periodontol* **21**: 107–12.

Pedrazzoli V, Kilian M, Karring T, Kirkegaard E (1991) Effect of surgical and non-surgical periodontal treatment on periodontal status and subgingival microbiota. *J Clin Periodontol* **18**: 598–604.

Pernu HE, Pajari UH, Lanning M (1996) The importance of regular dental treatment in patients with cyclic neutropenia. Follow-up of 2 cases. *J Periodontol* **67**: 454–9.

Pindborg JJ, Bhat M, Devanath KR et al. (1966) Occurrence of acute necrotizing gingivitis in South Indian children. *J Periodontol* **37**: 14–19.

Plagmann H-C, Kocher T, Kuhrau N, Caliebe A (1994) Periodontal manifestation of hypophosphatasia. A family case report. *J Clin Periodontol* **21**: 710–16.

Prichard JF, Ferguson DM, Windmiller J, Hurt WC (1984) Prepubertal periodontitis affecting the deciduous dentition and permanent dentition in a patient with cyclic neutropenia. A case report and discussion. *J Periodontol* **55**: 114–22.

Ram D, Bimstein E (1994) Subgingival bacteria in a case of prepubertal periodontitis, before and one year after extractions of the affected primary teeth. *J Clin Pediatr Dent* **19**: 45–7.

Rayner JA (1992) A dental health education programme, including home visits, for nursery school children. *Br Dent J* **172**: 57–62.

Renvert S, Wikström M, Dahlén G et al. (1990) Effect of root debridement on the elimination of *Actinobacillus actinomycetemcomitans* and *Bacteroides gingivalis* from periodontal pockets. *J Clin Periodontol* **17**: 345–50.

Roberts MW, Atkinson JC (1990) Oral manifestations associated with leukocyte adhesion deficiency: a five year case study. *Pediatr Dent* **12**: 107–11.

Roe DE, Braham PH, Weinberg A, Roberts MC (1995) Characterization of tetracycline resistance in *Actinobacillus actinomycetemcomitans*. *Oral Microbiol Immunol* **10**: 227–32.

Saarela MH, Dogan B, Alaluusua S, Asikainen S (1999) Persistence of oral colonization by the same *Actinobacillus actinomycetemcomitans* strain(s). *J Periodontol* **70**: 504–9.

Saxén L, Asikainen S (1993) Metronidazole in the treatment of localized juvenile periodontitis. *J Clin Periodontol* **20**: 166–71.

Saxén L, Asikainen S, Kanervo A et al. (1990) The long-term efficacy of systemic doxycycline medication in the treatment of localized juvenile periodontitis. *Arch Oral Biol* **35**: 227S–229S.

Sbordone L, Ramaglia L, Gulletta E, Iacono V (1990) Recolonization of the subgingival microflora after scaling and root planing in human periodontitis. *J Periodontol* **61**: 579–84.

Seow WK, Bartold PM, Thong YH (1998) Cohen syndrome with neutropenia-induced periodontitis managed with granulocyte colony-stimulating factor (G-CSF): case reports. *Pediatr Dent* **20**: 350–4.

Sheiham A (1966) An epidemiological survey of acute ulcerative gingivitis in Nigerians. *Arch Oral Biol* **11**: 937–42.

Shulman JD, Wells LM (1997) Acute ethanol toxicity from ingesting mouthwash in children younger than 6 years of age. *Pediatr Dent* **19**: 405–8.

Silness J, Löe H (1964) Periodontal disease in pregnancy. II. Correlation between oral hygiene and periodontal condition. *Acta Odontol Scand* **22**: 121–35.

Sjödin B, Matsson L (1994) Marginal bone loss in the primary dentition. A survey of 7–9-year-old children in Sweden. *J Clin Periodontol* **21**: 313–9.

Sjödin B, Matsson L, Unell L, Egelberg J (1993) Marginal bone loss in the primary dentition of patients with juvenile periodontitis. *J Clin Periodontol* **20**: 32–6.

Skach M, Zábrodsky, Mrklas L (1970) A study of the effect of age and season on the incidence of ulcerative gingivitis. *J Periodont Res* **5**: 187–90.

Slots J, Rosling BG (1983) Suppression of the periodontopathic microflora in localized juvenile periodontitis by systemic tetracycline. *J Clin Periodontol* **10**: 465–86.

Slots J, Ting M (1999) *Actinobacillus actinomycetemcomitans* and *Porphyromonas gingivalis* in human periodontal disease: occurrence and treatment. *Periodontol 2000* **20**: 82–121.

Socransky SS, Haffajee AD, Ximenez-Fyvie LA et al. (1999) Ecological considerations in treatment of *Actinobacillus actinomycetemcomitans* and *Porphyromonas gingivalis* periodontal infections. *Periodontol 2000* **20**: 341–62.

Spektor MD, Vandesteen GE, Page RC (1985) Clinical studies of one family manifesting rapidly progressive, juvenile and prepubertal periodontitis. *J Periodontol* **56**: 93–101.

Stevens AW, Cogen RB, Cohen-Cole S, Freeman A (1984) Demographic and clinical data associated with acute necrotizing ulcerative gingivitis in a dental school population. *J Clin Periodontol* **11**: 487–93.

Tinoco EMB, Beldi MI, Campedelli F et al. (1998) Clinical and microbiological effects of adjunctive antibiotics in treatment of localized juvenile periodontitis. A controlled clinical trial. *J Periodontol* **69**: 1355–63.

Tuan M-C, Nowarzi H, Slots J (1999) Clinical and microbiologic study of apically positioned flaps, with and without osseous surgery. *J Periodontol* **70**: 347.

Van der Velden U, Abbas F, Armand S et al. (1993) The effect of sibling relationship on the periodontal condition. *J Clin Periodontol* **20**: 683–90.

Van Winkelhoff AJ, Van der Velden U, De Graaff J (1987) Microbial succession in recolonizing deep periodontal pockets after a single course of supra- and subgingival debridement. *J Clin Periodontol* **15**: 116–22.

Van Winkelhoff AJ, Rodenburg JP, Goené RJ et al. (1989) Metronidazole plus amoxicillin in the treatment of *Actinobacillus actinomycetemcomitans* associated periodontitis. *J Clin Periodontol* **16**: 128–31.

Van Winkelhoff AJ, Tijhof CJ, de Graaff J (1992) Microbiological and clinical results of metronidazole plus amoxicillin therapy in *Actinobacillus actinomycetemcomitans*-associated periodontitis. *J Periodontol* **63**: 52–7.

Von Troil-Lindén B, Saarela M, Mättö J et al. (1996) Source of suspected periodontal pathogens re-emerging after periodontal treatment. *J Clin Periodontol* **23**: 601–7.

Waldrop TC, Anderson DC, Hallmon WW et al. (1987) Periodontal manifestations of the heritable Mac-1, LFA-1, deficiency syndrome. *J Periodontol* **58**: 400–16.

Wang NJ, Holst D (1995) Individualizing recall intervals in child dental care. *Commun Dent Oral Epidemiol* **23**: 1–7.

Wennström A, Wennström J, Lindhe J (1986) Healing following surgical and non-surgical treatment of juvenile periodontitis. A 5-year longitudinal study. *J Clin Periodontol* **13**: 869–82.

12
Behavior management

Stephen Shusterman

Pediatric dentists are fully versed in behavioral management of children. However, in many cases children with periodontal problems will be treated by the family dentist, an oral surgeon, or a periodontist. Periodontal treatment may be a challenge to any patient, adult or child. So what, then, is expected from the dentist to whom a child is referred for mucogingival surgery or merely periodontal evaluation? How should a dentist, who is performing periodontal treatment on children, manage the child's behavior? A dentist who is treating children can reasonably be required to be knowledgeable in the area of psychosocial growth and development and, more importantly, to be sensitive and caring in the presentation of the diagnosis and the completion of the treatment plan.

It is not the purpose of this chapter to create a pediatric specialist from the dentist treating children's periodontal problems, but rather to provide a simplified framework for managing the behavior of the child undergoing treatment (McKnight-Hanes et al., 1993).

Children who undergo treatment for gingival, mucogingival, or periodontal problems must be capable of focusing, following direction, understanding and coping with the possibility of postoperative discomfort, and contributing to the ensuing maintenance program designed to assure future periodontal health. Thoughtful selection of patients is the best assurance of an appropriate treatment outcome. For example, patients with learning difficulties who are treated with phenytoin (diphenylhydantoin) or are fed directly by gastric tube, may not be capable of maintaining the improved gingival height and contour following gingivoplasty, and therefore may not appreciably benefit from the procedure. In such cases it may be wise for the dentist to delay referral, focus on behavioral modification and home hygiene maintenance programs, and manage the periodontal treatment superficially so that the dentition and oral health will not further deteriorate before definitive treatment is possible.

Behavioral management menu

Behavioral management techniques include a wide range of approaches, from verbal methods (no restraint), to the use of a mouth prop (minimal restraint), and finally to general anesthesia in the operating room (the ultimate and total restraint). Most school-age children will have developed the cognitive skills necessary for understanding and retrieval of information (Cole and Cole, 1993), and therefore should respond favorably to an age-appropriate explanation. Conscious sedation or general anesthesia may be appropriate behavioral modifiers for some children when treatment is expected to be uncomfortable or tedious (e.g., gingivoplasty for gingival hyperplasia); this approach, however, may not be ideal for assuring future behavior, which is important for long-term periodontal health.

Management choices may be more easily understood when presented in menu form. These menu options are listed in order from the least authoritative (those requiring explanation and no restraint) to the most restraining and least interactive (general anesthesia). At the same time, they move from those that are most acceptable to parents to those that may be least acceptable; although for more urgent treatment, parents are more likely to accept methods involving restraint (Fields et al., 1984).

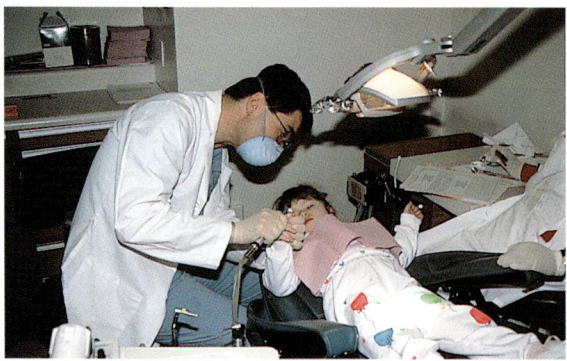

Figure 12.1

The dentist demonstrates the prophylaxis cup on the dental handpiece on the child's finger, while speaking directly to the child and attempting to maintain eye contact.

Tell—show—do

"Tell, show, and do" is the most commonly used management approach for children of all ages and is well accepted by most parents. In this approach, the dentist explains the procedure in easily comprehensible terms, demonstrates it in a non-invasive and simplified manner (Figure 12.1), and then begins treatment in a smooth, uninterrupted progression while maintaining the child's attention. It is important to establish both eye contact and direct communication with the child; instructions relayed through a parent may divert or confuse the child. For example, a dentist attempting the periodontal evaluation of a lower anterior mucogingival defect would explain to the child that he or she is going to look at the area of concern and measure the length of the (attached) "gum" (the extent of the gingival dehiscence) with a "special ruler" (periodontal probe). When injecting local anesthetic solution, the dentist should first use topical anesthesia ("sleepy butter on a paintbrush [swab]"), explain the discomfort of the injection ("pinch") and the feeling to be expected after the injection takes effect ("fuzzy and fat"). The explanation, demonstration, and injection follow without delay. Words that evoke unpleasant feelings, such as "needle," "shot," "hurt," "cut," etc., should be avoided.

Positive reinforcement

Positive reinforcement is one of the most important elements in behavioral modification (Pinkham, 1995). The dentist who frequently sees very young children for their first dental experience, and perhaps the first manipulation of the oral cavity, holds the key to establishing self-confidence in these patients. Some aspect of behavior or cooperation must be praised, no matter how unacceptable the actual behavior is. Praise is offered for the most minimal cooperation obtainable, such as a brief glimpse of the dentition. It is usually followed by a reward, and all dentists who treat children should keep prizes (rings, bracelets, stickers, balloons, etc.) in their offices as an acknowledgment of the child's "help." These rewards are automatic at the conclusion of the visit and are not contingent on cooperation.

As part of a periodontal treatment plan, positive reinforcement may be even more important. In this case, we must not only enlist patient cooperation at the chairside, but also in the home care program to follow. The level of understanding or the willingness to commit the effort may be more difficult to establish in a child; thus, each tentative step towards maintenance of a graft site or gingivoplasty should be acknowledged and any necessary modification explained in a constructive manner. Emphasis should be placed on accomplishment, even if the perception is that the effort was minimal or completely ineffective.

Distraction

Every dentist should make a conscious effort to divert the child's attention from the treatment being performed. The language used by the dentist and assistant as they ask for instruments or suction should avoid words that may be frightening ("knife", "needle", "suture", etc.), and the instruments passed should avoid the patient's direct view. Given the opportunity to focus on any of these, even adult patients may succumb to fears or uncertainties.

Distractions that are practical at the chairside for children range from hand-held radios with earphones to hand-held games (Figure 12.2),

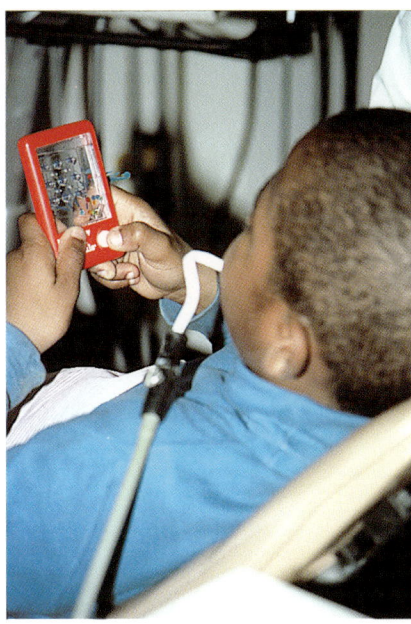

Figure 12.2

A hand-held game being used by the child as a distraction aid during administration of topical fluoride.

stuffed animals, or video presentations. Hand-held video games or mirrors may be useful during demonstrations or preparation, but may interfere with treatment. Furthermore, a mirror used to watch a bloody surgical field being prepared for a graft may become counterproductive. Kuhn has reviewed distraction and other methods of behavioral management, and has presented the "contingent distraction" which allows the patient a diversion in return for cooperative behavior (Kuhn and Allen, 1994). Anything that diverts the child's attention is useful in assuring successful treatment, but the actual method of distraction should be thoughtfully chosen after considering content, theme, and sound levels, to avoid parental concerns as well as to protect the office ambience.

Voice control

Modulation of the dentist's voice, either in tone or volume, is another simple method used to gain the child's attention and subsequent cooperation. Again, the dentist must speak directly to the child. The dentist should speak in soft, controlled tones, repeating the same phrases, as necessary. By raising your voice, you may telegraph your own lack of patience or increasing frustration. As parents, many of us are careful to avoid raised voices when speaking with our children, and are even more sensitive about others "yelling" at our kids. Lastly, if that raised voice filters out to the reception area, waiting patients may perceive a frazzled, frustrated practitioner; one they would rather not entrust with their child's dental care.

Some dentists advocate the use of loud tones as an aversive stimulus following unacceptable and disruptive behavior, and there is some evidence to confirm that disruptive behavior stops and the dentist is more able to maintain cooperative behavior. Shouting at the child has not been demonstrated to create a greater level of apprehension in follow-up evaluations (Greenbaum et al., 1990). In fact, the level of apprehension ("arousal") in children who received shouted commands was lower than in children who received commands in normal tones. These studies demonstrated that it was not what was said, but rather how it was said. Given that some dentists have only brief encounters with children, this method of behavioral management may be effective in calming fearful patients and in avoiding the necessity for pharmacological behavioral management.

Parental presence

The issue of parental presence has often been debated among pediatric dentists. In the past parents were routinely excluded, but parenting and attitudes toward participation in treatment have changed, and today a parent's presence is considered appropriate involvement in the child's care (Pinkham, 1991). Certainly, in the case of very young children, many practitioners agree that treatment should not be undertaken without the supportive presence of a parent (Rayman, 1987; Pinkham, 1991).

In lending support to their child, it is important that parents understand the parameters of their interaction during treatment. They should be encouraged to ask appropriate questions and to accurately relate their child's health history before the treatment. Lengthy parent–dentist discussions in the treatment room should be avoided as they may place pressure on the dentist's schedule and efficiency and thereby adversely affect the child's cooperation. During treatment, parents must remain silent (Rayman, 1987), assuring the child of their presence (by holding a hand or even a foot), but allowing the dentist to control behavior, request compliance, adjust positions, or conduct conversation. There is nothing more disconcerting than the parent who cannot resist the temptation to repeat each request or comment made to the child, e.g., "open wide," the parent repeats "open wide, say ahhh. . .". Soon the child's attention is lost; the child will respond only to the parent and, even worse, adopt the apprehension or fear telegraphed by the parent. If the child loses control, sobs inconsolably and reaches toward the parent, the dentist's ability to complete treatment may also be lost.

In the USA today, more than 70% of mothers work outside the home (Hoffman, 1989) and many children live with a single parent or an alternative caregiver (Hetherington et al., 1989). Many children start day-care or preschool at an early age and are therefore more comfortable with people outside the home. Stranger anxiety is a normal expectation in the psychosocial development of the child, but today it is modified by the widespread interactions with alternative caregivers. In an early stage of social development, Erikson (1963) stated that if a parent generally meets the infant's needs, a sense of trust, rather than mistrust, is developed. Despite the acceptance of "strangers," young children trust their parents first, and therefore parents should be involved in the discussion of treatment and the support of their children. They must receive a full explanation of risks, benefits, and costs to assure that their parental consent is fully informed.

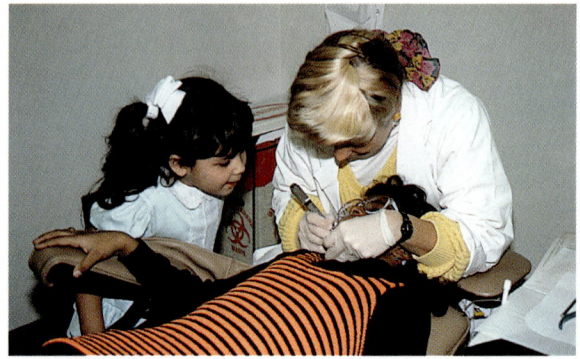

Figure 12.3

A child observing another child during the fitting of an appliance as an example of live modeling.

bays to assure the presence and support of other children. They may manage their schedules to reduce the possibility that a child who behaves adversely may influence another who is cooperative and calm. This type of support can be duplicated by pre-visit conditioning with introductory brochures, tapes, or a website. Information should describe office procedures, provide a look at the operative setting, and show pictures of the staff. If such material can be presented through the eyes of another child, it may be more supportive than text presented on an adult level.

Live modeling is an option open to dentists who have multi-chair bays or may have several child patients in the office at the same time (Kuhn and Allen, 1994). The opportunity to observe another child undergoing treatment has been shown to be effective in obtaining cooperative behavior (Figure 12.3), while at the same time improving the cooperation of the child being observed. Although this approach is helpful in shaping behavior, it is unlikely to be an option for the periodontist or dentist seeing children infrequently. It may be in that dentist's interest to group paediatric appointments, so that several children are present in the office at one time.

Role modeling

Children are supported by the presence of other children undergoing similar treatment. Pediatric dentists usually design multi-chair treatment

Time out

Time and the ability to translate our knowledge into technical accomplishments are the dentist's

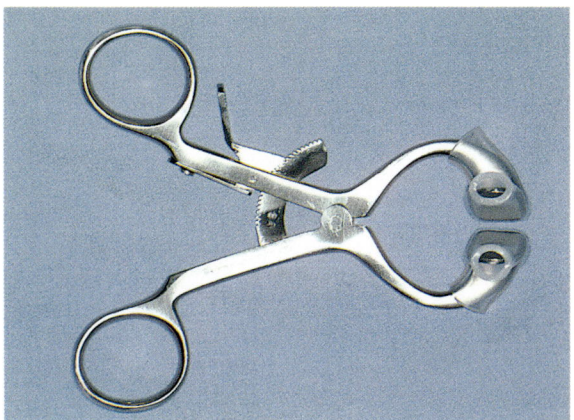

Figure 12.4

The Molt mouth prop, demonstrating its scissors-like ratcheted opening capability.

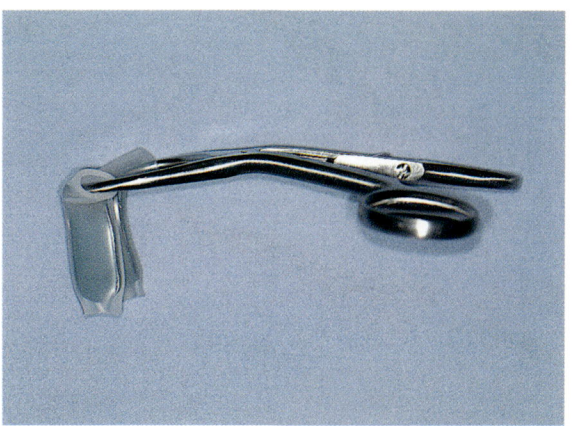

Figure 12.5

The Molt mouth prop viewed on its side to demonstrate the vinyl-protected arms to engage the dentition. Vinyl coverings may be removed, sterilized, and replaced.

greatest assets. It should come as no surprise that one of the newer concepts in behavioral modification is therefore underemployed by the dentist. "Time out" periods are perceived as procrastination, incurring costs which are in many cases non-reimbursable. However, "time out" can allow children to compose themselves and the dentist to re-evaluate his or her approach and personal demeanor.

"Contingent escape" is a modification of the "time out" described by Kuhn and Allen (1994). In this scenario, the child is allowed a pause contingent on cooperative behavior. Many dentists would choose this form of time out on the basis that it rewards good behavior rather than allowing an unruly child to control the treatment.

Physical restraint

Physical restraint is a clear escalation in aversive behavioral management techniques and may be employed to control a less cooperative child. These aversive techniques are disliked by parents, but limited applications may be beneficial to both dentist and child.

The simplest form of physical restraint is the use of a mouth prop. The Molt prop (Figures 12.4 and 12.5), a scissors-like prop which fits over the dental arch and is ratcheted open, may stabilize the dentition and allow greater access for the dentist. The child is told that we have a "pillow" to rest their teeth on and, after opening and introduction of the prop, is asked to bite on the plastic-covered arms. Again, the mouth prop steadies the dentition, relieves the child of straining to remain open (or simply tiring) and prevents injury to dentist or patient due to inadvertent bite closure.

Physical restraint of limbs with such devices as papoose boards, Velcro wraps, or hand over mouth (HOM), are now perceived as unacceptable by most parents and may be construed as assault in a legal sense. Many parents use the paradigm of child-rearing described by Mead (1978) as "prefigurative". In this method, little is based on traditional authoritative direction; rather, the parent continually experiments in an attempt to find a method that works. This parent is unlikely to accept the dentist's use of an authoritative approach. The HOM technique, in which the dentist's hand is placed over the patient's mouth to mute crying and to gain the child's attention (McTigue, 1984), is taught only by a few pediatric dental educators. In a variation of this technique, the airway was also restricted, but this is rarely used today. If the HOM method of behavioral management is chosen, parents must be fully informed and must consent to its use (Klein, 1987). Furthermore, the treatment plan should be reconsidered and the appropriateness of periodontal treatment reassessed in the face of the need for restraining techniques.

Pharmacological methods

A lengthy discussion of pharmacologically mediated behavior is beyond the scope of this chapter. However, to the extent that nitrous oxide/oxygen analgesia is capable of reducing a child's anxiety and modifying the threshold for discomfort, it is a useful adjunct to periodontal therapy. Nitrous oxide and oxygen alone may be used without the need for extensive monitoring of vital signs. It should be used at levels that assure adequate oxygenation and the dentist must be a careful observer to assure a patent airway and appropriate responsiveness. Child-sized and scented inhalers, with appropriate scavenging systems, are available commercially, and can be introduced to the child and parent as a safe and useful adjunct to comfortable treatment.

Nitrous oxide/oxygen analgesia may be combined with other drugs to produce a state of conscious sedation (American Academy of Pediatric Dentistry, 1999). This is a controlled, pharmacologically induced, minimally depressed level of consciousness that retains the patient's ability to maintain a patent airway independently and continuously, and to respond appropriately to physical stimulation or verbal commands. The goals of sedation are to facilitate the provision of quality care, minimize the extremes of disruptive behavior, promote a positive psychological response, promote patient welfare and safety, and to return the patient to a physiological state where safe discharge is possible. Oral agents that are commonly used include chloral hydrate, hydroxyzine, and meperidine. These are often used in combination with nitrous oxide and oxygen and are used to provide varying levels of conscious sedation. Five levels have been defined. Level 1 refers to mild sedation (anxiolysis) and, since the patient remains interactive, requires only clinical observation. Level 2 is an interactive level which is a minimally depressed level of consciousness

where the child's eyes are generally opened. The child is able to respond appropriately to verbal commands. The only monitoring that is necessary is a pulse oximeter. In level 3, however, the patient is non-interactive and arousable only with mild or moderate stimulation. At this level, pulse oximetry, a precordial stethoscope to monitor heart rate and respirations, and a blood pressure cuff are required, and must be monitored and recorded by a colleague trained in basic life support techniques. A "crash cart" with appropriate instruments and drugs must be kept nearby for emergency resuscitation, and a dedicated recovery area must be available. Deep sedation (level 4), where the patient's ability to maintain a patent airway independently and to respond purposefully to physical stimulation or verbal commands is diminished, requires the attendance of a third person trained in advanced cardiac life support methods and additional equipment such as capnography, an electrocardiograph, and a defibrillator. Such a deep level of sedation may not be appropriate for many dental practices, and may lead to the choice of general anesthesia (level 5) administered by a trained anesthesiologist in a fully equipped surgical setting.

General anesthesia is the ultimate sedation technique. Pediatric dentists, understanding the risks, usually reserve general anesthesia for patients who meet the following criteria: pre-cooperative age (under about 3 years), overwhelming caries (necessity for multiple restorations and/or extractions), and physical or mental challenges that preclude dental care in the usual chairside setting. With that in mind, dentists treating periodontal disease in children should reserve this form of management for the severely compromised patient requiring extensive treatment who cannot tolerate chairside treatment using any other method of behavioral management. The treating dentist must also be certain that the patient and the family will be capable of maintaining the health of the dentition following the surgical procedure. Periodontal treatment extensive enough to require this level of sedation should not be undertaken without the assurance that postoperative gingival health can be maintained and that the exposed dentition will be functional and not at greater risk of dental caries.

Local anesthesia will be required for any chairside surgical procedure, and is perceived by

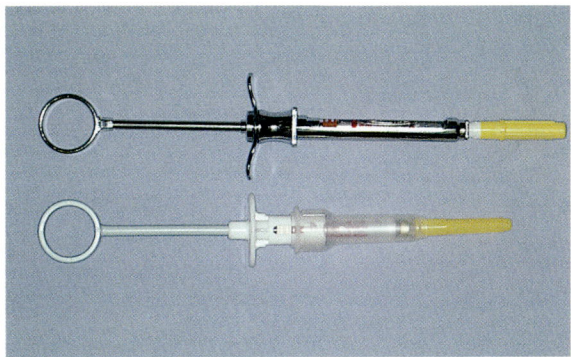

Figure 12.6

The Monoject disposable syringe (Sherwood Medical, St. Louis, MO, USA), compared with the reusable stainless steel syringe for administration of local anesthetic solutions.

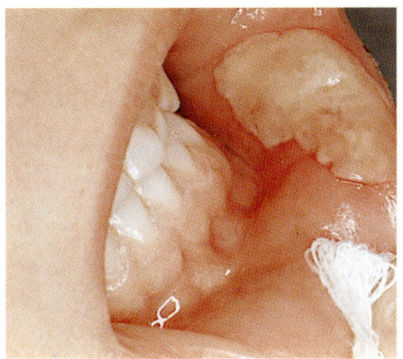

Figure 12.7

Traumatic lesion on the inner surface of the lip and cheek approximately 24 hours after local anesthetic injection. Some children, especially younger children, test the anesthetized area by pinching or chewing it. The result is an elevated white or gray lesion on the surface, which if removed, reveals a raw, bleeding ulcer. Swelling may be present. Treatment is palliative to reduce discomfort and maintain hygiene; antibiotic therapy is not necessary. The lesion will resolve spontaneously in 7–10 days.

most children as the most fear-inducing part of treatment. Any discussion of behavioral modification must, therefore, include injection techniques. To minimize discomfort, injection of a local anesthetic solution should always be preceded by the application of a topical anesthetic agent such as benzocaine-containing compounds (e.g., Hurricaine Gel) or EMLA, a percutaneous medicament containing lidocaine (lignocaine) 2.5% and prilocaine 2.5% in a cream. Topical agents must be left in contact with the mucous membrane long enough to assure surface anesthesia to mask the needle penetration. Infiltration of local anesthetic solution is acceptable for many maxillary procedures, but, if block injection is required, the dentist must be aware of the more inferior position of the inferior alveolar nerve in the mandible of young children. The maximum safe dose of local anesthetic drug for a child must not be exceeded (e.g., 4 mg/kg for lidocaine). Disposable syringes (Figure 12.6) which avoid the more threatening appearance of stainless steel are preferred. Needles large enough to permit aspiration of red blood cells (27 gauge) permit a more comfortable injection. It is important to note that the after-effects of local anesthesia (numbness and puffiness) may be very disturbing to children. Children who test the anesthetic by biting or pinching their lips or cheeks may cause severe ulcerations and postoperative discomfort (Figure 12.7). Parents

should be advised beforehand that close observation of the child following treatment will be necessary to prevent this traumatic sequela, particularly in very young children.

Conclusion

Understanding of behavioral management options is essential for dentists treating children with periodontal disease. In planning treatment, the primary care dentist and the periodontist must be certain of their ability to achieve and maintain treatment objectives. In gaining that assurance, chairside non-pharmacological methods of behavioral management, depending on language and behavioral milestones, offer the best opportunity for long-term oral health.

References

American Academy of Pediatric Dentistry (1999) Reference Manual. *Pediatr Dent* **21**: 68–73.

Cole M, Cole SR (1993) *The Development of Children*. New York: Scientific American.

Erikson EH (1963) *Childhood and Society*, 2nd edn. New York: WW Norton.

Fields HW, Machen JB, Murphy MG (1984) Acceptability of various behavior management techniques relative to types of dental treatment. *Pediatr Dent* **6**: 199–203.

Greenbaum PE, Turner C, Cook EW (1990) Dentists' voice control: effects on children's disruptive behavior. *Health Psychol* **9**: 546–58.

Hetherington EM, Stanley-Hagan M, Anderson E (1989) Marital transitions; a child's perspective. *Am Psychol* **44**: 303–12.

Hoffman LW (1989) Effects of maternal employment in the two-parent family. *Am Psychol* **44**: 283–92.

Klein A (1987) Physical restraint, informed consent and the child patient. *ASDC J Dent Child* **55**: 121–2.

Kuhn BR, Allen KD (1994) Expanding child behavior management technology in pediatric dentistry: a behavioral science perspective. *Pediatr Dent* **16**: 13–17.

McTigue DJ (1984) Behavioral management in children. *Dent Clin North Am* **28**: 81–93.

McKnight-Hanes C, Myers DR, Dushku JC, Davis HC (1993) The use of behavior management techniques by dentists across practitioner type, age, and geographic region. *Pediatr Dent* **15**: 267–71.

Mead M (1978) *Culture and Commitment: The New Relationships Between the Generations in the 1970s*. New York: Columbia University Press.

Pinkham JR (1991) An analysis of the phenomenon of increased parental participation during the child's dental experience. *ASDC J Dent Child* **58**: 458–63.

Pinkham JR (1995) Personality development; managing behavior of the cooperative preschool child. *Dental Clin North Am* **39**: 771–86.

Rayman MS (1987) Parent observation: inviting a parent to accompany his/her child into the treatment room can be rewarding for everyone. *J Calif Dent Assoc* **15**: 20–4.

PART VI

Areas of special interest

13

Malocclusion, orthodontic intervention, and gingival and periodontal health

Enrique Bimstein and Adrian Becker

The intimate relationship between malocclusion, orthodontic treatment, and gingival and periodontal health, needs to be carefully understood, since it has a direct bearing on the longevity of the dentition. It is essential to identify patients who have gingival and periodontal diseases—or are at risk of developing them—to establish a comprehensive treatment strategy. In some cases, this requires teamwork involving the orthodontist, the pediatric dentist, and the periodontist to monitor all aspects of the oral health before, during, and after a course of orthodontic therapy.

The complexity of the interplay between gingival and periodontal health, malocclusion, and orthodontic treatment is at least partly responsible for the wide disparity of reported views on this subject. These may be firstly attributed to a simplistic approach to a complex multifactorial cause-and-effect relationship. Biologic factors are never isolated in vivo. The clinician should be aware of all the factors operating in a particular case and their relative importance, as they influence the diagnosis, treatment regimen and outcome. Secondly, reported studies are difficult to compare because of variations in:

- population characteristics (age, gender, type of malocclusion, and ethnicity)
- diagnostic criteria of malocclusion and of gingival and periodontal disease
- treatment characteristics (type of appliance, direction and magnitude of the orthodontic force and length of treatment, retention or follow-up periods)
- group or individual variation.

The findings of clinical research in groups of individuals show general trends within the particular experimental group examined. This does not mean that conclusions from these findings may be applied automatically to every patient. Care must be taken to address individual needs.

In addition, caution must be exercised in interpreting case reports. It is important to remember these reports are distinctly individual insights related to a particular patient, which may have been published because of the peculiarity of the condition or because of an unusual, exceptional, or even unique approach to treatment. This may have been the reason it was accepted for publication and may make it inappropriate to adopt as a model for routine clinical practice.

Malocclusion in relation to gingival and periodontal health

The presence of such factors as gingival inflammation, inadequate width of attached gingiva (Figure 13.1a), root resorption, and deficient alveolar bone height may be seen in association with a single misplaced tooth or in general malocclusion. This may lead one to assume a direct cause-and-effect relationship between malocclusion and gingival and periodontal diseases. An orthodontist may justify aiming at ideal dental alignment and occlusion on the assumption of therapeutic effects on gingival and periodontal health. However, individuals with obvious malocclusion and little or no associated gingival and periodontal diseases may be frequently seen (Figure 13.1b).

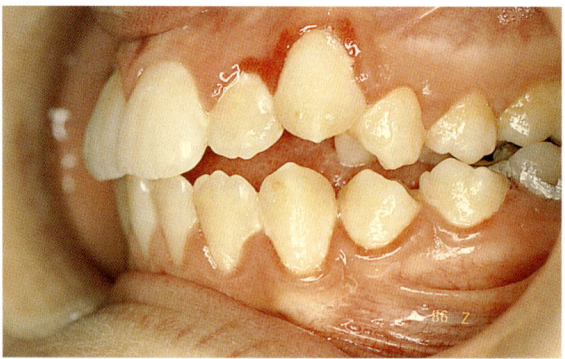

a

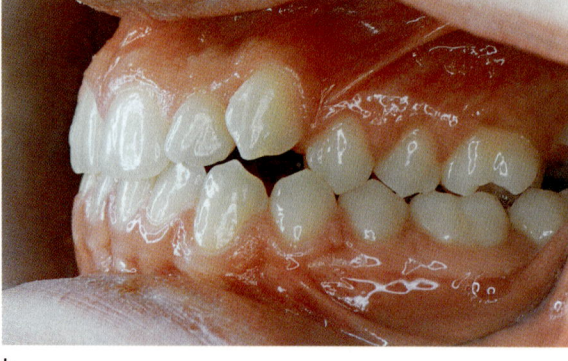

b

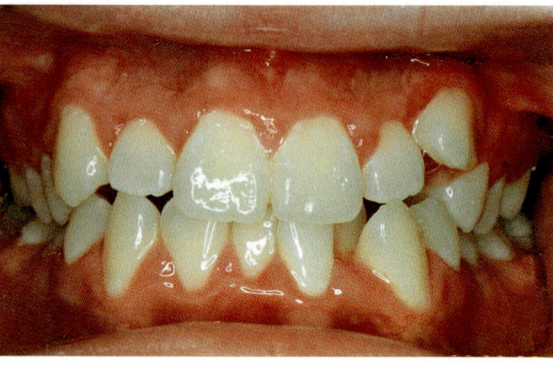

c

Figure 13.1

(a) Gingival disease adjacent to malaligned teeth. Plaque accumulation has already caused decalcification in several cervical areas of the teeth crowns. A carious cavity has been treated with an amalgam restoration in the buccal surface of the mandibular first permanent molar. (b) Malaligned teeth with excellent gingival condition. No plaque accumulation is evident. (c) Gingivitis associated with crowding and extreme displacement and consequent poor oral hygiene. The ectopic maxillary canine erupted in the oral mucosa above the attached gingiva.

The reaction of the gingival and periodontal tissues to malocclusion spans a wide range, from the innocuous and transient to the severe and irreversible. This lack of uniformity is perplexing insofar as:

- class of occlusion (Angle), studied by sex and race, shows no consistent relation to inflammation and periodontal destruction (Geiger et al., 1972)
- no positive associations are found between crowding, spacing, periodontal destruction, and gingival inflammation (Geiger et al., 1974).
- there is no consistent relationship between crossbite and periodontal disease (Geiger and Wasserman, 1977).
- leaving a malocclusion untreated in the young patient does not appear to influence subsequent development or non-development of

periodontal disease in adulthood (Sadowsky and BeGole, 1981).

Effect of tooth malalignment or malocclusion on the gingival and periodontal tissues

Departure from ideal alignment and occlusion facilitates plaque accumulation and calculus formation, due to an altered oral environment, abnormal occlusal forces, food impaction, and poor gingival contour and/or alveolar bone architecture. Since bacterial plaque and its by-products are the main etiologic factors for gingival and periodontal diseases (Löe et al., 1964; Listgarten, 1986), it follows that the establishment and progress of these diseases may be exacerbated by

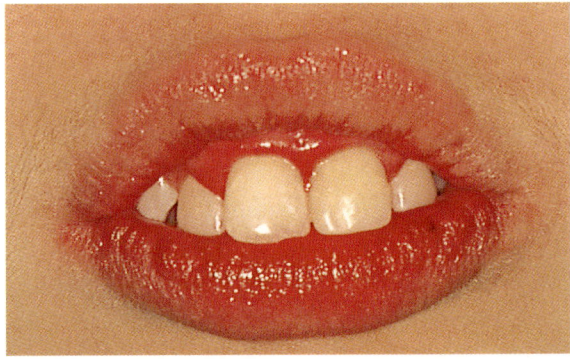

a

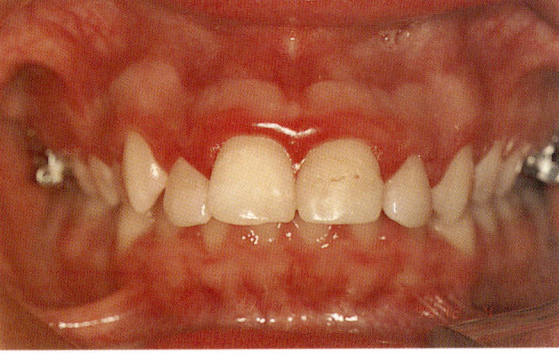

b

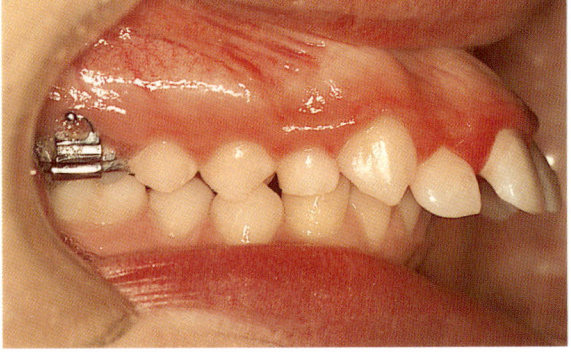

c

Figure 13.2

(a) Resting posture of incompetent lips displaced much labial gingiva. (b) Desiccated, inflamed and swollen gingivae of patient in (a). (c) Lateral view to show the extreme overjet and an over-retained deciduous canine.

such conditions and, conversely, that good oral hygiene may preserve gingival and periodontal health. Malocclusion is therefore not so much a primary etiologic factor as a contributory factor, insofar as it facilitates plaque accumulation.

Crowding (Paunio, 1973; Ingervall et al., 1977), increased overjet and overbite (Geiger et al., 1973; Geiger and Wasserman, 1976; Davies et al., 1988), crossbite (Harrison et al., 1991; Al-Jasser and Hashim, 1995), open bite, inadequate or poor lip seal, and mouth breathing (Machtei et al., 1990; Wagaiyu and Ashley, 1991), and tooth rotations (Peretz and Machtei, 1996) have all been related to periodontal disease.

Crowding

Crowding may adversely affect the health of the gingiva (Figure 13.1c) and the periodontium if:

- dental irregularity creates inaccessible corners between and around the teeth which lead to plaque accumulation
- teeth displaced from the line of the arch receive their occlusal load non-axially, leading to a lateral force component each time the teeth come together
- interproximal contacts are poor—the intercuspation of opposing teeth may cause food impaction
- ectopic teeth erupt through the oral mucosa rather than within the band of attached gingiva.

Increased overjet and overbite

It has been reported that the damaging influence of an increased overjet exceeds that of an increased overbite, although the two frequently

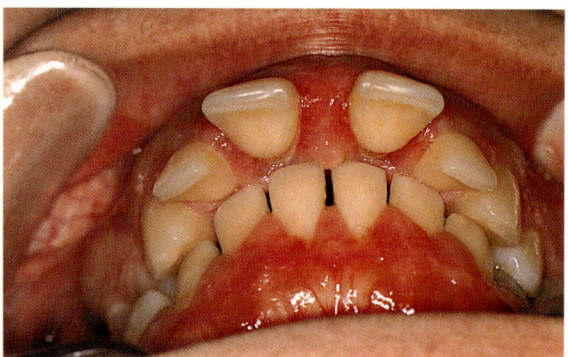

Figure 13.3

Deep overbite with direct trauma to the gingiva by the mandibular teeth.

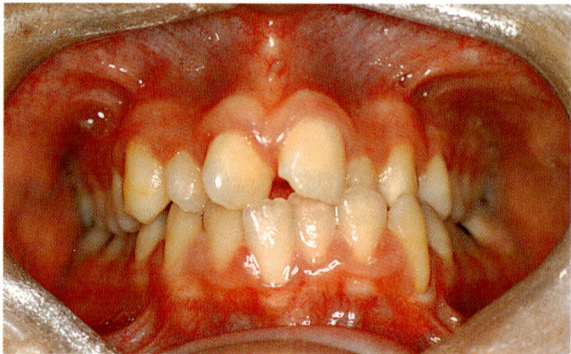

Figure 13.4

Crossbite affecting the right central maxillary and mandibular incisors. Note a similar crossbite of the left canines, associated with severe gingival recession whose etiology must include the frenal attachment adjacent to the mandibular canine.

occur together. A normal overbite and overjet relationship is accompanied by fair to good lip cover and a lower lip that controls the incisal edges of the maxillary incisors. Under these normal conditions the anterior oral seal during swallowing is produced by the two lips coming into light contact. The presence of an increased overjet (Figure 13.2) is accompanied (and generated) by an abnormal seal, which may be produced by the lower lip contracting behind the upper incisor teeth, with or without the involvement of a forward tongue posture. In these circumstances, the upper lip will play no part in the involuntary reflex behavior that forms the seal and an enlarged overjet will be present. Inadequate lip cover and an abnormal anterior oral seal often reduce the capacity for natural food clearance from the area, leading to food debris and plaque accumulation, particularly in the labial gingival area of the maxillary incisors.

A deep overbite (Figure 13.3) brings the mandibular incisal edges in contact with the cervical part of the upper incisors or with the gingiva itself, causing direct trauma. This may lead either to inflammation due to food impaction, or to ulceration due to direct and blunt trauma from the opposing teeth.

Crossbite

Opposing anterior teeth that occlude in crossbite (Figure 13.4) will often show gingival recession,

more gingival inflammation, and greater pocket depths than adjacent, correctly related teeth. Crossbite is often brought about by teeth that have erupted ectopically and, as such, have reduced width or absence of keratinized attached gingiva and—particularly in the lower incisor region—a reduced amount of labial alveolar bone, with gingival recession evident.

It has been proposed that a self-perpetuating circle may occur in cases of gingival recession, in which gingival recession facilitates plaque accumulation, which causes inflammation, producing further gingival recession. Clinical experience suggests additional factors such as exposed sensitive cementum and gingival bleeding as reasons for the patient to avoid brushing the area.

Open bite, lip seal, and mouth breathing

In anterior open bite (Figure 13.5), the incisor teeth do not come into occlusal function at any time. There is no incisal guidance, the patient rarely protrudes the mandible in function, and virtually all productive masticatory activity occurs in the posterior areas of the dentition. Accordingly, a stagnant and partially dehydrated plaque collection exists around the anterior teeth, accumulating with succeeding meals. This

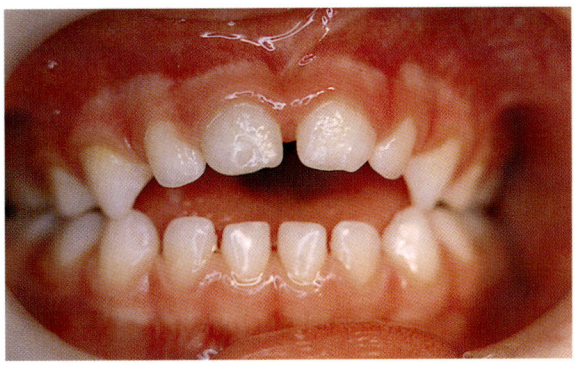

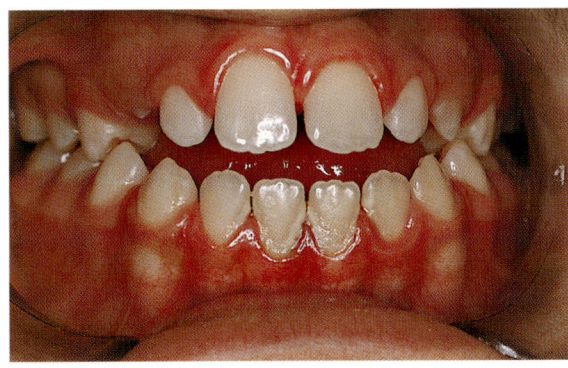

a

b

Figure 13.5

(a) Anterior open bite in the primary dentition showing gingival inflammation with plaque. (b) Anterior open bite in the permanent dentition showing gingival inflammation with plaque and calculus.

could account for the occurrence of a more hyperplastic type of gingivitis in open bite cases and for the longer clinical crowns that these patients exhibit, which may be the result of more significant recession.

Individuals who breathe predominantly through the mouth have many more sites with plaque accumulation and gingival inflammation than do nose breathers. Similar patterns are found with poor lip seal and reduced lip coverage. However, when mouth breathing, lip seal, and lip coverage are assessed separately, only mouth breathing and lip coverage are found to be potent factors, exhibiting a higher number of sites with plaque. The ill-effects of mouth breathing appear to be seen more on the palatal side while poor lip coverage largely affects the labial side. The relationship between gingivitis and plaque in mouth breathers is dependent not only on the amount of plaque, but also on plaque composition and alterations in the response of the tissues to the plaque.

A word of caution is needed in relation to a confusion that exists generally, regarding the terms used here. Mouth breathing and open mouth posture are *not* the same thing. The fact that the lips are open does not mean that the child is breathing through the mouth, since, in addition to the anterior oral seal, the mouth also has a posterior oral seal. The posterior seal is formed between the dorsum of the tongue and the soft palate and it effectively prevents mouth breathing. A minority of patients are true mouth breathers (Vig, 1979) and this is usually due to severe chronic nasal obstruction. To differentiate between open mouth posture and true mouth breathing, the actual movement of expired air should be tested. This is probably done most simply by noting the movement of a wisp of cotton wool held beneath each of the nares and then close to the lips to detect the stream of air, or by using a mouth mirror which will steam up from the expired air. Unfortunately, many clinicians—dentists and ear, nose and throat surgeons alike—and researchers diagnose mouth breathing on the basis of an open mouth posture alone.

Rotations

Mild rotations of individual teeth are not usually associated with a deterioration in the health of the gingiva, but when the rotation is severe there is evidence that the height of the investing alveolar bone will be reduced.

In exceptional circumstances malocclusion may lead to increased mechanical forces that exceed the tolerance of the periodontal tissues—in other words, occlusal traumatism. Significant damage may be caused to the periodontal tissues, specifically when dental plaque accumulation and occlusal trauma occur together.

Dental plaque in relation to malocclusion

The patient with "straight teeth" has fewer potential stagnation areas and this will facilitate the maintenance of a plaque-free state. An individually planned oral hygiene regimen will be needed for more irregular dentitions, to achieve the same aim. To illustrate this point, Sadowsky and BeGole (1981) found that the periodontal condition in a group of patients with marked malocclusion, but with a high level of oral hygiene, was equivalent to that of a parallel group of orthodontically treated patients with similarly high oral hygiene levels.

Clinical awareness and common sense must guide the clinician in recommending treatment to prevent the vicious circle of plaque accumulation, disease, pain, and further plaque accumulation. Oral hygiene techniques must be adapted to gingival morphology and tooth position and to the child's comprehension and manual skills. Furthermore, the clinician must avoid teaching a style of tooth brushing that is overzealous in its use of force and inadequate in technique.

Control of gingival inflammation is also an important factor in the treatment of isolated gingival recession of teeth with or without crossbite. Gingival contour is enhanced and frenal involvement may decline when control of gingival inflammation is sustained (Powell and McEniery, 1982; Persson and Lennartsson, 1986; Bimstein et al., 1988; Bimstein, 1989; Andlin-Sobocki et al., 1991). For this purpose, the clinician must be aware that abnormal gingival morphology, a high frenum attachment, or a shallow buccal or lingual sulcus or tooth angulation and occlusion (Figures 13.1a, c, 13.2–13.4, 13.6), may hinder oral hygiene procedures (Bimstein et al., 1988). The topic of attached gingiva is discussed in Chapter 4.

The effect of orthodontic treatment on periodontal tissues

There are conflicting data regarding the effect of orthodontic treatment on the periodontal tissues: reported effects vary from beneficial, through innocuous, to deleterious.

Potential benefits

Improvement of width of attached gingiva

Eruption of teeth, in a normal faciolingual position, takes place with the investing tissues modifying the width of the keratinized gingiva and alveolar bone height. These structures also respond to orthodontic alteration in the functional environment of the teeth (Ainamo and Ainamo, 1978; Gazit and Lieberman, 1980; Coatam et al., 1981; Karring, 1982; Melsen et al., 1988; Harrison et al., 1991; Sanders, 1999).

Exhibiting a long clinical crown, incisor teeth in crossbite show a decrease in the discrepancy of gingival height with their adjacent teeth, following orthodontic treatment. This change is due more to an increase in crown length in the adjacent teeth than to a reduction in clinical crown length in the affected tooth (Harrison et al., 1991). Moreover, with a labially positioned tooth, the width of attached gingiva and bone thickness may increase when the tooth is moved lingually (Karring, 1982; Bimstein et al., 1990; Sanders, 1999). This increase, however, may be hindered by a simultaneous orthodontic intrusion of the mandibular incisors (Bimstein et al.,

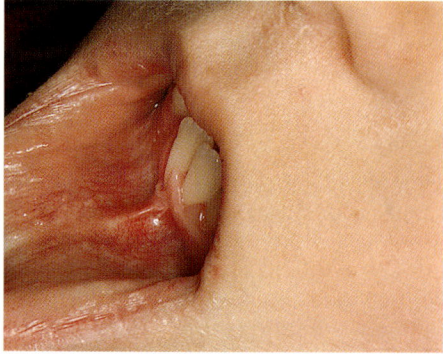

Figure 13.6

A high frenum attachment with a shallow buccal sulcus hinders the performance of adequate oral hygiene. With permission of *ASDC J Dent Child*, from Bimstein et al., 1988.

1990) or lingual tipping of mandibular incisors, a movement that tips their roots labially, thinning both alveolar bone and soft tissues (Sperry et al., 1977).

Inducement of bone formation

Orthodontic therapy may help to solve periodontal problems by inducing bone formation (Polson et al., 1984). This improvement in the health of the periodontium may enhance the prognosis for periodontally compromised teeth and the success of the orthodontic treatment itself, since an increase in periodontal support is crucial for the prevention of relapse (Sjølien and Zachrisson, 1973; Hollender et al., 1980; Sharpe et al., 1987).

Siting preparation margins supragingivally and re-establishing biologic width in teeth with subgingival or subcrestal margins

In overerupted teeth, the distance from the cementoenamel junction to the alveolar bone crest remains unchanged. The bone follows the tooth and a constant relationship between the height of the alveolar bone and the cemento-enamel junction is maintained (Baxter, 1967). This principle has been put to use in applying adjunctive orthodontics to restorative treatment.

Forced eruption offers the potential for salvaging isolated teeth in which caries, trauma, or iatrogenesis have destroyed the clinical crown to a level apical to the crestal bone (Figure 13.7). In these cases the orthodontic treatment brings the fractured, diseased, or prepared margins of the neck of the tooth more coronally, to re-establish the biologic width, facilitate impression-taking, achieve adequate etching on enamel or dentine, control hemorrhage, maintain periodontal health, and restore function and appearance (Ingber, 1976; Stern and Becker, 1980; Bielak et al., 1982). The clinician must be aware that forced eruption may be accompanied by an increase in the keratinized gingiva while the mucogingival junction remains unaltered (Reitan, 1967; Atherton, 1970). However, it will result in a smaller diameter of the apically tapered root being positioned in the unchanged mesiodistal

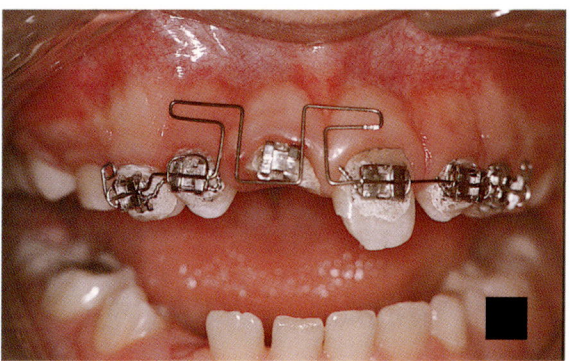

a

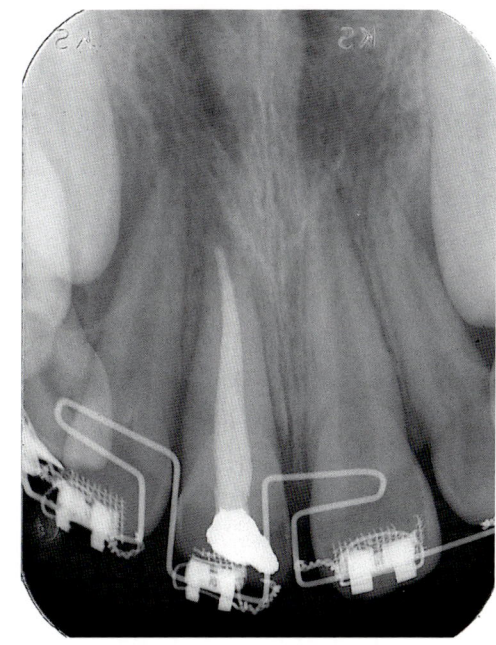

b

Figure 13.7

(a) Tooth with a crown–root subgingival fracture caused by a traumatic injury. (b) Anterior pericapical radiograph of the area in (a).

space between the adjacent teeth, which the restored crown must ultimately occupy. The radiographic appearance of the crestal bone will show uneven margins (Ingber, 1976).

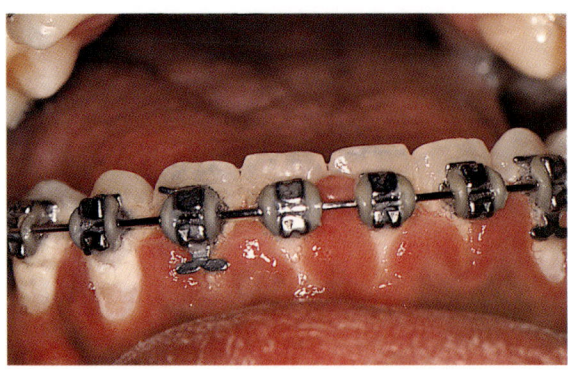

a

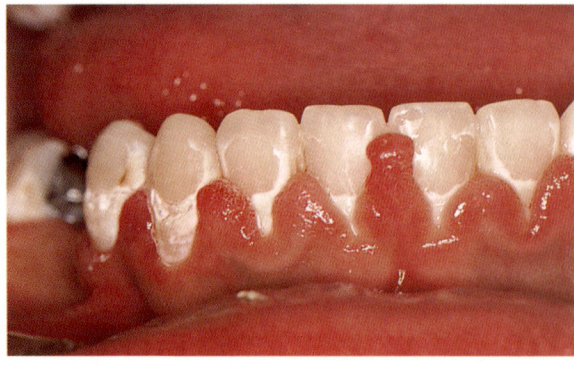

b

Figure 13.8

Obvious absence of oral hygiene, severe hypertrophic gingivitis, gingival recession, widespread decalcification and early caries lesions (a) in the presence and (b) after removal of orthodontic appliances.

Closure of spaces

Orthodontic therapy may help to solve periodontal disease complications by closing spaces of extracted teeth (McLain et al., 1983).

Harmful effects

Gingival and periodontal changes related to orthodontic treatment are, in general, transient with no permanent damage. Loss of attachment and alveolar bone loss are known to occur during orthodontic treatment, but are reported to be temporary (Sjølien and Zachrisson, 1973; Zachrisson and Alnaes, 1974; Alstad and Zachrisson, 1979). However, if lengthy orthodontic treatment continues in the sustained absence of oral hygiene, gingival and periodontal damage takes place, not to mention frank caries (Figure 13.8). The deleterious effects include gingivitis, gingival hyperplasia (Figure 13.9a), marginal periodontitis, gingival recession mostly at extraction areas, loss of attachment, interdental clefts (Figure 13.9b), mostly at the vestibular aspects of extracted mandibular first premolar sites, reduced width of keratinized gingiva, and marginal bone and apical root resorption (Figure 13.9c) (Pearson, 1968; Zachrisson and Zachrisson, 1972; Sjølien and Zachrisson,1973;

Zachrisson and Alnaes, 1973; Kloehn and Pfeifer, 1974; Robertson et al., 1977; Dorfman,1978, Hollender et al., 1980; Sharpe et al., 1987). Some of these may undermine the stability of the orthodontic result, particularly where there is a reduction in bone support or the presence of gingival clefts and recession.

Periodontitis

Exaggerated plaque accumulation during orthodontic treatment may facilitate the formation of localized, deep anaerobic pockets in which periodontal pathogens may flourish, and the situation may deteriorate rapidly into a more serious condition (Ericson et al., 1977; Sinclair et al., 1987; Huser et al., 1990; Paolantonio et al., 1999). The gingiva initially becomes inflamed, owing to the presence of stagnating plaque. Later, the patient complains of pain and bleeding. Clinical examination may then reveal a hemorrhagic gingiva and a pocket that extends to the furcation.

Gingival recession and clefts

Teeth with adequate attached gingiva occasionally develop localized recession during orthodontic treatment. It has generally been assumed that

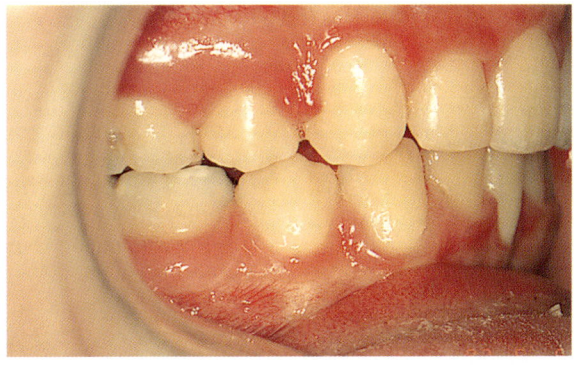

a

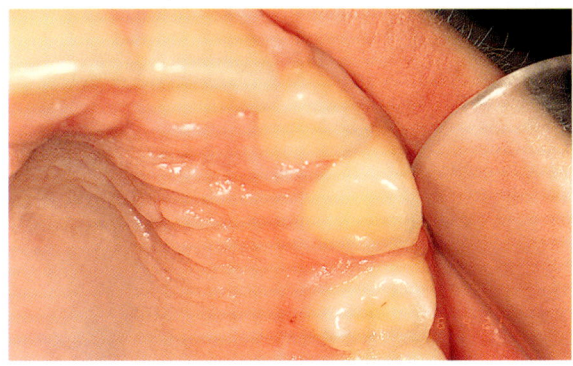

b

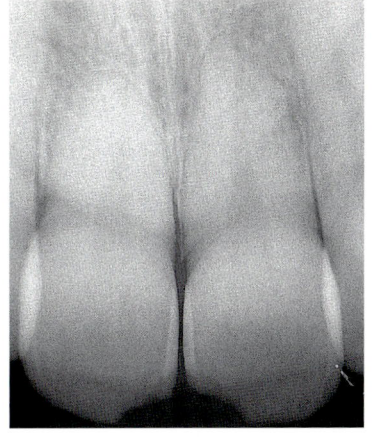

c

Figure 13.9

(a) On completion of orthodontic treatment there is loss of attachment at the mandibular right central incisor and mild hypertrophic gingivitis elsewhere. (b) Interdental cleft at the slightly reopened extraction site of the first premolar, between the maxillary canine and second premolar. (c) Apical root resorption evident after orthodontic treatment. Tooth fractures are unrelated to the root resorption.

this is associated with excessive forces that hinder the repair and remodeling of the alveolar bone. It is, however, more likely that the direction and extent of movement have forced the tooth through the cortical plate, while the remaining gingival attachment appears relatively free of inflammation, such as when a molar with wide and divergent roots is moved into a narrow (dimensionally inadequate) premolar alveolar zone (Geiger, 1980). Furthermore, where teeth are extracted as part of the treatment, the orthodontic closure of the extraction spaces may give rise to gingival invagination or clefting (Figure 13.9b), in the immediate area (Robertson et al., 1977).

Controversy exists over the need for an adequate zone of attached gingiva before tooth movement. Where the labial tissue is thin, especially if the orthodontist plans to move the tooth labially, it appears logical that the labial tissue should be augmented (Sanders, 1999). On the other hand, the absence of keratinized gingiva alone is not an indication for its surgical enhancement has been reported:

- There were no differences between a control group and an orthodontic treatment group in the prevalence of mucogingival problems or in moderate to severe periodontal disease, 12–35 years after orthodontic treatment (Sadowsky and BeGole, 1981). However, the orthodontic group had a greater prevalence of mild to moderate periodontal disease in the maxillary posterior and mandibular anterior regions of the mouth.
- Areas with narrow keratinized gingival tissues appear to remain stable over an 18-year period (Freedman et al., 1999).
- Teeth with minimal widths of keratinized gingiva (less than 2 mm) may withstand orthodontic forces, even when there is moderate inflammation and fair to poor oral hygiene (Coatam et al., 1981).

- If recession is found to progress, in general or during orthodontic treatment, then surgical augmentation may be necessary (Newman et al., 1994; Freedman et al., 1999).
- Surgical intervention does not guarantee success. Among orthosurgical patients, the risk of recession increased when genioplasty was combined with mandibular advancement, at sites in which the keratinized gingiva and underlying bone appeared thin (Fousshee et al., 1985). In addition, preorthodontic gingival grafting does not necessarily decrease postorthodontic gingival recession (Ngan et al., 1991).

Root resorption

Tooth support is measured by the length of root that is invested with alveolar bone. Loss of attachment and crestal alveolar bone will reduce this support. So, too, will loss of root length by resorption (Figure 13.9c). Root resorption generated by orthodontic treatment has a wide range of severity and very different and locally acting factors have been implicated.

- Interrupted force results in less root resorption than does the application of continuous force (Acar et al., 1999). On the other hand, Owman-Moll et al. (1996a, b) found no relation between frequency or severity of force and root resorption, indicating great individual variation in the relation between tooth movement and root resorption.
- Incisor intrusion together with lingual root torque is strongly related to external root resorption. In contrast, distal bodily retraction, extrusion, or lingual crown tipping have a lesser or no effect (Parker and Harris, 1998; Horiuchi et al., 1998).
- Root approximation to the palatal cortical bone during orthodontic treatment has a significant effect on the appearance of root resorption (Horiuchi et al., 1998).
- Intrusion forces may cause root resorption (Kucukkeles and Okar, 1994).
- Root resorption has also been found to occur in relation to general factors, including chronic inflammation and infections, such as asthma, chronic periodontal disease and juvenile arthritis (Davidovitch et al., 1995).

That orthodontic treatment is directly associated with root resorption in many cases is no longer in question, and it is true to say that resorption occurs more severely in the maxillary anterior region and in the teeth adjacent to a closed extraction space, when space closure has been performed (Sjølien and Zachrisson, 1973). The resorptive process almost invariably stops when orthodontic forces are removed at the end of treatment (Brezniak and Wasserstein, 1993). Many studies of resorption have been undertaken and almost as many conflicting results have been seen, and this is in part due to the criteria for diagnosing root resorption, the type of appliance used, force applied, extent of tooth movement, duration of active treatment, and dental age. The risk of root resorption appears to be especially great when root torque is applied (Morse, 1971; Goldson and Henrikson, 1975). The work of Levander and Malmgren has pointed to the blunt apex, the apically bent root, and the pipette-shaped root as the most likely to become resorbed (Levander and Malmgren, 1988, 1998; Levander et al., 1994, 1998a, b). Periapical radiographs are to be taken at the half year mark after initiation of orthodontic treatment, to check for root resorption. If none is seen, then subsequent resorption is unlikely to occur during the rest of the treatment. Should resorption be diagnosed, a 2–3 month break in the application of force is recommended (Levander and Malmgren, 1988, 1998; Levander et al., 1994, 1998a, b).

Reduction in alveolar bone height

Despite the expectation of alteration in the alveolar bone height during orthodontic treatment, several studies indicate no significant detrimental effect (Kloehn and Pfeifer, 1974; Baxter, 1967; Polson and Reed, 1984). Moreover, bone loss due to apparently damaging "jiggling" forces regenerates after discontinuation of the forces (Karring, 1982).

Follow-up

The effect of orthodontic treatment on the periodontal tissues is not limited to the duration of active treatment but continues after its completion, although a degree of uncertainty prevails regarding the short-term and long-term effects on the periodontium. Thus, an unintentional thinning out of the mucosa or narrowing of the alveolar bone thickness during treatment by expansion, retraction, or torque may predispose the patient to future recession which may be aggravated by mechanical irritation, periodontitis, or traumatic occlusion (Zachrisson, 1978).

Factors that may undermine the potential benefit of orthodontic treatment

With excellent oral hygiene and in the absence of periodontal disease, proper orthodontic therapy causes no significant long-term effects on periodontal attachment and bone levels. Conversely, in patients with active periodontitis, orthodontic movement may accelerate the disease progress, even when oral hygiene is practiced (Sanders, 1999).

The placement of orthodontic appliances of all types juxtaposes physical obstacles to the external surfaces of the teeth, which interfere with the natural food slew-ways or pathways that permit masticated food to move smoothly over the buccal and lingual surfaces and away from the teeth. The interference thus created traps for food around the appliance, keeping it in close contact with the teeth and gingival tissues. In these circumstances, inflammation of these tissues will rapidly occur and will be considerably worse than any pretreatment condition (Figures 13.10a, b). Conversely, and in the light of these possible dangers, patients with a newly fitted orthodontic appliance may overzealously perform oral hygiene procedures, leading to trauma of the gingiva and teeth with resulting recession (Ainamo et al., 1986). The inflammation that is abetted and encouraged by the placement of appliances varies and is complicated by such factors as oral hygiene compliance, innate factors of the patient, and treatment characteristics.

Oral hygiene

The effectiveness of a patient's home oral hygiene may improve during orthodontic treatment;

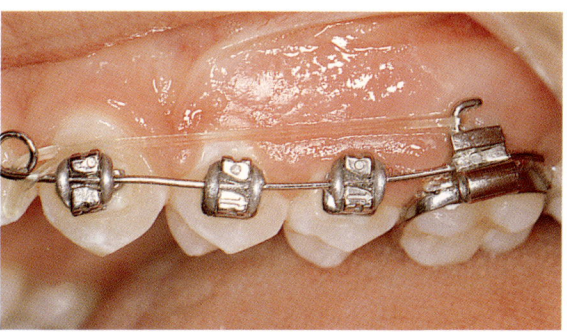

a

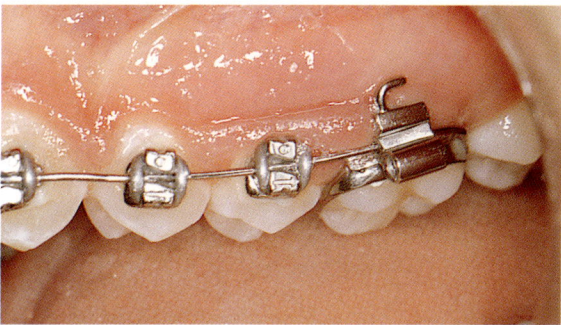

b

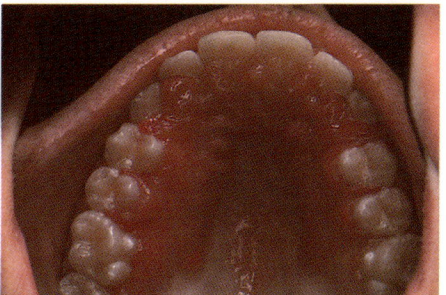

c

Figure 13.10

(a) The molar band carries a bulky triple tube and hook assembly which has caused marked inflammation of the gingiva. The elastic module is partially covered by the excessive gingival tissue and may have been a contributory cause. (b) Removal of the elastic module shows the severity of the lesion. Spontaneous resolution of the condition may be expected following removal of the appliance and accompanying oral hygiene. (c) Palatal and gingival inflammation due to lack of oral hygiene under a maxillary acrylic retainer.

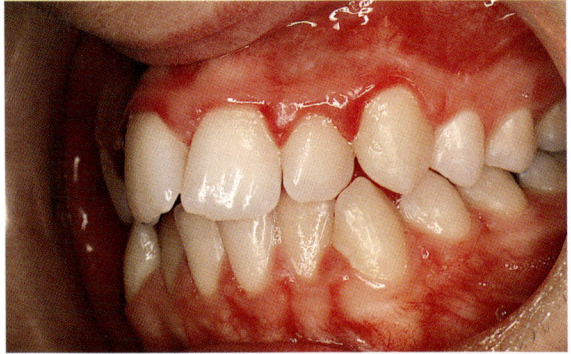

a

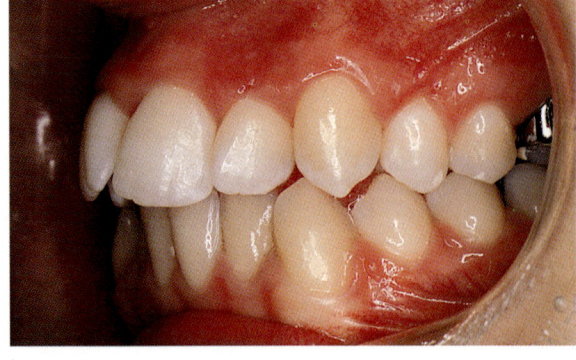

b

Figure 13.11

(a) A regular tooth brusher with inadequate technique shows gingival inflammation at first orthodontic examination. (b) Resolution of gingival condition occurred within 3 weeks after oral hygiene improved, allowing initiation of orthodontic treatment. (c) Gingival condition at the completion of orthodontic treatment.

c

however, an increase in gingival inflammation and probing depths, and gingival hyperplasia have been reported (Zachrisson and Zachrisson, 1972; Kloehn and Pfeifer, 1974; Kornhauser et al., 1996). Eventually, the successful outcome of the treatment will facilitate plaque control leading to a reduction in gingival inflammation and hyperplasia, mostly in the first 48 hours following appliance removal and continuing to decrease during the retention period (Zachrisson and Zachrisson, 1972; Kloehn and Pfeifer, 1974; Kornhauser et al., 1996). Moreover, once the orthodontic appliances are removed, some patients may have better plaque control and less gingival inflammation than their untreated fellows, having derived benefit from their orthodontic experience (Alstad and Zachrisson, 1979).

Even with good oral hygiene an increase in periodontal pathogens in orthodontic patients is observed. Different forms of orthodontic appliance, such as removable appliances and bonded retainers, produce comparable levels of inflammation of the periodontal tissues, but in different ways (Heier et al., 1997). At the gingival area closest to orthodontic bands, bonded attachments, or bonded retainers, the microbial composition of plaque is altered (Sinclair et al., 1987; Huser et al., 1990). Noteworthy is the fact that changes in microbial composition are restricted to subgingival plaque in the immediate area of the orthodontic appliance and do not affect the microbiologic condition of the whole mouth (Paolantonio et al., 1999). A removable appliance may nurse a low-grade inflammation of a wide area of the palatal mucosa and of the gingiva on the palatal side of the teeth, which are covered by the acrylic base (Figure 13.10c). It should be emphasized, therefore, optimizing oral hygiene before orthodontic treatment begins and conserving it during treatment will increase the possibilities of a successful outcome (Figure 13.11). In any case in which oral hygiene compliance is not achieved, the orthodontic appliances must be removed and treatment discontinued (Figure 13.12; see also Figure 13.8).

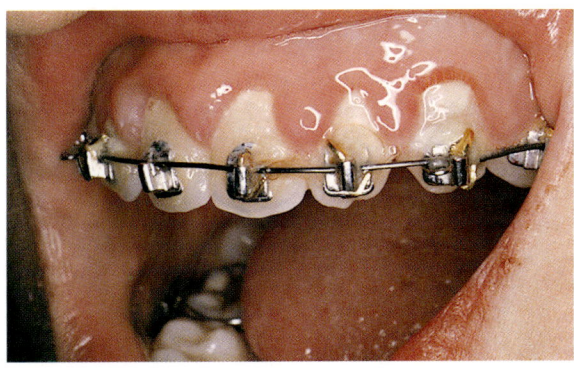
a

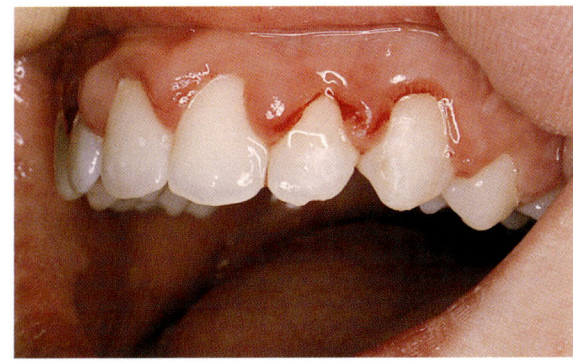
b

Figure 13.12

(a) Severe gingival reaction to obvious plaque accumulation around fixed appliances. (b) Immediately after removal of appliances and prophylaxis.

Innate factors

Innate factors may be:

- strictly local, referring to a specific area of the mouth, a pre-existing disease condition, or traumatic injury
- systemic, such as a hereditary predisposition for periodontal disease, reaction to dental materials, or general health status
- personal, such as age, gender, and ethnicity.

In patients with such predisposing factors routine oral hygiene may not be enough and additional or more meticulous antiplaque measures should be adopted. Oral hygiene techniques should be adapted to the patient's age, manual skill and dexterity, occlusal characteristics, and individual susceptibility to periodontal disease.

Treatment characteristics: type of appliance

Removable and fixed appliances

Removable appliances are capable only of tipping movements, which are achieved relatively quickly. In contrast, fixed appliances are used to perform root uprighting and torqueing movements, intrusive and extrusive movements and rotations, in addition to tipping movements. This means that they are more intimately involved in applying multidirectional forces over the entire interface between the root and the surrounding tissues, more intensively, and for a longer period. It is therefore not surprising that more root resorption is found with the use of fixed appliances (Morse, 1971; Sjølien and Zachrisson, 1973; Goldson and Henrikson, 1975).

Removable appliances comprise an acrylic base, with a fitting surface closely adapted to the palatal area of the maxilla and to the lingual side of the mandible. They are held in place by clasps and carry expansion screws and springs for the movement of individual or groups of teeth. Even the most accurately fitting appliances will collect food underneath them during meals and will retain and protect this food accumulation against natural clearance by the tongue and cheeks. The patient must be instructed to specifically, but lightly, brush these areas of mucosa and the corresponding fitting surface of the acrylic base, in order to avoid soft tissue inflammation and decalcification of the covered surfaces of the teeth.

Archwires are the means of applying forces to the teeth, through the agency of the bonded brackets of a fixed appliance. With the newer developments in superelastic nickel and titanium alloys, the loops and hooks that used to be bent into stainless steel archwires may now largely be avoided. Nevertheless, loops are still needed in many instances, creating problems of food accumulation and stagnation.

When fixed or removable appliances are first placed, the patient must be taught an individual method of brushing that takes into account the specific malocclusion and the complications the appliance presents. A single-tufted brush should be used to negotiate areas where a regular toothbrush may not reach, specifically the labial and interproximal gingival areas, and fluoride rinses may be advisable.

Banded versus bonded tubes

In clinical practice today—presumably because of their perceived greater reliability—bands are still largely used to carry a tube attachment on the buccal aspect of a molar tooth, in preference to bonded tubes. Compared with a healthy pretreatment baseline, both bonded tubes and cemented bands with tubes are associated with increased plaque accumulation and resultant gingival inflammation. However, with bands the gingival reaction is more exaggerated during the treatment period. Additionally, for many months after removal of the appliances, the previously banded molars retain their periodontal disadvantage, with more gingival inflammation and attachment loss than those that carried a bonded tube (Figure 13.10a, b). There is also evidence to support the thesis that, given the same overall conditions, adolescents are more affected than older patients (Boyd and Baumrind, 1992).

Allergies

Nickel is an important cause of allergic contact dermatitis and produces more allergic reactions than all other dental materials combined. Most orthodontic wires contain nickel, including all the stainless steel materials and the superelastic nickel–titanium alloys, at a high enough level to evoke manifestations of allergic reactions in the oral cavity. It seems that one in four patients will have a positive nickel patch test; most of these are female. Some patients may become

sensitized during the treatment itself (Bass et al., 1993), and allergy due to the constituents of the bonding agent (Hutchinson, 1994; Sohoel et al., 1994) should not be overlooked. Several cases of individuals exhibiting allergic reactions to nickel during orthodontic treatment due to the nickel-containing wires have been reported (Veien et al., 1994; Al-Waheidi, 1995; Janson et al., 1998; Kim and Johnson, 1999). In these cases the dermatitis is expected to clear completely after removal of the appliances (Veien et al., 1994). Hypersensitivity has also been reported and related to potassium dichromate (Veien et al., 1994).

Nickel allergy will generally be first discovered at the time of placement of the orthodontic appliances. Once it has been confirmed, the appliances should be removed. The orthodontic trade market is today replete with nickel-free materials, and the use of titanium or epoxy-coated wires (Kim and Johnson, 1999) and gold-plated or porcelain brackets should be considered in order to overcome the problem.

It is rare to come across an allergy to the acrylic base plate used in removable orthodontic appliances, including functional appliances and retainers (Figure 13.13). In such cases it is important to confirm the accuracy of the diagnosis and to distinguish it from the much more common inflammation caused by improper oral hygiene (see Figure 13.10c). It should be remembered that removable appliances that are worn full-time collect food debris, much of which remains as a thin film of plaque covering the fitting surface of the acrylic and on that area of the palatal mucosa covered by the plate. Unless specifically instructed to brush the mucosal area, few patients will realize the importance of doing so. The resultant hypertrophic inflammation is easily confused with an allergic reaction (Figures 13.10c, 13.13c, d).

Iatrogenic damage from rubber bands

Case reports have described severe localized periodontal destruction caused by rubber bands placed directly on the teeth to close a diastema. The roots of the teeth taper towards the apex, and a rubber band around the cervical area of two adjacent teeth will tend to move along the root surface, eventually causing a "bloodless

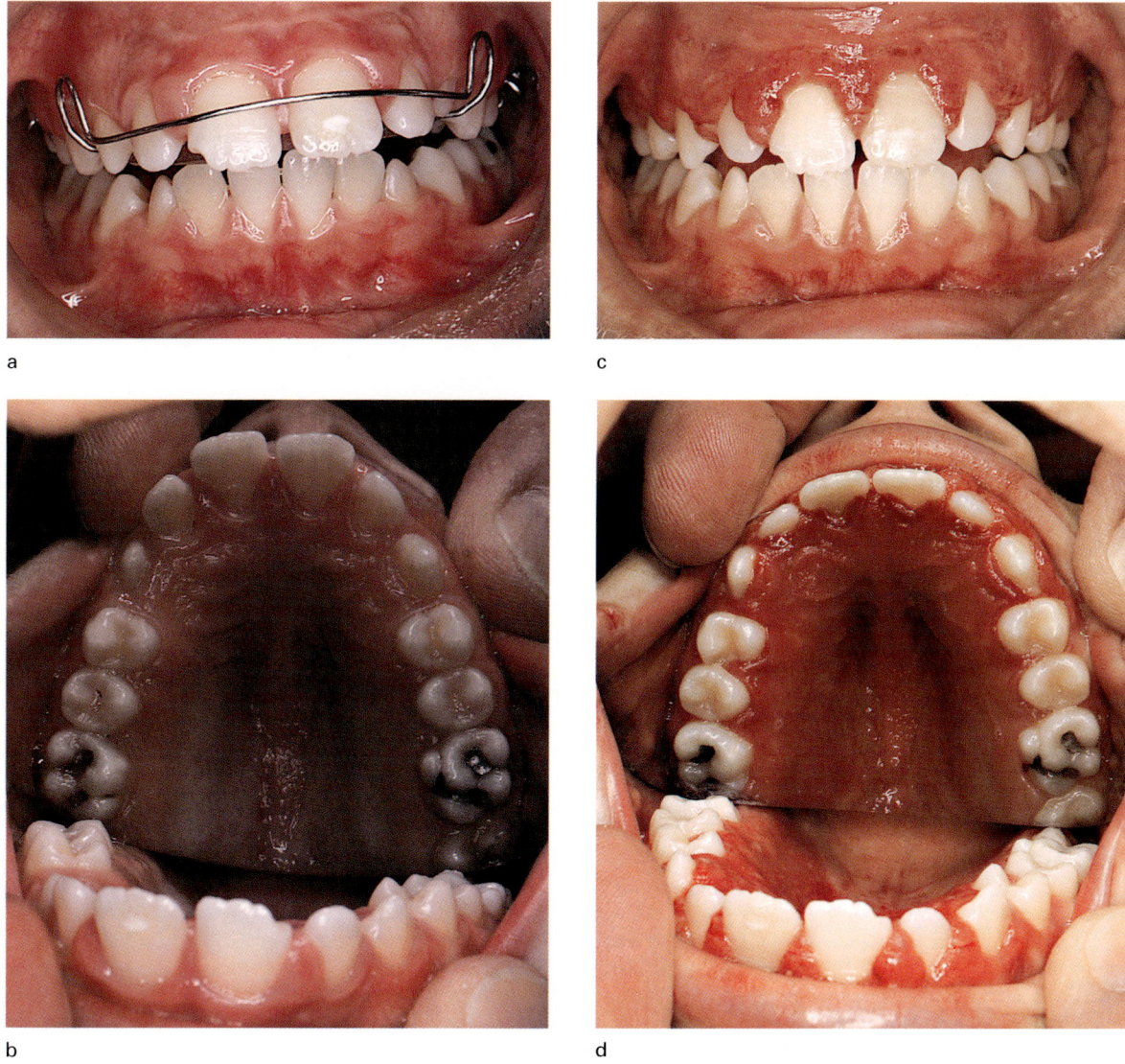

a

c

b

d

Figure 13.13

(a) Orthodontic removable appliance with acrylic base at date of insertion. (b) Occlusal view of the palate before treatment. (c) Allergic reaction despite good oral hygiene. (d) Occlusal view of the palate with allergy mucosal inflammation.

extraction" of the teeth concerned—see Figure 1.5b, c (Zilberman et al., 1976).

Extraction

Orthodontic treatments that include extraction of dental units and movement of adjacent teeth into the extraction sites can lead to attachment loss, bone loss, gingival clefts, gingival recession, and root resorption. In second premolar extraction cases and in terms of the effects on the periodontium, it seems to matter little if the teeth are extracted after their eruption or if they are surgically enucleated before they erupt. The gingival health, pocket depth, and loss of attachment of the adjacent mandibular first molars and first premolars, both clinically and radiographically, are similar. Some constriction of the alveolar process may be observed in about half the cases, both after routine extraction and after surgical enucleation. Only the radiographically measured distance from the cementoenamel junction to the bone margin on the proximal surfaces adjacent to the extracted tooth was somewhat greater after extraction than after surgical enucleation (Wisth, 1975).

Force

Teeth with adequate attached gingiva occasionally develop localized recession during orthodontic treatment. This has been attributed to excessive forces that have prevented the repair and remodeling of the alveolar bone (Geiger, 1980). The large forces produced by rapid (suture-splitting) palatal expansion have been shown to create a slight degree of attachment loss and some loss of alveolar bone height, particularly in older patients (Greenbaum and Zachrisson, 1982). Similarly, it is largely believed that excessive orthodontic force will increase the risk of root resorption (Reitan, 1974), although in more recent studies excessive orthodontic forces appeared not to increase the severity of root resorption (Owman-Moll et al., 1996a, b).

Direction and extent of movement

Even in controlled tooth movement where expansion is avoided, some types of movement may be more detrimental to the periodontium than others. Animal experiments have shown that extensive tipping and intrusive forces in a dentition with a high plaque index may result in plaque becoming located subgingivally, converting gingivitis into a destructive periodontitis. On the other hand, orthodontic forces moving animal teeth bodily under the same conditions do not seem to generate this adverse change. Moreover, similar orthodontic forces in plaque-free teeth do not result in the formation of infrabony pockets (Ericson et al., 1977).

Ectopic and impacted teeth

Impaction of maxillary central incisors occurs in a small but significant number of children and

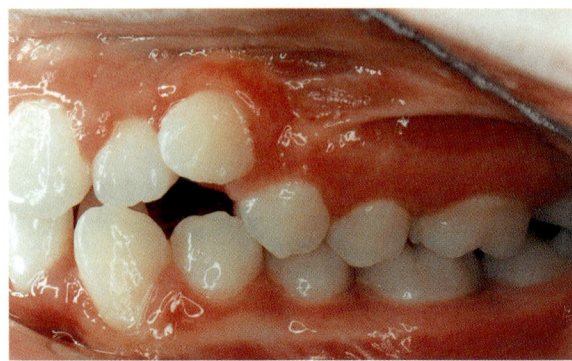

Figure 13.14

An ectopic maxillary canine erupting in the oral mucosa above the attached gingiva.

the most common cause is the existence of some form of physical obstruction, such as an unerupted supernumerary tooth or odontome. Ectopic positioning of the tooth bud may account for a small number of cases and trauma may result in a deformed or dilacerated tooth, which may also not erupt (Becker, 1998). In these cases, the surgical removal of the obstruction may result in spontaneous eruption, although often additional orthodontic traction forces are needed to bring the exposed tooth into place.

Usually because of crowding, but sometimes due to primary tooth germ displacement, maxillary canine teeth may erupt on the labial side of the ridge in an ectopic position above the line of the attached gingiva (Becker, 1998)—see Figures 13.1a, c, 13.4, 13.14. Such teeth develop a poor quality of attachment, which consists of a thin and delicate oral mucosa. This may also occur when a buccally impacted tooth is surgically exposed, using a minimal circular incision to remove the mucosa overlying the tooth. While early clinical examination (before the tooth erupts) will allow a preventive approach to the problem, this is rarely practicable. It should be remembered that the clinical feature that first convinces the patient to approach the orthodontist may well be the ectopic tooth itself (Becker, 1998).

Nevertheless, if the potentially affected tooth is recognized sufficiently early, the provision of space by orthodontic treatment will often allow the tooth to migrate distally and finally erupt close to its place in the dental arch, surrounded by attached gingiva. Failing this, the tooth may be exposed using an apically repositioned periodontal flap, which places attached gingiva on its buccal aspect (Vanarsdall and Corn, 1977). Alternatively, the tooth may be exposed, an attachment placed, and then orthodontically drawn through the fully closed and resutured full flap (McBride, 1979; Vermette et al., 1995) that had been sited in the wide band of attached gingiva.

Teeth that erupt normally and achieve full alignment in the occlusal plane will generally have a normal periodontium and alveolar bone height. Impacted teeth may sometimes erupt spontaneously when sufficient space is made for them in the dental arch and when the orientation of an adjacent tooth is favorably altered. However, many of these teeth are more stubborn, and require surgical and often orthodontic assistance to bring about their eruption. Simple exposure will encourage the more superficial ones to erupt spontaneously, at which point orthodontic appliances may be placed to complete their alignment. Impacted teeth that are more deeply sited or lie in difficult locations relative to adjacent teeth will usually demand surgical exposure, the bonding of an attachment, and the application of extrusive force. These three procedures each have the potential to inflict varying degrees of damage on the tooth and its surrounding tissues, either at the time of exposure or as the tooth passes through the surrounding hard and soft tissues, from a position within the alveolar bone to its final erupted place in the dental arch (Hansson and Linder-Aronson, 1972; Wisth et al., 1976; Becker et al., 1983; Kohavi et al., 1984a, b).

The path to a good periodontal outcome

The path to a good periodontal outcome from operative treatment is fraught with many obstacles. The factors involved and the decisions that need to be made include the following.

Surgical considerations

These include:

- tooth accessibility (Becker, 1998; Jacobs, 1999)
- the degree of exposure that is performed, including whether the flap is reduced, how much of the follicle is removed, and whether this has been taken down to the level of the cementoenamel junction (Vanarsdall and Corn, 1977; Becker et al., 1983; Kohavi et al., 1984a, b)
- how much bone is removed (Crescini et al., 1994)
- whether the attachment is bonded immediately or some weeks subsequently (Becker et al., 1996)
- whether the wound is fully sutured back (primary closure), or whether the patency of the exposure is maintained by more radical tissue removal (follicle, bone, and flap tissue), with the use of a pack (MacDonald and Yap, 1986; Vermette et al., 1995; Burden et al., 1999).

Bonding considerations

Problems of bonding procedure include:

- acid damage from inadvertent spillage of etchant on the tissues (Becker, 1998)
- poor bonding technique causing bond failure and the need to re-expose.

Orthodontic attachment considerations

Problems may arise from the bonded attachment themselves:

- the use of a large bracket (instead of a small, low-profile eyelet or button) causing gingival irritation as the tooth emerges through the gingiva (Becker et al., 1996)
- poor attachment placement resulting in unnecessary rotational movement which will need later derotation.

Traction

Traction difficulties include:

- irritation from the traction wire, gold chain or elastic thread being pulled against the surgical flap or the exposure margins

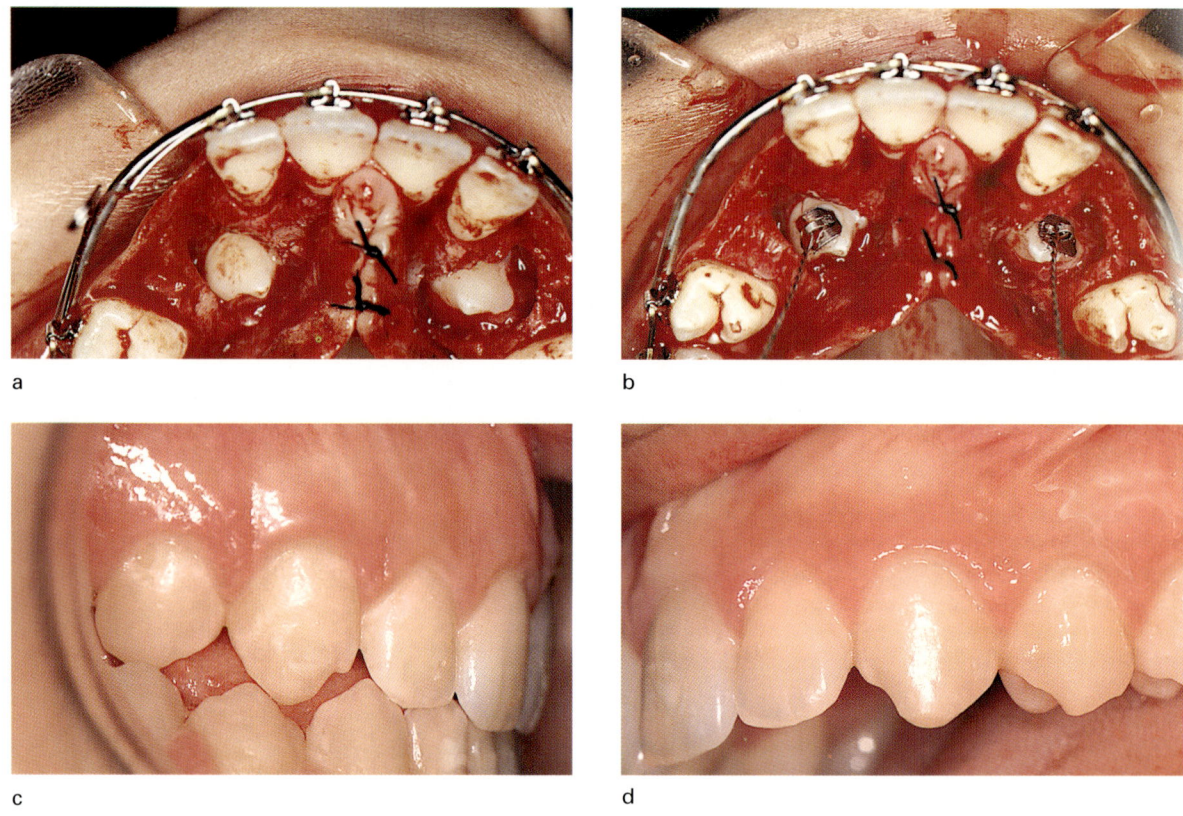

a

b

c

d

Figure 13.15

Bilateral palatal impaction of the maxillary canines. Orthodontic treatment has aligned the teeth and opened spaces in the arch for the impacted teeth. (a) A wide flap has been reflected and the impacted teeth are clearly visible, exposed only enough to provide a minimal bonding surface. (b) Eyelet attachments are bonded to each tooth, following which full flap closure was performed, with the pigtail ligature from the eyelet drawn through the palatal tissue. (c, d) The canines have been aligned and show an excellent gingival contour and appearance, indistinguishable from any other tooth.

- excessive force application
- force applied in the wrong direction, which can occur when the orthodontist has misjudged the position of the unseen impacted tooth, either through not being present at the surgical exposure or because of careless radiographic positional diagnosis.

Finishing

The orthodontist must consider whether torque-ing and uprighting movements of the tooth will be necessary. The need to perform these movements on previously impacted teeth has

been shown to worsen their periodontal prognosis (Kohavi et al., 1984b).

Advances in treatment

Because of serious shortcomings in orthodontic technique in former years, much reliance was placed on radical surgical procedures to resolve the more difficult impactions. The loss of much soft and hard tissue achieved an orthodontic alignment with a very deficient periodontal condition (MacDonald and Yap, 1986; Kohavi et al., 1984b). However, with the development of acid-etch bonding and newer methods of

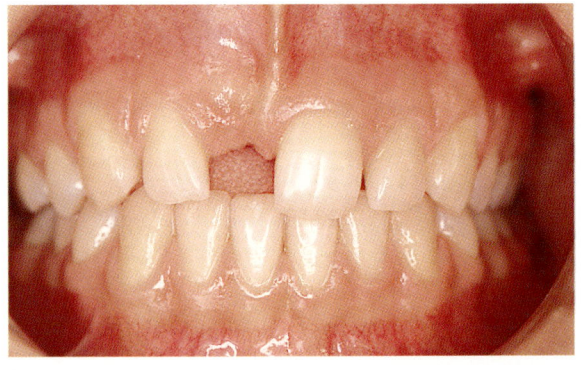

a

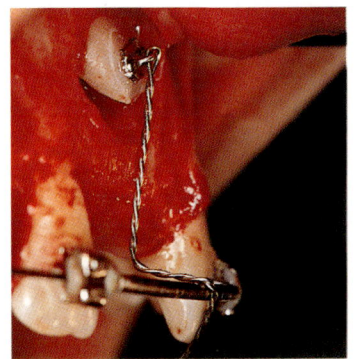

b

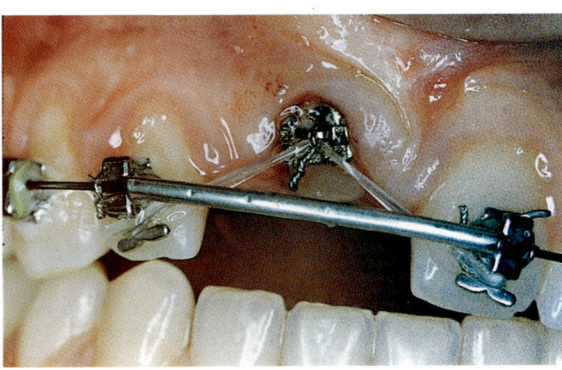

c

d

Figure 13.16

An impacted maxillary central incisor. (a) There is inadequate space for the impacted tooth and a deviated maxillary dental midline. (b) Following space opening, a labial flap has been raised from the crest of the ridge, to include attached gingiva. The height of the impacted tooth is evident and an eyelet attachment is placed at the time of exposure. (c) The surgical flap has been fully replaced and sutured, with only the pigtail ligature visible through the sutured edges. (d) Elastic module traction has partially erupted the incisor. (e) The gingival condition of the previously impacted tooth seen 1 year after treatment is indistinguishable from that of its neighbor.

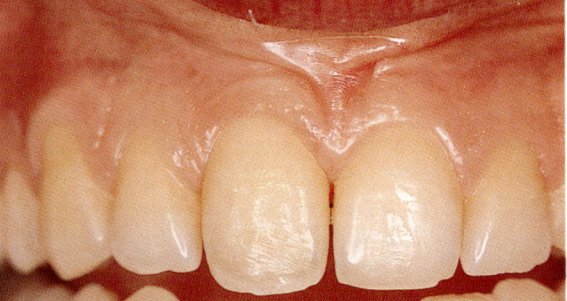

e

mechanotherapy (Kornhauser et al., 1996; Becker, 1998), the most modest of exposures is now possible, involving minimal tissue damage, with full flap replacement and primary healing, even with the most difficult of impactions (Figures 13.15 and 13.16), with correspondingly improved periodontal outcomes (Heaney and Atherton, 1976; Wisth et al., 1976; Odenrick and

Modeer, 1978; Becker et al., 1983; Boyd, 1984; Kohavi et al., 1984a, b; Crescini et al., 1995; Vermette et al., 1995).

In routine orthodontic practice, most impactions treated using orthodontic and surgical methods are relatively mild, with the tooth lying close to the mucosal surface. In these cases, there may be little periodontal advantage in fully closing the flap over the surgically exposed impacted tooth (Burden et al., 1999). Improvements in radiographic imaging, with the use of views taken at right angles and computerized tomographic scanning, have permitted accurate three-dimensional representation of the position and orientation of unerupted teeth. A classification of maxillary canines according to their position in the maxilla (Becker, 1998), and hence in accordance with the complexity of their mechanotherapeutic resolution, is now available. This classification provides the operator with guidance as to an appropriate treatment approach, and forecasts the periodontal outcome of the proposed treatment.

Conclusions

A wide spectrum of reaction of periodontal tissues to malocclusions and orthodontic treatments is possible, ranging from beneficial to innocuous, deleterious but transient, and to severe and irreversible.

Essentially malocclusion and orthodontic treatments are not primary etiologic factors for gingival and periodontal diseases, but rather contributory factors insofar as they facilitate plaque accumulation. Therefore, any potentially deleterious effect on the periodontium may be alleviated by an adequate oral hygiene regimen, adapted to the individual case.

The orthodontic treatment plan and the completion and follow-up of the treatment itself should take account of the gingival and periodontal characteristics of each patient. An innate tendency to develop gingival and periodontal diseases or allergic reactions may hinder orthodontic treatment.

Orthodontic treatment changes the morphology of the periodontal tissues and should be performed within the limits of tolerance of the tissues. This varies between individuals, and irreversible iatrogenic complications may be caused despite a good oral hygiene regimen.

References

Acar A, Canyurek U, Kocaaga M, Erverdi N (1999) Continuous vs. discontinuous force application and root resorption. *Angle Orthod* **69**: 159–63.

Ainamo A, Ainamo J (1978) The width of attached gingiva on supraerupted teeth. *J Periodont Res* **13**: 194–8.

Ainamo J, Paloheimo L, Norbland A, Mertomaalt H (1986) Gingival recession in schoolchildren aged 7, 12, and 17 years of age in Espoo, Finland. *Commun Dent Oral Epidemiol* **14**: 283–6.

Al-Jasser N, Hashim H (1995) Periodontal findings in cases of incisor cross-bite. *J Clin Pediatr Dent* **19**: 285–7.

Alstad S, Zachrisson BU (1979) Longitudinal study of the periodontal condition associated with orthodontic treatment in adolescents. *Am J Orthod* **76**: 277–86.

Al-Waheidi EM (1995) Allergic reaction to nickel orthodontic wires: a case report. *Quintess Int* **26**: 385–7.

Andlin-Sobocki A, Marcusson A, Persson M (1991) 3–year observations on gingival recession in mandibular incisors in children. *J Clin Periodontol* **18**: 155–9.

Atherton JD (1970) The gingival response to orthodontic tooth movement. *Am J Orthod* **58**: 179–86.

Bass JK, Fine H, Cisneros GJ (1993) Nickel hypersensitivity in the orthodontic patient. *Am J Orthod Dentofac Orthop* **103**: 280–5.

Baxter DH (1967) The effect of orthodontic treatment on alveolar bone adjacent to the cemento enamel junction. *Angle Orthod* **37**: 35–47.

Becker A (1998) *The Orthodontic Treatment of Impacted Teeth*. London: Martin Dunitz.

Becker A, Kohavi D, Zilberman Y (1983) Periodontal status following the alignment of palatally impacted canine teeth. *Am J Orthod* **84**: 332–6.

Becker A, Shpack N, Shteyer A (1996) Attachment bonding to impacted teeth at the time of surgical exposure. *Eur J Orthod* **18**: 457–64.

Bielak S, Bimstein E, Eidelman E (1982) Forced eruption: the treatment choice for subgingivally fractured permanent incisors. *ASDC J Dent Child* **49**: 186–90.

Bimstein E (1989) Non-surgical treatment of pseudo-recession in children and adolescents. *Am J Dent* **2**: 25–7.

Bimstein E, Machtei E, Becker A (1988) The attached gingiva in children: diagnostic, developmental and orthodontic considerations for its treatment. *ASDC J Dent Child* **55**: 351–6.

Bimstein E, Crevoisier R, King D (1990) Changes in the morphology of the buccal alveolar bone of protruded mandibular permanent incisors secondary to orthodontic alignment. *Am J Orthod Dentofac Orthop* **97**: 427–30.

Boyd RL (1984) Clinical assessment of injuries in orthodontic movement of impacted teeth. II. Surgical recommendations. *Am J Orthod* **86**: 407–18.

Boyd RL, Baumrind S (1992) Periodontal considerations in the use of bonds or bands on molars in adolescents and adults. *Angle Orthod* **62**: 117–26.

Brezniak N, Wasserstein A (1993). Root resorption after orthodontic treatment. II. Literature review. *Am J Orthod* **103**: 138–46.

Burden D, Mullally BH, Robinson SN (1999) Palatally ectopic canines: closed eruption versus open eruption. *Am J Orthod* **115**: 634–39.

Coatam GW, Behrents RG, Bissada NF (1981) The width of keratinized gingiva during orthodontic treatment: its significance and impact on periodontal status. *J Periodontol* **52**: 307–13.

Crescini A, Clauser C, Giorgetti R et al. (1994) Tunnel traction of infraosseous impacted maxillary canines. A three-year periodontal follow up. *Am J Orthod Dentofac Orthop* **105**: 61–72.

Davidovitch Z, Godwin SL, Park Y-G et al. The etiology of root resorption in orthodontic treatment. In: McNamara JA (ed.) *The Management of Unfavorable Sequelae*. Craniofacial Growth Series, no. 31. pp. 93–117. Michigan: Center for Human Growth and Development. University of Michigan.

Davies TM, Shaw WC, Addy M, Dummer PM (1988) The relationship of anterior overjet to plaque and gingivitis in children. *Am J Orthod* **93**: 303–9.

Dorfman HS (1978) Mucogingival changes resulting from mandibular incisor tooth movement. *Am J Orthod* **74**: 286–97.

Ericson I, Thilander B, Lindhe J, Okamoto H (1977) The effect of orthodontic tilting movements on the periodontal tissues of infected and non-infected dentitions in dogs. *J Clin Periodont* **4**: 278–93.

Freedman A, Green K, Salkin LM et al. (1999) An 18-year longitudinal study of untreated mucogingival defects. *J Periodontol* **70**: 1174–6.

Foushee DG, Moriaty JD, Simpson DM (1985) Effects of mandibular orthognathic treatment on mucogingival tissues. *J Periodontol* **56**: 727–33.

Gazit E, Lieberman M (1980) Occlusal and orthodontic considerations in the periodontally involved dentition. *Angle Orthod* **50**: 346–9.

Geiger AM (1980) Mucogingival problems and the movement of mandibular incisors: a clinical review. *Am J Orthod* **78**: 511–27.

Geiger AM, Wasserman BH (1976) Relation of occlusion and periodontal disease. IX. Incisor inclination and periodontal status. *J Periodontol* **46**: 99–110.

Geiger AM, Wasserman BH (1977) Relation of occlusion and periodontal disease. X. Relation of cross-bite to periodontal status. *J Periodontol* **48**: 785–9.

Geiger AM, Wasserman BH, Thompson RH, Turgeon LR (1972) Relation of occlusion and periodontal disease. V. Relation of classification of occlusion to periodontal status and gingival inflammation. *J Periodontol* **43**: 554–60.

Geiger AM, Wasserman BH, Turgeon LR (1973) Relation of occlusion and periodontal disease. VI. Relation of anterior overjet and overbite to periodontal destruction and gingival inflammation. *J Periodontol* **44**: 150–7.

Geiger AM, Wasserman BH, Turgeon LR (1974) Relation of occlusion and periodontal disease. VIII. Relation of crowding and spacing to periodontal destruction and gingival inflammation. *J Periodontol* **45**: 43–9.

Goldson L, Henrikson CO (1975) Root resorption during Begg treatment. A longitudinal roentgenologic study. *Am J Orthod* **68**: 55–66.

Greenbaum KR, Zachrisson BU (1982) The effect of palatal expansion therapy on the periodontal supporting tissues. *Am J Orthod* **81**: 12–21.

Hansson C, Linder-Aronson S (1972) Gingival status after orthodontic treatment of impacted upper canines. *Trans Eur Orthod Soc* **48**: 433–41.

Harrison RL, Leggott PJ, Kennedy DB et al. (1991) The association of simple anterior crossbite to gingival discrepancy. *Pediatr Dent* **13**: 296–300.

Heaney TG, Atherton JD (1976) Periodontal problems associated with the surgical exposure of unerupted teeth. *Br J Orthod* **3**: 79–85.

Heier EE, De Smit AA, Wijgaerts IA, Adriaens PA (1997) Periodontal implications of bonded versus removable retainers. *Am J Dentofac Orthop* **112**: 607–16.

Hollender L, Rönnerman A, Thilander B (1980) Root resorption, marginal bone support and clinical crown length in orthodontically treated patients. *Eur J Orthod* **2**: 197–205.

Horiuchi A, Hotokezaka H, Kobayashi K (1998) Correlation between cortical late proximity and apical root resorption. *Am J Orthod Dentofac Orthop* **114**: 311–18.

Huser MC, Baehni PC, Lang R (1990) Effects of orthodontic bands on microbiologic and clinical parameters. *Am J Orthod Dentofac Orthop* **97**: 213–18.

Hutchinson I (1994) Hypersensitivity to an orthodontic bonding agent. A case report. *Br J Orthod* **21**: 331–3.

Ingber JS (1976) Forced eruption: Part II. A method of treating nonrestorable teeth. Periodontal and restorative considerations. *J Periodontol* **47**: 203–16.

Ingervall B, Jacobson L, Nyman SA (1977) A clinical study of the relation between crowding of teeth, plaque and gingival condition. *J Clin Periodontol* **4**: 214–22.

Jacobs SG (1999) Localization of the unerupted maxillary canine: how to and when to. *Am J Orthod Dentofac Orthop* **115**: 314–22.

Janson GR, Dainesi EA, Consolaro A et al. (1998) Nickel hypersensitivity reaction before, during and after orthodontic therapy. *Am J Orthod Dentofac Orthop* **113**: 655–60.

Karring T (1982) Bone regeneration in orthodontically produced alveolar bone dehiscences. *J Periodont Res* **17**: 309–15.

Kim H, Johnson JW (1999) Corrosion of stainless steel, nickel-titanium, coated nickel-titanium, and titanium orthodontic wires. *Angle Orthod* **69**: 39–44.

Kloehn JS, Pfeifer JS (1974) The effect of orthodontic treatment on the periodontum. *Angle Orthod* **44**: 127–34.

Kohavi D, Zilberman Y, Becker A (1984a) Periodontal status following the alignment of buccally ectopic maxillary canine teeth. *Am J Orthod* **85**: 78–82.

Kohavi D, Becker A, Zilberman Y (1984b) Surgical exposure, orthodontic movement, and final tooth position as factors in periodontal breakdown of treated palatally impacted canines. *Am J Orthod* **85**: 72–7.

Kornhauser S, Schwartz Z, Bimstein E (1996) Changes in the gingival structure of maxillary permanent teeth related to the orthodontic correction of simple anterior crossbite. *Am J Orthod Dentofac Orthop* **110**: 263–8.

Kucukkeles N, Okar I (1994) Root resorption and pulpal changes due to intrusive force. *J Marmara Univ Dent Fac* **2**: 404–8.

Levander E, Malmgren O (1988) Evaluation of the risk of root resorption during orthodontic treatment: a study of upper incisors. *Eur J Orthod* **10**: 30–8.

Levander E, Malmgren O (1998) Long-term follow-up of maxillary incisors with severe apical root resorption. *Eur J Orthod* **20**: 427.

Levander E, Malmgren O, Eliasson S (1994) Evaluation of root resorption in relation to two orthodontic treatment regimes: a clinical experimental study. *Eur J Orthod* **16**: 223–8.

Levander E, Bajka R, Malmgren O (1998a) Early radiographic diagnosis of apical root resorption during orthodontic treatment: a study of maxillary incisors. *Eur J Orthod* **20**: 57–63.

Levander E, Malmgren O, Stenback K (1998b) Apical root resorption during orthodontic treatment of patients with multiple aplasia: a study of maxillary incisors. *Eur J Orthod* **20**: 427–34.

Listgarten MA (1986) Pathogenesis of periodontitis. *J Clin Periodontol* **13**: 418–25.

Löe H, Theilade E, Jensen SB (1964) Experimental gingivitis in man. *J Periodontol* **36**: 177–87.

MacDonald F, Yap WL (1986) The surgical exposure and application of direct traction of unerupted teeth. *Am J Orthod* **89**: 331–40.

Machtei EE, Zubery Y, Bimstein E, Becker A (1990) Anterior open bite and gingival recession in children and adolescents. *Int Dent J* **40**: 396–401.

McBride LJ (1979) Traction—a surgical/orthodontic procedure. *Am J Orthod* **76**: 287–99.

McLain JB, Proffit WR, Davenport RH (1983) Adjunctive orthodontic therapy in the treatment of juvenile periodontitis: report of a case and review of the literature. *Am J Orthod* **83**: 290–8.

Melsen B, Agerbaek N, Eriksen J, Terp S (1988) New attachment through periodontal treatment and orthodontic intrusion. *J Orthod Dentofac Orthop* **94**: 104–16.

Morse PH (1971) Resorption of upper incisors following orthodontic treatment. *Dent Pract* **22**: 21–35.

Newman GV, Goldman MJ, Newman RA (1994) Mucogingival orthodontic and periodontal problems. *Am J Orthod Dentofac Orthop* **105**: 321–7.

Ngan PW, Burch JG, Wei SHY (1991) Grafted and ungrafted labial recession in pediatric orthodontic patients: effects of retraction and inflammation. *Quintess Int* **22**: 103–11.

Odenrick L, Modeer T (1978) Periodontal status following surgical-orthodontic alignment of impacted teeth. *Acta Odontol Scand* **36**: 233–6.

Owman-Moll P, Kurol J, Lundgren D (1996a) Effects of a double orthodontic force magnitude on tooth movement and root resorptions. An intra-individual study in adolescents. *Eur J Orthod* **18**: 141–50.

Owman-Moll P, Kurol J, Lundren D (1996b) The effects of a four-fold increased orthodontic force magnitude on tooth movement and root resorptions. An intra-individual study in adolescents. *Eur J Orthod* **18**: 287–94.

Paolantonio M, Festa F, di Placido G et al. (1999) Site specific subgingival colonization by Actinobacillus actinomycetemcomitans in orthodontic patients. *Am J Orthod Dentofac Orthop* **115**: 423–8.

Parker RJ, Harris EF (1998) Directions of orthodontic tooth movements associated with external root resorption of the maxillary central incisor. *Am J Orthod Dentofac Orthop* **114**: 677–83.

Paunio K (1973) The role of malocclusion and crowding in the development of periodontal disease. *Int Dent J* **23**: 470–5.

Pearson LE (1968) Gingival height of lower central incisors, orthodontically treated and untreated. *Angle Orthod* **38**: 337–9.

Peretz B, Machtei EE (1996) Tooth rotation and alveolar bone loss. *Quintess Int* **27**: 465–8.

Persson M, Lennartsson B (1986) Improvement potential of isolated gingival recession in children. *Swed Dent J* **10**: 45–51.

Polson AM, Reed BE (1984) Long-term effect of orthodontic treatment on crestal alveolar bone levels. *J Periodontol* **55**: 28–34.

Polson A, Caton J, Polson AP et al. (1984) Periodontal response after tooth movement into infrabony defects. *J Periodontol* **55**: 197–202.

Powell RN, McEniery TM (1982) A longitudinal study of isolated gingival recession in the mandibular central incisor region of children aged 2–8 years. *J Clin Periodontol* **9**: 357–64.

Reitan K (1967) Clinical and histologic observations on tooth movement during and after orthodontic movement. *J Am Orthod* **53**: 721–45.

Reitan K (1974) Initial tissue behavior during apical root resorption. *Angle Orthod* **44**: 68–82.

Robertson PB, Schultz LD, Levy BM (1977) Occurrence and distribution of interdental gingival clefts following orthodontic movement into bicuspid extraction sites. *J Periodontol* **48**: 232–5.

Sadowsky C, BeGole EA (1981) Long-term effects of orthodontic treatment on periodontal health. *Am J Orthod* **80**: 156–72.

Sanders NL (1999) Evidence-based care in orthodontics and periodontics: a review of the literature. *J Am Dent Assoc* **130**: 521–7.

Sharpe W, Reed B, Subtelny JD, Polson A (1987) Orthodontic relapse, apical resorption, and crestal alveolar bone levels. *Am J Orthod Dentofac Orthop* **91**: 252–8.

Sinclair PM, Berry CW, Bennet CL, Israelson H (1987) Changes in gingiva and gingival flora with bonding and banding. *Angle Orthod* **57**: 271–8.

Sjølien T, Zachrisson BU (1973) Periodontal bone support and tooth length in orthodontically treated and untreated persons. *Am J Orthod* **64**: 28–37.

Sohoel H, Gjerdet NR, Hensen-Pettersen A, Ruyter IE (1994) Allergenic potential of two orthodontic bonding materials. *Scand J Dent Res* **102**: 126–9.

Sperry TP, Speidel TM, Isaacson RJ, Worms FW (1977) The role of dental compensations in the orthodontic treatment of mandibular prognathism. *Angle Orthod* **47**: 293–9.

Stern N, Becker A (1980) Forced eruption: biological and clinical considerations. *J Oral Rehab* **7**: 395–402.

Vanarsdall RL, Corn H (1977) Soft-tissue management of labially positioned unerupted teeth. *Am J Orthod* **72**: 53–64.

Veien NK, Borchorst E, Hattel T, Laurberg G (1994) Stomatitis or systemically-induced contact dermatitis from metal wire in orthodontic materials. *Cont Dermat* **30**: 210–3.

Vermette ME, Kokich VG, Kennedy DB (1995) Uncovering labially impacted teeth: apically positioned flap and closed-eruption technique. *Angle Orthod* **65**: 23–32.

Vig PS (1979) Respiratory mode and morphological types: some thoughts and preliminary conclusions. In: McNamara J (ed.) *Clinical Alteration of the Growing Face*. Craniofacial Growth Series, no 9. pp. 233–50. Michigan: Center for Human Growth and Development. University of Michigan.

Wagaiyu EG, Ashley P (1991) Mouthbreathing, lip seal and upper lip coverage and their relationship with gingival inflammation in 11–14 year-old children. *J Clin Periodontol* **18**: 698–702.

Wisth J (1975) Periodontal status of neighboring teeth after orthodontic closure of mandibular extraction sites. *Scand J Dent Res* **83**: 307–13.

Wisth PJ, Nordeval K, Boe OE (1976) Periodontal status of orthodontically treated impacted canines. *Angle Orthod* **46**: 69–76.

Zachrisson BU (1978) Clinical interrelation of orthodontics and periodontics. In: *Proceedings of the International Conference of Orthodontics*, Philadelphia, 1978.

Zachrisson BU, Alnaes L (1973) Periodontal condition in orthodontically treated and untreated individuals. I. Loss of attachment, gingival pocket depth and clinical crown height. *Angle Orthod* **43**: 402–11.

Zachrisson BU, Alnaes L (1974) Periodontal condition in orthodontically treated and untreated individuals. II. Alveolar bone loss. *Angle Orthod* **44**: 48–55.

Zachrisson S, Zachrisson BU (1972) Gingival condition associated with orthodontic treatment. *Angle Orthod* **42**: 26–34.

Zilberman Y, Shteyer A, Azaz, B (1976) Iatrogenic exfoliation of teeth by the incorrect use of orthodontic elastic bands. *J Am Dent Assoc* **93**: 89–93.

14
Dental implants

David Kohavi

Endosseous osseointegrated implants are increasingly used to replace missing teeth. The high success rates (Zarb and Schmitt, 1993) and the improvement in surgical and prosthetic techniques make it the treatment of choice in a variety of clinical situations, both in adults and in young patients. The outcome of implant therapy depends on the amount and quality of bone (Jaffin and Berman, 1991), on correct combined surgical and prosthetic treatment design, and on the precise placement of the implant and restoration. There are very few systemic conditions that limit implant placement in the general population (Tanner, 1997). In the adolescent, skeletal development must also be considered. Early clinical documentation on implants in younger patients has mainly focused on ectodermal dysplasia patients (Bergendal et al., 1991; Guckes et al., 1991; Smith et al., 1993; Cronin et al., 1994; Ledermann et al., 1993).

Advances in implant design and operator skills have allowed patients with congenitally missing teeth or traumatic tooth loss to be candidates for treatment. Two different treatment approaches have emerged. The first emphasizes the preservation of the bony ridge, even around the deciduous teeth, by early implant insertion, although this practice may necessitate later surgical intervention for correction of malaligned implants. The second approach tries to prevent damage to the bone by postponing implant insertion until growth is complete. New and successful bone augmentation techniques are used prior to implant insertion, or simultaneously with it, to create sufficient bone volume around the implant to meet prosthetic and esthetic demands.

Growth of the facial skeleton

Most of the limitations of implant therapy in children and adolescents are due to developmental processes. Growth patterns of different parts of the maxilla and mandible determine the timing and the outcome of the treatment. In the mandible (Bjork, 1969) the pattern of growth is characterized by an upward and forward curving growth in the condyles, with absence of growth in the anterior aspect of the bone; this results in forward rotation of the mandible. The center of rotation may be located in the center of the joint, at the incisal tips of the mandibular anterior teeth, or in the mandibular body in the premolar area. These types of mandibular rotational growth increase the height of the posterior alveolus. The overall result is that the mandible rotates in relation to the maxilla as it grows. In the maxilla (Bjork and Skieller, 1977), the main part of the growth is associated with the sutural lowering of the bony corpus. This growth is almost double that of the lowering of the floor of the orbit. In addition, the appositional growth in height of the alveolar process is about one-third greater than the increase in height of the alveolar process, as seen in relation to the nasal floor. The vertical maxillary growth is caused by these changes and this results in downward and forward growth, with a varying degree of vertical rotation. The horizontal diameter of the maxilla is increased as a result of growth in the median suture. This growth is greater in the posterior part than in the anterior. This results in a transverse rotation of the two maxillae, causing the lateral segments of the maxilla to move more laterally in the posterior part than in the anterior part. Thus, the distance between the molars increases more during growth than the distance between the canines, while the length of the dental arch becomes reduced in the mid-sagittal plane.

Implant placement in the developing facial skeleton

Animal studies

Odman et al. (1991) and Thilander et al. (1992) examined the effect of implant insertion on the alveolar bone and adjacent teeth in young growing pigs. Screw-type implants were inserted in the maxillary primary lateral incisor area, the mandibular primary canine area, the mandibular primary first premolar area, and the mandibular primary second premolar area on the opposite side. Six of the 20 implants (30%) that were inserted failed to integrate. In the premolar regions with erupting adjacent teeth, crater-like marginal defects were present, essentially burying the implants. This was not discerned in the animal that lost the implant in this region. Furthermore, the implants were found to be located lingual to the adjacent teeth. In the canine and lateral incisor areas where vertically erupting teeth were lacking, no defects were found around the implants. Both authors concluded that osseointegrated implants behave like ankylosed teeth during development of the dentition in the growing pig, and that the implants do not move together with the erupting adjacent teeth. These animal studies indicate that because of the different growth rate of parts of the jaws, no single guideline can be used for implant placement.

Clinical reports

The early human clinical reports agree with the results of the animal studies reported by Odman et al. (1991) and Thilander et al. (1992). In the human, several problems occurred as a consequence of the developmental process. For example, in studies using ceramic implants the failure rate was high, being greatest in children less than 11 years old (Scholz and d'Hoedt, 1984; Frisch et al., 1990; Oesterle et al., 1993). Esthetic problems and implant fractures occurred frequently. However, in these early implants, it is not clear to what extent the use of fragile ceramic materials and the surgical techniques contributed to the high failure rate. In a later study following refining of osseointegration methods, Ledermann et al. (1993) in their 7 year follow-up study reported a 90% success rate. However, several shortcomings of the use of implants in children emerged. There was a shortening of implant-borne crowns, resulting from the continued eruption of the adjacent natural teeth to their final positions, which was accompanied by cratering in the alveolar bone adjacent to the implants following the eruption of the adjacent teeth. Shortening of the implant-borne crown was also reported by Johansson et al. (1994), who placed an implant in a child aged 12 years 3 months. As in the Ledermann study, Johansson noted, in a 4.5 year follow-up, substantial marginal bone loss where the implant had been inserted close to the tooth. Westwood and Ducan (1996) described another case in a boy aged 15 years 4 months, in whom an implant was inserted to replace the congenitally missing maxillary left second premolar immediately after the removal of the retained primary molar. A radiograph taken 48 months following implant placement revealed bone resorption due to the skeletal growth in the floor of the antrum. The resorption exposed the apical end of the implant in the sinus.

Recommendations as to the appropriate age for implant treatment can be summarized as follows. Most of the clinical reports (Ledermann et al., 1993; Bergendal et al., 1996; Westwood and Ducan, 1996) recommend limiting the treatment to children who are nearing or have achieved complete alveolar bone growth. Bergendal et al., (1991) added that only in rare cases of total aplasia, as in ectodermal dysplasia, should treatment with implants be advocated in childhood. Johansson et al. (1994) suggested that with careful and optimal placement of the implant, taking into consideration the further development of the jaws, implants could be inserted in growing adolescents. This issue of treatment time is discussed below.

Indications

The two main reasons for edentulous spaces in children are trauma, and the congenital absence of deciduous and permanent teeth. Although these clinical situations have several common characteristics, the therapeutic approaches differ. Congenitally missing teeth may be associated with other disorders of the stomatogenic system that affect treatment, while the management of trauma is usually confined to the injured region. Both conditions present a special challenge in planning and carrying out treatment, because they involve several dental disciplines that dictate the sequence, timing, and methods of the treatment.

Congenitally missing teeth

Based on the 1996 Consensus Conference on Oral Implants in Young Patients (Koch et al., 1996), the following definitions are used in this chapter:

- *hypodontia* is the absence of one to five permanent teeth
- *oligodontia* is the absence of six or more permanent teeth
- *anodontia* is the absence of all permanent teeth.

The incidence rates given for congenital absence range from 0.3% to 13.6% (not taking third molars into account). Oligodontia is a much rarer disorder, with an incidence rate of 0.08%. Anodontia is found in an even smaller percentage. Upper laterals, second premolars, and the lower incisors are the most common missing teeth. There is no difference between males and females. Special attention should be given to children with ectodermal dysplasia; these patients have higher prevalence of oligodontia and aplasia, and have special psychological and prosthetic needs.

Ectodermal dysplasia is a group of rare inherited disorders that affect various tissues of ectodermal origin. The mode of inheritance varies among the different disorders. The most common form of ectodermal dysplasia is hypohidronic ectodermal dysplasia, which most severely affects the hair, nails, teeth, and skin. Males are more often and more severely affected than females. The transmission is from the female carrier, who usually appears normal and unaffected. The oral abnormalities are the absence of most, if not all, of the permanent and/or primary teeth. The teeth that are present are usually malformed: anterior teeth have conical crowns, and posterior teeth have a reduced occlusal table. In rare cases, one or both arches are totally edentulous. The most striking abnormality that may affect future implant treatment is that the alveolar process does not develop in the absence of teeth, and therefore is missing in the edentulous spans. Even in areas with teeth, these patients exhibit poor alveolar ridge development. This may be a problem if implant treatment is prescribed in a case of tooth loss; for review, see Gorlin et al. (1990) and Tape and Tye (1995). Several studies (Sarnat et al., 1953; Hamano et al., 1980) demonstrated that the lack of teeth did not affect the growth of the body of the mandible. However, the anterior growth of the maxilla was reduced in cases of anodontia, not only because of the absence of teeth, but also because of early prosthetic replacement and chronic rhinitis conditions due to allergic disorders, which are common in these patients.

Guckes et al. (1998) examined the pattern of permanent teeth present in 52 individuals with ectodermal dysplasia and severe hypodontia who were referred for treatment with dental implants. They found that the maxillary central incisors, maxillary and mandibular first molars, and the maxillary canines are the most conserved teeth in severe hypodontia. They also suggest that because of the frequently missing permanent mandibular anterior teeth, these patients may be good candidates for implant treatment.

Treatment considerations

Alternative treatment

Traditional treatment of edentulous areas in children and adolescents included temporary restorations in nature, such as removable partial dentures and cemented prostheses with minimal tooth preparation (Hobkirk and Brook, 1980). At a later stage fixed restorations, sometimes with combination of removable dentures, were constructed. In many cases implant treatment is an alternative; it precludes the necessity to prepare intact teeth, and prevents mucosal inflammation, which is almost inevitable with acrylic-based partial dentures.

Treatment of hypodontia

The maxillary lateral incisors and first premolars are the most commonly missing teeth (Schalk-van der Weide et al., 1992; Kjaer et al., 1994), and hence these areas need special attention during treatment planning. These two locations exhibit different growth patterns, and early implant treatment may jeopardize the outcome. In the upper laterals early insertion will result in submerged implants and restorations, causing esthetic problems and bone deficiency in the adjacent teeth. Early insertion in the location of the upper premolar may result in loss of the bony implant support. This is due to the coronal movement of the maxillary sinus during development. This movement is accompanied by bone resorption in the floor of the antrum, exposing the ankylosed implant to the antrum. The Guckes et al. (1998) study may be helpful in formulating protocols for prosthetic treatment of individuals with hypodontia and oligodontia.

Treatment of oligodontia

Two implant approaches for the treatment of oligodontia have been described. The first (Ledermann et al., 1993; Durstberger et al., 1999) advocates the placement of implants in adolescent patients because the alveolar ridge formed during the eruption of the deciduous teeth can often be used as a host site. However, a severe malposition of the implants must be anticipated, depending on the location of treatment and the age of the patient. In some of these cases, further treatment is needed after completion of growth. This may consist of the removal of malposed implants or even segmental repositioning of the bone. In the second approach, treatment is postponed until the patient has completed or nearly completed growth (Kohavi, 1999). The absence of the alveolar ridge may be aggravated

by resorption, as was found by Ostler and Kokich (1994), who studied changes in ridge width over time in patients with congenitally missing mandibular second premolars, and found that ridge width decreased almost 30% during a period of 6 years. Further resorption may be caused by the difficulty (due to continuous growth) of fitting dentures. Because of the lack of development and the time-dependent resorption, there is a need for correction by planned surgical intervention aimed at bone augmentation.

Multidisciplinary approach

Bergendal et al. (1996) presented a multidisciplinary approach to oral rehabilitation using implants in children and adolescents with hypodontia and oligodontia. Representatives from the dental specialties of orthodontics, pediatric dentistry, oral surgery, prosthodontics, and radiology made up the team. A preliminary long-term treatment plan was established for the patient at the age of 8–10 years, as well as a detailed plan for the coming years. Using this approach, the issues to be discussed by the group are: early considerations on permanent therapy; esthetic considerations; control of vertical dimension; pattern of facial growth; dentoalveolar growth; optimal placement of existing teeth; and intermediate appliances to replace missing teeth. At a later stage the issues of preserving the alveolar ridge for implant insertion and the stages of the implant therapy are discussed, as well as the clinical considerations and the treatment changes from early diagnosis at the age of 8 years to the end of treatment. At 8 years old, children with missing incisors are examined radiographically to determine the extent of the hypodontia. The initial treatment consists of information and prophylaxis. At age 10–14 years the alveolar growth and the eruption of the maxillary canines are observed. Orthodontic treatment is aimed at correcting the position of the incisors and deep bite. This is also the time for composite recontouring of anterior teeth. At age 12–14 years, the facial and alveolar growth are examined as well as the bone mass and quality in edentulous areas. The position of the future abutment teeth in relation to the edentulous areas is determined, and the possibility of implant treatment is considered. Extensive orthodontic treatment is carried out to achieve the rehabilitation goals and to correct the malocclusion. The retention phase continues up to the age of final growth. At the end of facial growth, a tomographic assessment is made and a decision taken on the final prosthetic therapy alternatives. Temporary prosthetic appliances, implant surgery, and definitive prosthetic therapy are accomplished. This multidisciplinary team approach provides the optimal treatment. The involvement of the prosthodontist and the surgeon during the early stages when the decisions to move the abutment teeth are made shortens the overall orthodontic treatment time, and makes treatment more definitive. This team approach should be adopted also in the treatment of trauma cases.

Treatment of aplasia

Since the congenital absence of teeth results in minimal bone support for removable dentures, the retention provided by the implants is essential for successful treatment. Clinical documentation in adults supports the efficacy of restoring a partial or completely edentulous mandible using an implant-supported denture anchored in the anterior mandible. This treatment has to be considered in view of the growth pattern of the anterior mandibular region, the prosthetic needs, and the temporary alternative treatment in each individual.

The consequences of using implants in very young patients was described by Guckes et al. (1997). In a 3-year-old boy diagnosed with ectodermal dysplasia, four implants were inserted in the mandible and two in the maxilla. Five months following the insertion second-stage surgery was performed. One maxillary implant failed to integrate and was removed. Prosthetic treatment consisted of a conventional maxillary denture and mandibular overdenture supported by two cast gold bars, which were separated in the midline. The patient was followed for 4 years, and the dentures were remade or relined to accommodate the eruption of two maxillary teeth and overall growth.

During the 4 years of follow-up the patient experienced remarkable growth. However, the relative position of the mandibular implants remained unchanged as growth took place mainly in the rami and condyles. This is consistent with the mandibular growth described by Bjork (1969). Encouragingly, the rotation of the mandible that accompanies growth did not cause a significant problem relative to the angulation of implants and the prosthetic occlusal plane. The unloaded single maxillary implant did not move with the downward and forward growth of the maxilla, and was positioned at the end of the follow-up in close proximity to the floor of the nose. With further significant growth anticipated, this implant could present a significant complication to the patient.

This young patient was referred to Guckes for possible participation in an ongoing protocol (with the implants already inserted by the oral surgeon). The most significant issue raised by this case is whether treatment of a young child using implants is indicated and prudent, and if so, when. Besides the psychological benefit in young children of restorative treatment using a lower denture supported by implants, there is the theoretical possibility that implant-supported restorations have a positive effect on craniofacial growth and development. This assumption is based on limited evidence in adults demonstrating that the increase in function at load on the mandible following treatment with implant-supported restorations may be associated with an increase in the mass of the mandible (Taylor and Helfrick, 1989; Oikarien and Siirila, 1992; Davarpanah et al., 1997).

Traumatic tooth loss

Various statistics have shown that avulsion (total displacement of tooth out of its socket) following traumatic injuries is relatively infrequent, ranging from 0.5% to 16% of traumatic injuries in the permanent dentition. The maxillary central incisors are the most frequently avulsed teeth, while the lower jaw is seldom affected. Avulsion of teeth occurs most often in children aged 7–9 years, when the permanent incisors are erupting. Most frequently, avulsion involves a single tooth, but multiple avulsions are occasionally encountered. Fractures of the alveolar socket wall are often associated with avulsion (Andreasen and Andreasen, 1994).

After the tooth is lost, an almost certain sequela is the rapid resorption of alveolar bone. In many cases, only a very thin crestal bony lamella remains after healing of the alveolus, with clinically obvious horizontal and vertical depressions. In a young patient missing an anterior tooth, the operator may find implant insertion in the proper anatomical position difficult or impossible, because of inadequate bone volume. This situation worsens with time because of continuous resorption and relative growth of the adjacent alveolar bone around the teeth.

Treatment considerations

Timing of surgical treatment

An important factor in the implant treatment plan is the availability of bone. Massive loss of alveolar bone following tooth avulsion or extraction is common. New and predictable bone augmentation techniques allow compensation for bone reduction while waiting for completion of growth.

In cases of localized ridge augmentation, the amount of initial bone volume and its shape dictate whether implant insertion and bone augmentation will be performed simultaneously (Becker et al., 1994; Buser et al., 1994). The indications for this approach are sufficient bone volume to achieve initial implant stability and a predictably high success rate for the augmentation. When bone volume and shape do not allow for initial stability, a staged approach can be adopted, in which the bone is initially augmented, the results are evaluated, and the implant is then inserted. The first stage, bone regeneration, may last 8–10 months. The second stage, implant integration, may take an additional 6–8 months. The effect of growth on the augmented bone is not clear and there is a paucity of information concerning bone regeneration procedures in growing patients (Zoolo and Ferreria, 1994). This technique involves biological considerations other than implant treatment. A regenerated or grafted site will probably demonstrate the same developmental pattern as the adjacent tissues. Clinical decisions on when to start implant treatment after avulsion are dependent not only on the timing of implant insertion, but also on bone regeneration procedures. When most of the horizontal and vertical bony walls of the extraction site are lost, augmentation procedures as a measure to reduce the deficiency may be considered even in preadolescents (author's unpublished data). Currently a long-term study is examining the benefit of this treatment.

Clinical report of trauma in a preadolescent patient

Case 1—preparatory bone augmentation procedure

A 9-year-old boy presented with pain and inflamed tissue around the right central incisor (Figure 14.1a). Eight months earlier, the tooth had been avulsed and subsequently replanted. A radiograph taken on examination (Figure 14.1b) revealed that almost the entire root was resorbed. A wide radiolucency occupied the space of the periodontal ligament. Upon periodontal probing it was also evident that the tooth had lost almost all its support. The right lateral incisor had not erupted, while the left lateral incisor was almost completely erupted. Following treatment of the acute phase, examination confirmed that the tooth prognosis was hopeless and that the buccal bony wall was missing. The main concern in the treatment plan was that following the extraction the palatal thin bony wall would also be resorbed, leaving the extraction site with vertical and horizontal bony deficiencies that would preclude the possibility of a future simple augmentation procedure. Incisions for the extraction were planned to allow an augmentation procedure at the same appointment. Upon flap reflection it was evident that the buccal bone had been completely resorbed and that the lateral incisor crown had emerged from the bone without communicating with the resorbed area (Figure 14.1c).

Indeed, the remaining palatal wall was thin, and an augmentation procedure using Bio-oss (Geistlich AG, Wolhusen, Switzerland) and a membrane (Gore-Tex, WL Gore, Flagstaff, Ariz., USA) was performed (Figure 14.1d). Care was taken to confine the augmentation procedure to

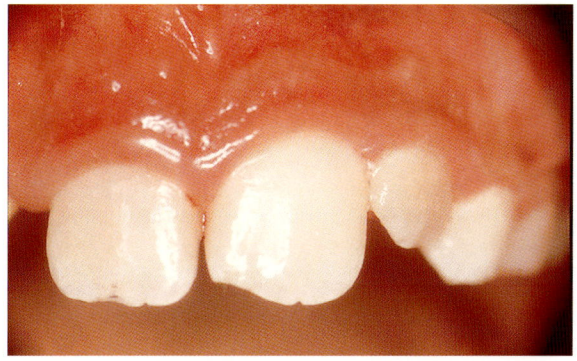

a

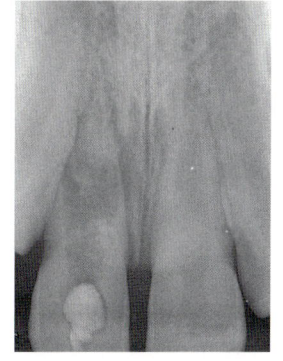

b

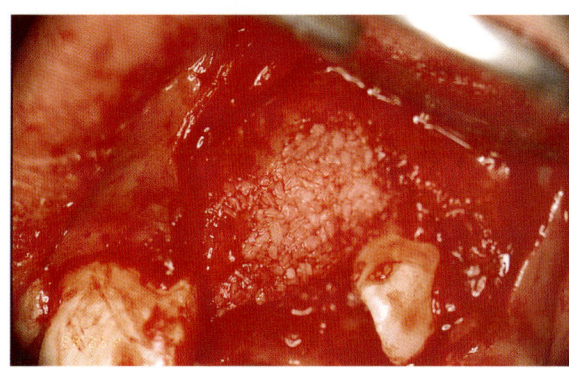

c

d

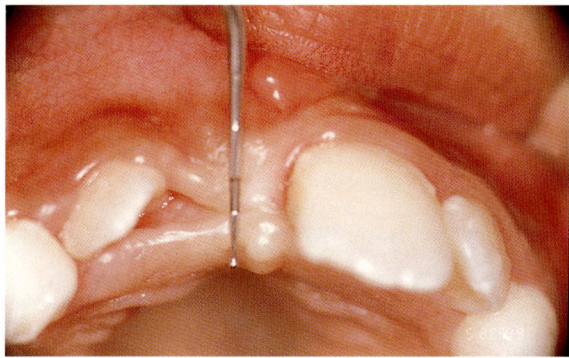

e

Figure 14.1

(a) The right central incisor was avulsed and subsequently replanted. Eight months later the tissue was inflamed and the tooth was painful. (b) A radiograph taken at the time of examination revealed that almost the entire root was resorbed. A wide radiolucency occupied the space of the periodontal ligament. (c) Upon flap reflection, it became evident that the buccal bone had been completely resorbed and that the lateral incisor crown emerged from the bone without communication with the resorbed area. (d) The extraction defect was filled with Bio-oss. This area would be covered by the membrane. Care was taken to confine the augmentation procedure to the defect without involving the erupting lateral incisor in the surgical procedure. (e) Six months later, clinical follow-up revealed good healing with a wide edentulous area between the left central and the erupting right lateral incisors.

the defect without involving the erupting lateral incisor in the surgical procedure. Six months later, follow-up revealed good healing with a wide edentulous area between the left central and the right lateral incisors (Figure 14.1e).

Although this case presents an experimental procedure, it demonstrates the need for early involvement in the treatment of trauma in preadolescence. The early augmentation reduces the damage of both the trauma and the rapid

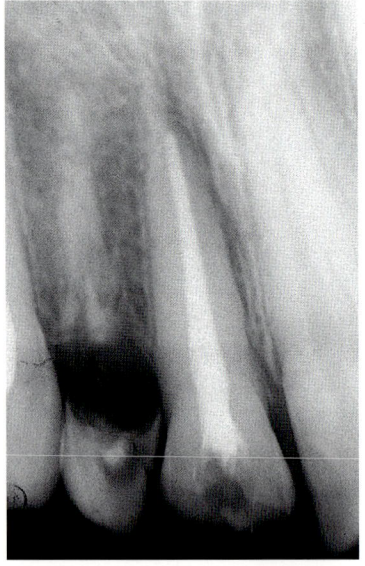

a

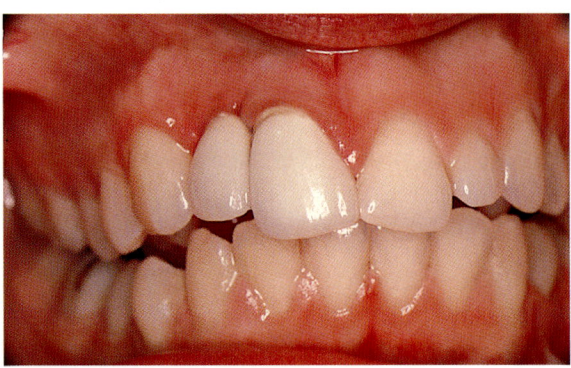

c

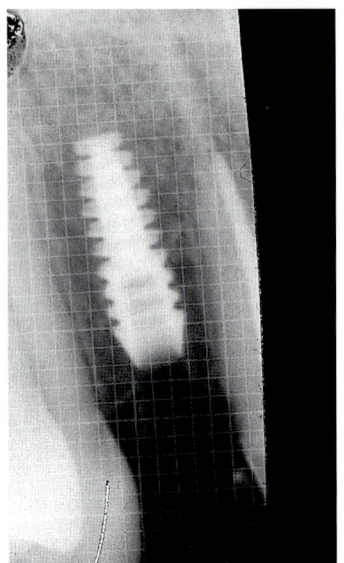

b

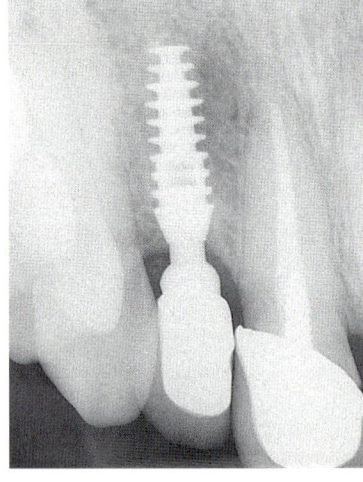

d

Figure 14.2

(a) Radiograph taken on examination, 5 years after avulsion and reimplantation. The entire root surface of the maxillary right lateral incisor has been replaced by bone. Localized areas of surface resorption can be seen along the mesial aspect of the maxillary right central incisor. Radiolucent areas are not evident, indicating that there is no loss of bone. (b) Radiograph of the implant area 6 months following insertion. (c) Two separate ceramometal crowns supported by the maxillary right central incisor, and an implant replacing the lateral incisor. (d) Follow-up radiograph at 7.5 years. Note that the location of the apical part of the implant in relation to the apices of the adjacent teeth has not changed. The coronal part of the implant reveals healthy bone tissue, without any sign of excessive bone loss.

resorption of the alveolar bone following the extraction. A clinical trial is under way to assess the benefit of such early preventive augmentation procedures in trauma cases, in reducing bone loss during the active growth. Despite early successes in this procedure, caution must be exercised in preventing damage to erupting teeth.

Clinical reports of trauma in adolescent patients

The following reports illustrate three cases of missing teeth in young patients. The sequence and timing of bone augmentation and implant treatment are described.

Case 2—implant placement where sufficient bone is diagnosed

A 16-year-old girl presented with a mobile maxillary right lateral incisor crown which was attached only by soft tissue. Five years earlier, the maxillary right lateral incisor and maxillary right central incisor had been avulsed and subsequently replanted. Radiographic examination (Figure 14.2a) revealed that the entire root surface of the lateral incisor was replaced by bone, leaving only root canal material. There were no radiolucencies noted. A normal periodontal ligament space was evident on the distal aspect of the central incisor. On the mesial aspect, localized areas of surface resorption along the roots were observed. It was also evident that sufficient bone was available for an implant. Manual examination under local anesthesia revealed that the width of the alveolar bone was adequate for a narrow implant. Considering the 5 years that had elapsed since replantation, the resorption on the central incisor was diagnosed as self-limiting. Treatment involved the placement of temporary crowns on the central incisor and lateral incisor as a cantilever, followed by an implant-supported single tooth restoration on the lateral incisor and a ceramometal restoration on the central incisor. During the surgical preparation of the implant bed, the gutta-percha was removed without perforation of the buccal bony plate, and an implant (Driskel Bioengineering, Ohio, USA) was inserted. Six months after insertion, in a second surgical procedure, the implant was exposed. A radiograph (Figure 14.2b) and clinical examination showed that integration had taken place, and the abutment was connected. Two separate crowns were then prepared (Figure 14.2c). It is evident from the follow-up radiograph, taken 7.5 years later, that the location of the implant in relation to the adjacent teeth had not changed

(Figure 14.2d). Thus, there was no eruption of alveolar bone or teeth after implant insertion. The coronal part of the bone surrounding the implant neck revealed bone loss of about 1 mm, which is considered a normal rate of resorption around implants.

In this case the diagnosis was replacement resorption without inflammation. The available bone volume was adequate, and as this kind of root resorption does not damage the alveolar bone, implant treatment was started upon cessation of growth.

Case 3—implant placement where the amount of bone is in doubt

A 16-year-old girl presented with a mobile maxillary right central incisor. Clinical examination showed a fistula and inflammation of the soft tissue surrounding the tooth. Four years earlier, the central incisor had been avulsed due to traumatic injury, and replanted. Since then attempts were made to resolve the inflammation by a series of root canal treatments. A radiograph revealed replacement resorption along the two sides of the root, as well as internal and inflammatory resorption (Figure 14.3a). The tooth was extracted (Figure 14.3b) and a removable partial denture was used as a temporary restoration. From the manual examination it was not clear if the bone width was sufficient to prevent dehiscence and to permit correct positioning of the implant. Three months following extraction, the future implant site was evaluated using computerized tomography (CT). A cross-sectional image (Figure 14.3c) demonstrated adequate width and length. However, the quality of the tissue at the extraction site was poor. After a further 3 months, an implant (Mark II, Biocare, Gotenborg, Sweden) was inserted. Ten months later, at second-stage surgery, the implant was exposed. A radiograph (Figure 14.3d) and clinical examination showed that integration had occurred. The abutment was connected and a ceramometal crown was constructed (Figure 14.4e).

In this case the diagnosis was replacement resorption with inflammation. It was not clear if the inflammation had left a sufficient volume of bone for implant insertion. An additional diagnostic means, CT, was used to clarify whether a regenerative procedure was necessary.

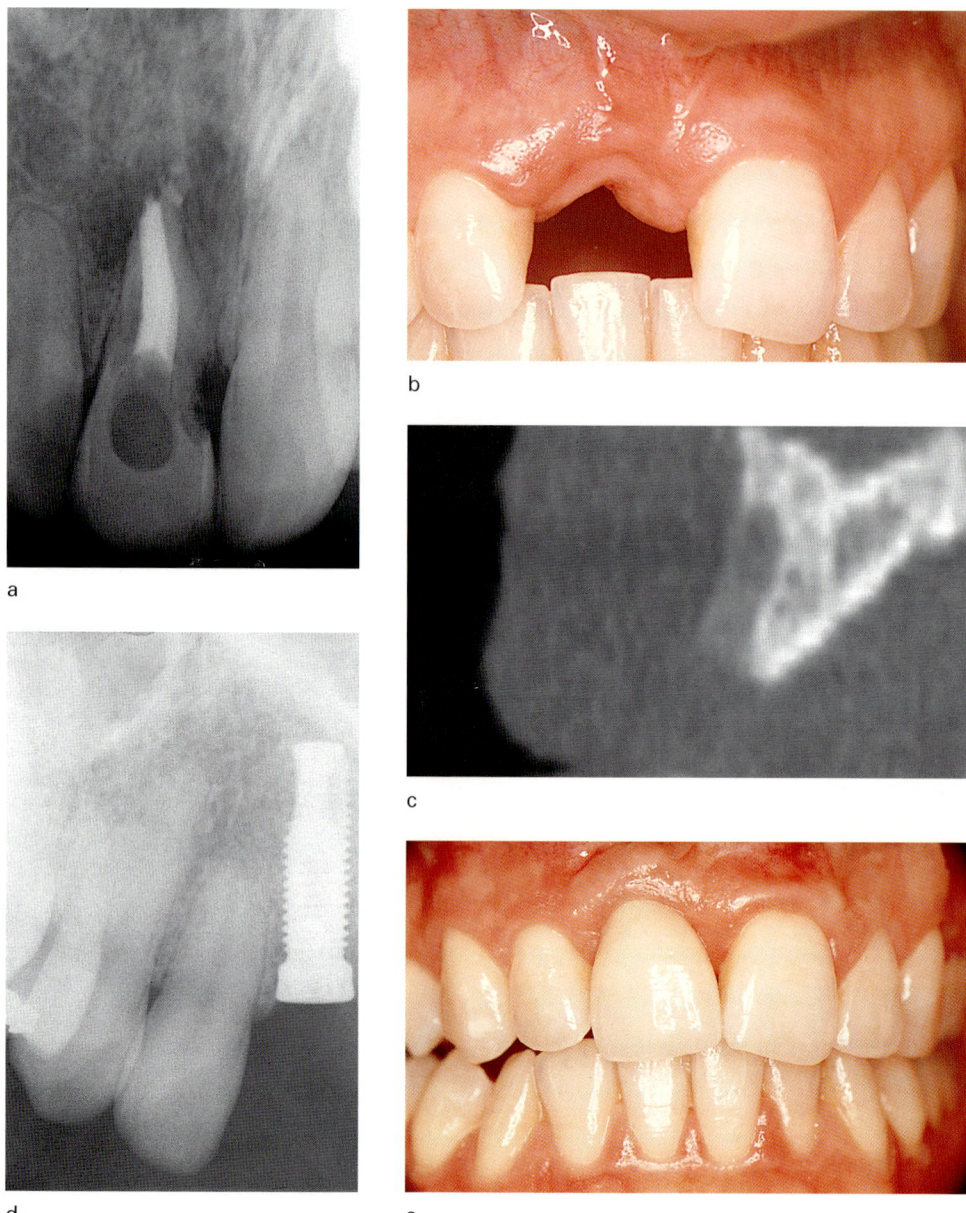

Figure 14.3

(a) Radiograph taken 4 years following replantation, in a patient aged 16.5 years. Replacement resorption along the two sides of the roots as well as internal and inflammatory resorption are evident on the maxillary right central incisor. (b) Clinical view of the right upper central incisor area. The tooth was extracted 4 years after replantation because of continuous inflammation. (c) Cross-sectional image, obtained by reformatted computerized tomography, used to diagnose the available bone remaining after inflammation and extraction. The adequate bone length and width show that the inflammatory resorption did not destroy the entire buccal bone. However, the bone at the site of extraction site (arrows) is not yet mature. (d) Radiograph taken 6 months following implant insertion. The implant has integrated and there is no sign of the previous pathological condition. (e) Implant-supported ceramometal restoration on maxillary right central incisor.

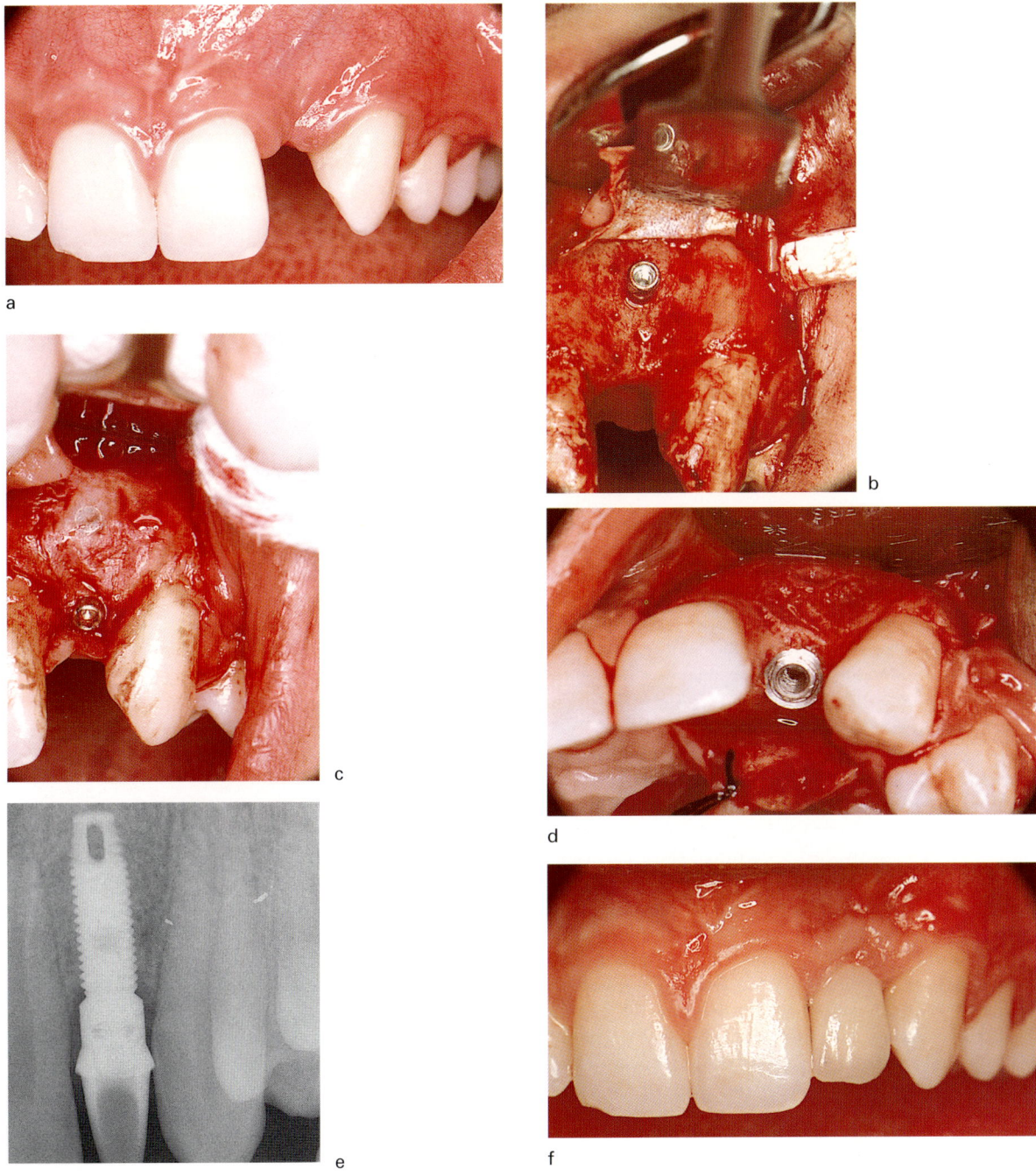

Figure 14.4

(a) Close view of the missing lateral incisor area. The soft and hard buccal tissues are depressed, indicating the extent of bone loss. (b) Upon flap reflection, only a thin palatal alveolar plate remained after the extraction of the upper left lateral incisor. The supporting screw and membrane are already prepared. (c) Ten months following the augmentation procedure; when the flap was raised and the membrane was removed, it was evident that hard tissue had filled the previous gap. (d) The augmented bone is allowing an ideal position for the implant. (e) Implant-supported ceramometal restoration on maxillary left lateral incisor. (f) A follow-up radiograph taken 34 months after completion of the restoration revealed that the integration was maintained without any changes in the relation between the implant and adjacent teeth.

Examination revealed limited but sufficient bone volume and implant treatment was initiated after cessation of growth. If the CT scan had demonstrated insufficient bone volume, a regenerative procedure could have been started before cessation of growth, thus decreasing the time involved in the overall treatment by 8–10 months.

Case 4—implant placement requiring augmentation

A 15-year-old boy presented with a mobile maxillary left lateral incisor. Clinical examination showed inflamed soft tissue surrounding the tooth. Six months earlier the lateral incisor had been avulsed due to traumatic injury, and replanted. A periapical radiograph revealed severe bone loss around the tooth. Four weeks following extraction, oral examination showed that the soft and hard buccal tissues were depressed (Figure 14.4a); horizontal probing revealed that only a thin palatal plate remained. Two separate procedures were planned: a regenerative one, followed by implant insertion. On flap reflection during the regenerative procedure, it was obvious that the buccal plate was missing (Figure 14.4b). An expanded polytetrafluoroethylene (e-PTFE) membrane (Gore-Tex, WL Gore, Flagstaff, Ariz., USA) and demineralized, freeze-dried bone (Pacific Coast Tissue Bank, Calif., USA) were used to augment the bone. Healing was uneventful. Two weeks following surgery, a temporary partial denture was constructed. Ten months later, when a flap was raised and the membrane was removed, it was evident that hard tissue had filled the previous gap (Figure 14.4c). A screw-type implant was then inserted (Biocare, Gotenborg, Sweden) (Figure 14.4d). Clinical and radiographic examinations revealed that the implant was integrated and a ceramometal crown was constructed (Figure 14.4e). A follow-up radiograph taken 34 months following completion of the restoration revealed that the integration was maintained without any changes in the relation between the implant and adjacent teeth (Figure 14.4f).

In this case, clinical examination unequivocally demonstrated that owing to the amount of bone loss a regenerative procedure prior to implant insertion would be required. This procedure was started 1 year before the cessation of growth,

thus saving substantial time. This case illustrates not only the importance of early referral for surgical evaluation, but also that healing is not affected by the young age of the patient, and confirms the value of the regeneration technique in the growing patient.

Orthodontic applications of dental implants

Anchorage—one of the fundamental aspects of orthodontics—can be reliably achieved using osseointegrated implants. Implants introduced by Wehrbein et al. (1996a) and manufactured by Orthosystem (Institut Straumann, Waldenburg, Switzerland) consist of a one-piece titanium fixture with a screw-type endosseous implant body, 4 mm and 6 mm in length, and an abutment. Clamp-caps provide attachment of square orthodontic wires to the abutment. Wehrbein et al. (1996b) reported on a pilot study, in which one fixture (6 mm in length) was inserted into the mid-sagittal anterior palatal region in each of six adult patients with Angle class II malocclusion (distocclusion 7–8 mm, overjet approximately 9 mm). The treatment plan included extraction of the first maxillary premolars and retraction of the anterior teeth based on maximum anchorage of the posterior teeth without using compliance-dependent anchorage aids such as headgear or class II elastics. Because of the design of the implant, only one simple surgical procedure was required for insertion. Early results revealed no implant mobility or dislocation, favorable peri-implant soft tissue conditions, and achievement of treatment goals. Retrieval of the fixture and postoperative wound healing were uncomplicated. The advantage of this treatment modality is that no compliance-dependent extraoral anchorage was required, and the well-aligned mandibular dentition was not bonded to provide anchorage support.

Majzoub et al. (1999) examined, in an animal model, the effect of early orthodontic loading on the bone–implant interface. No differences could be found between the pressure and tension surfaces of the test implants relative to bone quality and density near the implant. Similarly, histological differences were not observed between the apical and coronal portions of test fixtures. No statistically significant difference in the percentage of bone-to-metal contact length fraction was found between test pressure surfaces, test tension surfaces, and unloaded control surfaces. This animal study suggests that short endosseous implants can be used as anchoring units for orthodontic tooth movement early in the healing period following insertion. Akin-Nergiz et al. (1998) also demonstrated that osseointegrated implants can resist continuous horizontal forces of at least 5 N (about 510 gm) over a period of several months.

Conclusion

The successes and the failures of the past have paved the path for modern implant treatment in children and adolescents. The challenge to operators now is the correct analysis of the many options of new surgical and restorative techniques and their adaptation to the treatment of the young individual receiving care. Psychological, social, economic, medical, and developmental factors are involved in the consideration of implant treatment. Each young patient's need is different. The psychological profile of the child and the parents, developmental stage, and implant location are the critical factors in planning treatment. In patients with only a few missing teeth, the implant treatment should be completed after termination of the alveolar growth. However, because the anterior part of the mandible terminates its main growth at a very early age, treatment here can be performed earlier without the risk of malposed implants at the end of growth. In patients with oligodontia, two treatment options are available. If severe psychological problems might be alleviated by correction of the dentition, early intervention should be considered. The European groups that support early treatment feel that it is justified by the temporary gain of function and alveolar bone preservation, despite the fact that implant positioning at growth completion could necessitate surgical correction. The second option is to take advantage of the growth period to correct the malpositioned teeth by orthodontics, and to start the surgical phase later. If treatment is carefully timed, augmentation procedures can be started approximately 1 year before the anticipated cessation of growth, substantially reducing overall treatment time. The drawback of the augmentation techniques is the unpredictable results in cases with severe vertical bone loss. With the future improvement of vertical ridge augmentation techniques, the urgency of ridge preservation by early implant placement, with all its disadvantages, will be replaced by the options of carefully planned treatment, without the need for surgical corrections of malposed implants. In cases of anodontia where complete tooth agenesis calls for improved denture retention, insertion of a few implants in the mandibular anterior region appears to be of a great functional and psychological value. Despite the agreement between researchers and operators on how implants relate to the growing bone, there are different opinions as to how to use this knowledge to benefit young patients. Whichever treatment approach is chosen by the professional team, they must exercise caution to prevent damage and avoid unnecessary treatment.

Acknowledgments

Cases 2–4 are published courtesy of *Pediatric Dentistry* and the American Academy of Pediatric Dentistry.

References

Akin-Nergiz N, Nergiz I, Schulz A et al. (1998) Reactions of peri-implant tissues to continuous loading of osseointegrated implants. *Am J Orthod Dentofac Orthop* **114**: 292–8.

Andreasen JO, Andreasen FM (1994) Avulsion. In: *Textbook and Color Atlas of Traumatic Injuries to the Teeth,* 3rd edn. Copenhagen: Munksgaard, p. 383.

Becker W, Becker BE, McGuire MK (1994) Localized ridge augmentation using absorbable pins and e-PTFE barrier membranes: a new surgical technique. Case reports. *Int J Periodont Res Dent* **14**: 49–61.

Bergendal T, Eckerdal O, Hallonsten AL et al. (1991) Osseointegrated implants in the oral habilitation of a boy with ectodermal dysplasia: a case report. *Int Dent J* **41**: 149–56.

Bergendal B, Bergendal T, Hallonsten AL et al. (1996) A multidisciplinary approach to oral rehabilitation with osseointegrated implants in children and adolescents with multiple aplasia. *Eur J Orthod* **18**: 119–29.

Bjork A (1969) Prediction of mandibular growth rotation. *Am J Orthod* **55**: 585–99.

Bjork A, Skieller V (1977) Growth of the maxilla in three dimensions as revealed radiographically by the implant method. *Br J Orthod* **4**: 53–64.

Buser D, Dula K, Hirt HP, Berthold H (1994) Localized ridge augmentation using guided bone regeneration. In: Buser D (ed.) *Implant Dentistry*. Chicago: Quintessence, pp. 189–233.

Cronin RJ, Oesterle LJ, Ranly DM (1994) Mandibular implants and the growing patient. *Int J Oral Maxillofac Impl* **9**: 55–62.

Davarpanah M, Moon JW, Yang LR et al. (1997) Dental implants in the oral rehabilitation of a teenager with hypohidrotic ectodermal dysplasia: report of a case. *Int J Oral Maxillofac Impl* **12**: 252–8.

Durstberger G, Celar A, Watzek G (1999) Implant-surgical and prosthetic rehabilitation of patients with multiple dental aplasia: a clinical report. *Int J Oral Maxillofac Impl* **14**: 417–23.

Frisch E, Pehrsson K, Engelke W et al. (1990) Beitrag zur problematic der implantation im oberkiefer-frontzahn bereich. *Z Zahnarztl Implantol* **6**: 108–10.

Gorlin RJ, Cohen MM, Levin LS et al. (1990) *Syndromes of the Head and Neck,* 3rd edn. Oxford University Press, pp. 451–6.

Guckes AD, Brahim J, McCarthy G et al. (1991) Using endosseous dental implants for patients with ectodermal dysplasia. *J Am Dent Assoc* **122**: 59–62.

Guckes AD, McCarthy GR, Brahim J (1997) Use of endosseous implants in a 3-year-old child with ectodermal dysplasia: case report and 5-year follow-up. *Pediatr Dent* **19**: 282–5.

Guckes AD, Roberts MW, McCarthy GR (1998) Pattern of permanent teeth present in individuals with ectodermal dysplasia and severe hypodontia suggests treatment with dental implants. *Pediatr Dent* **20**: 278–80.

Hamano Y, Nakata M (1980) Anodontia, part III. Retarded maxillofacial growth of anodontia with anhidrotic ectodermal dysplasia. *Japan J Pedodont* **18**: 618–27.

Hobkirk JA, Brook AH (1980) The management of patients with severe hypodontia. *J Oral Rehab* **4**: 289–98.

Jaffin RA, Berman CL (1991) The excessive loss of Branemark fixtures in type IV bone: a 5-year analysis. *J Periodontol* **62**: 2–4.

Johansson G, Palmqvist S, Svenson B (1994) Effects of early placement of a single tooth implant. A case report. *Clin Oral Impl Res* **5**: 48–51.

Kjaer I, Kocsis G, Nodal M, Chistensen LR (1994) Aetiological aspects of mandibular tooth agenesis—focusing on the role of nerve, oral mucosa, and supporting tissues. *Eur J Orthod* **16**: 371–5.

Koch G, Bergendal T, Kvint S, Johansson UB (1996). *Consensus Conference on Oral Implants in Young Patients*, Jonkoping, Sweden. Institute for Postgraduate Dental Education.

Kohavi D (1999) Sequence and timing of bone augmentation and implant insertion for the adolescent patient: three case reports. *Pediatr Dent* **21**: 57–63.

Kraut RA (1996) Dental implants for children: creating smiles for children without teeth. *Pract Periodont Aesthet Dent* **8**: 909–13.

Ledermann PD, Hassell TM, Hefti AF (1993) Osseointegrated dental implants as alternative therapy to bridge construction of orthodontics in young patients: seven years of clinical experience. *Pediatr Dent* **15**: 327–33.

Majzoub Z, Finotti M, Miotti F et al. (1999) Bone response to orthodontic loading of endosseous implants in the rabbit calvaria: early continuous distalizing forces. *Eur J Orthod* **21**: 223–30.

Odman J, Crondahl K, Lekholm U, Thilander B (1991) The effect of osseointegrated implants on the dento-alveolar development. A clinical and radiographic study in growing pigs. *Eur J Orthod* **13**: 279–86.

Oesterle LJ, Cronin RJ, Ranly DM (1993) Maxillary implants and the growing patient. *Int J Oral Maxillofac Impl* **8**: 377–87.

Oikarinen VJ, Siirila HS (1992) Reparative bone growth in an extremely atrophied edentulous mandible stimulated by an osseointegrated implant-supported fixed prosthesis: a case report. *Int J Oral Maxillofac Impl* **7**: 541–4.

Ostler MS, Kokich VG (1994) Alveolar ridge changes in patients congenitally missing mandibular second premolars. *J Prosthet Dent* **71**: 144–9.

Patrick D, Zosky R, Lubar R, Buchs A (1990) Tissue integration in oral, orthopedic and maxillofacial reconstruction. In: Laney WR, Tolman DE (eds). *The Longitudinal Clinical Efficacy of Core-vent Dental*

Implants in Partially Edentulous Patients: a 5–Year Report. Chicago: Quintessence, pp. 341–9.

Perrott DH, Sharma AB, Vargervik K (1994) Endosseous implants for pediatric patients. *Oral Maxillofac Surg Clin North Am* **6**: 79–88.

Sarnart BG, Brodie AG, Kubacki WH (1953) Fourteen-year report of facial growth in case of complete anodontia with ectodermal dysplasia. *Am J Dis Child* **86**: 163–9.

Schalk-van der Weide Y, Steen WH, Bosman F (1992) Distribution of missing teeth and tooth morphology in patients with oligodontia. *ASDC J Dent Child* **59**: 133–40.

Scholz F, d'Hoedt B (1984) Der frontzahnverlust im jugendlichen gebiss-therapiemoglichkeiten durch Implantate. *Dtsch Zahnarztl Z* **39**: 416–24.

Smith RA, Vargervik K, Kearns G et al. (1993) Placement of an endosseous implant in a growing child with ectodermal dysplasia. *Oral Surg Oral Med Oral Path* **75**: 669–73.

Takahashi T, Fukuda M, Yamaguchi T, Kochi S (1997) Use of endosseous implants for dental reconstruction of patients with grafted alveolar clefts. *J Oral Maxillofac Surg* **55**: 576–83.

Tape MW, Tye E (1995) Ectodermal dysplasia: literature review and case report. *Compendium* **16**: 524–8.

Taylor TD, Helfrick JF (1989) Technical considerations in mandibular ridge reconstruction with collagen/hydroxylapatite implants. *J Oral Maxillofac Surg* **47**: 422–5.

Tanner T (1997) Treatment planning for dental implants: considerations, indications, and contraindications. *Dent Update* **24**: 253–60.

Thilander B, Odman J, Crondahl K, Lekholm U (1992) Aspects on osseointegrated implants inserted in growing jaws. A biometric and radiographic study in the young pig. *Eur J Orthod* **14**: 99–109.

Wehrbein H, Merz BR (1998) Aspects of the use of endosseous palatal implants in orthodontic therapy. *Am J Orthod Dentofac Orthop* **114**: 292–8.

Wehrbein H, Glatzmaier J, Mundwiller U, Diedrich PJ (1996a) The Orthosystem—a new implant system for orthodontic anchorage in the palate. *Orofac Orthop* **57**: 142–53.

Wehrbein H, Merz BR, Diedrich P, Glatzmaier J (1996b) The use of palatal implants for orthodontic anchorage. Design and clinical application of the orthosystem. *Clin Oral Impl Res* **7**: 410–16.

Wehrbein H, Merz BR, Diedrich P (1999) Palatal bone support for orthodontic implant anchorage: a clinical and radiological study. *Eur J Orthod* **21**: 65–70.

Westwood RM, Ducan JM (1996) Implants in adolescents: a literature review and case reports. *Int J Oral Maxillofac Impl* **11**: 750–5.

Zarb GA, Schmitt A (1993) The longitudinal clinical effectiveness of osseointegrated dental implants in posterior partially edentulous patients. *Int J Prosthodont* **6**: 189–96.

Zoolo ML, Ferreria MO (1994) Ridge augmentation following extraction of replanted central incisor. *Endod Dent Traumatol* **10**: 94–7.

Index